GERIATRIC NURSING

A CONCEPTUAL APPROACH

GERIATRIC NURSING
A CONCEPTUAL APPROACH

EDITED BY

Desmond F. S. Cormack
RGN, RMN, DipN, Dip ED, MPhil, PhD
Reader in Nursing
Dundee College of Technology

**BLACKWELL
SCIENTIFIC PUBLICATIONS**
OXFORD LONDON EDINBURGH
BOSTON PALO ALTO MELBOURNE

© 1985 by
Blackwell Scientific Publications
Editorial offices:
Osney Mead, Oxford, OX2 0EL
8 John Street, London, WC1N 2ES
23 Ainslie Place, Edinburgh, EH3 6AJ
52 Beacon Street, Boston
  Massachusetts 02108, USA
667 Lytton Avenue, Palo Alto
  California 94301, USA
107 Barry Street, Carlton
  Victoria 3053, Australia

First published 1985

Set by Action Typesetting, Gloucester
Printed by Billing & Sons Ltd,
Worcester

DISTRIBUTORS

USA
  Blackwell Mosby Book Distributors
  11830 Westline Industrial Drive
  St Louis, Missouri 63141

Canada
  Blackwell Mosby Book Distributors
  120 Melford Drive, Scarborough
  Ontario M1B 2X4

Australia
  Blackwell Scientific Publications
   (Australia) Pty Ltd
  107 Barry Street, Carlton,
  Victoria 3053

British Library
Cataloguing in Publication Data

Geriatric nursing: a conceptual
approach
  1. Geriatric nursing
  I. Cormack, Desmond F. S.
  610.73'65   RC954

ISBN 0-632-01323-0

Contents

PART 2: GERIATRIC NURSING CONCEPTS

List of Contributors

Philip Barker
Clinical Nurse Consultant in Behaviour Therapy, Honorary Lecturer, Dundee and Angus College of Nursing and Midwifery

Desmond F.S. Cormack
RGN, RMN, DipN, DipEd, MPhil, PhD, Reader in Nursing, Dundee College of Technology

Ann Faulkner
SRN, RCNT,DipEd, MA, MLitt, PhD, Director of Communication in Nurse Education Project, Examiner for Chelsea College BN Course

Anne P. Kennedy
SRN, BSc(Hons), Research Associate, Department of Geriatric Medicine University of Manchester; Committee Member of British Standards Institute Technical Committee SGC/1

Maureen S. Macmillan
RGN, BA, Research Associate, Nursing Research Unit, University of Edinburgh; Coordinating Secretary, Edinburgh Medical Group

George J. McKenzie
RGN, RMN, RNT, CertNNN, BA, Lecturer in Nursing Studies, Dundee College of Technology; Examiner in Professional Studies for Nursing Degree Course, Edinburgh University

Ruth A. Schröck
SRN, RMN, RNT, DNS(Educ), MA, PhD, Head of Department of Health and Nursing, Queen Margaret College, Edinburgh; Deputy Chairman of the SNB and Chairman of its Postbasic Nursing Committee; member of the UKCC for Nursing, Midwifery and Health Visiting

Preface

The role of the nurse in monitoring and optimizing the health status of the elderly is crucial, as is her role in caring for the elderly person who is ill. The significant number of such people (aged 65 years or more) is increasing in all 'western' societies, as are the number of 'very old' people, those who are aged 75 years or more.

Nurses in virtually all specialist fields of work, both in community and in hospital, come into close and continuous contact with the elderly; *Geriatric Nursing: A Conceptual Approach* was written with them in mind. Additionally, it is offered as a text for use by all nurses in training, and by all post-basic nursing students who are studying a subject which includes considering the care of the elderly; health visiting, district nursing, geriatric nursing and community psychiatric nursing are examples.

This text should be used in addition to a range of 'medical' texts which will introduce readers to such subjects as surgery, medicine, psychiatry, ophthalmology and dermatology. In short, this is a nursing book which contains a number of references to medicine.

Four important assumptions, in which I firmly believe, underlie the general content of, and approach taken in, the following chapters.

First, there are no fundamental differences between a well person's potential nursing needs, and those of an ill person. Thus, a well person is adequately hydrated and oriented; an ill person may be dehydrated and disoriented. The range of concepts contained in Part 2 do, therefore, have an equal relevance to the well and ill person.

Second, there is no fundamental difference between the nursing needs of physically ill and mentally ill elderly persons. Thus, the potential range of nursing care strategies used by nurses for both groups of patients are the same. Indeed, whether patients have physical or non-physical nursing needs is often independent of whether they have a physical or psychiatric diagnosis.

Third, the range of potential nursing needs of each elderly person is *relatively* independent of his medical diagnosis.

Finally, there are no fundamental differences in the actual or potential nursing needs of an elderly person in the community as compared with one who has been institutionalized. Having said this, it is accepted that the type of nursing intervention and the manner in which it is organized, delivered and evaluated may differ in the two settings.

The three parts of *Geriatric Nursing: A Conceptual Approach* deal with 'The elderly', 'Geriatric nursing concepts' and 'Facilities for the elderly', respectively. The use of references and further reading lists throughout the text reflects the necessity to use it as a framework within which to study and understand the elderly and their nursing care requirements. Readers are encouraged and expected to make full use of the growing literature in this subject area. That literature and experience in caring for the elderly repeatedly underlines the need for teamwork, and for fully involving the patient, close relatives and a range of health care professionals in the decision-making process. This text, although written from a primarily nursing perspective, shares that view and attempts to take full account of the contributions of those other than nurses.

Working with the elderly, be they ill or well, offers us the opportunity to make the fullest possible use of our skills in both community and hospital settings. Furthermore, it offers us an ideal opportunity to practice holistic nursing and to use a variety of nursing models including the medical/ physical, psychotherapeutic, sociotherapeutic and behavioural approaches.

Apart from those instances when a patient of a specific gender is being discussed (Mrs X, for example) patients will be referred to as 'he' and nurses as 'she'. This arrangement will avoid the repeated and tedious use of he/she, him/her, and so on.

PART 1
THE ELDERLY

The eleven chapters of Part 1 introduce 'the elderly' in terms of who they are, their position in contemporary society, theories of ageing and the normal changes which accompany the ageing process. This part of the text 'sets the scene' for much of what follows, it seeks to identify the elderly as a special group who *are* different from other age groups. Chapter 4, 'Ageism', explores the notion of prejudice and stereotype as they apply to this group, and proposes strategies for reducing this phenomenon.

Chapter 8 focuses on the pathology of old age and on the diseases commonly experienced during this period. An understanding of Chapter 9 'Models of Care', 10 'Nursing Concepts' and 11 'The Geriatric Nursing Process' is a prerequisite for successful use of Part 2.

Chapter 1
The Elderly

For the purposes of this book the term 'elderly people' will relate to those people who are aged 65 years or more. Despite the fact that this definition is inappropriate in that it relates to a very diverse group of people, it is nevertheless felt necessary in order to give a focus to the text. The definition used will relate to a wide range of individuals who may be 'frail' and 65 years old, or relatively fit and 100 years old or more. It will also relate to very 'young' 70-year-olds, and apply equally to very 'old' 70-year-olds. The term, therefore, encompasses a large and heterogeneous group of people who have differing histories, experiences, needs and futures. Although the term 'the elderly' will be used to describe persons who have lived for 65 or more years, it should be remembered that it is being used for the convenience of the reader and writer; it must never be used to stereotype the group whom it is describing. They, like 'the young' or the 'middle aged' are individuals.

Despite the heterogeneous nature of this group, there are a number of attributes which they have a tendency to share. Indeed, if they did not have a number of features in common, it would be wrong to write a textbook relating to the care of 'the elderly'. Examples of these characteristics include the facts that the individual is almost certainly reaching the end of his physical existence, he will have more health problems than younger persons, he may have reached the end of a period of paid employment, and he is at risk of becoming increasingly alienated from many aspects of society because of the fact that he is old. Other shared attributes of people in this group are that they have spent much of their lifetime contributing to society, they have a wisdom and knowledge which only comes with age, they have few constraints imposed on how they spend their time, they are a stabilizing force in many societies and play a central role in preserving their culture.

The role and position of the elderly in some societies is very different from that of others. This book will view the elderly in terms of a 'Western' perspective. This position is taken in the belief that there are considerable similarities between the position of the elderly in Western European, North American and a number of other English-speaking countries. Additionally, it is the perspective with which the authors are familiar and which, in large part, is the concern of the intended readership. The extent to which this work can be applied to other cultures is a matter for individual readers and groups to decide, taking account of the fact that important similarities, as well as differences, exist; for example, increasing age increases the likelihood of death in all societies. Similarly, chronicity and multiple pathology are a feature of the elderly in *all* societies. Finally, all of the concepts dealt with in Part 2 are universally applicable.

HOW MANY PEOPLE ARE ELDERLY?

Not only do the elderly constitute an important subgroup of our population, they also form a relatively large proportion of it. Table 1.1 shows the distribution of the population by age groups in a typical Western country and illustrates actual and projected numbers. Table 1.2 contains the same information in percentage, rather than number, form. It can be seen that the number of people in the age group 65 to 74 years is relatively stable. However, a dramatic increase in the numbers of people aged 75 years or more is anticipated. It is reasonable to suppose that these figures, certainly as they relate to the elderly constituting an increasingly large proportion of the population, are to be found in Western societies generally. Thus, 9% of a typical population may be 'old' (65 to 74 years), whilst 5% of the population may be 'very old' (75 years or more). It can be seen that these figures represent many millions of elderly persons in the United Kingdom, and even larger numbers in other countries such as the United States of America.

WHERE ARE ELDERLY PEOPLE?

The majority of elderly people, probably in the region of 95%, are either living relatively independent lives in the privacy of their own homes or are living with relatives. However, this does not mean that they have *perfect* health. It is widely acknowledged that elderly people are more at risk, experience more frequent and longer term health care problems, and utilize a relatively larger proportion of health care facilities than the younger population. The concepts of *chronicity,* health problems of extended duration, and *multiple pathology,* multiple problems occurring at the same time, frequently apply to the elderly as individuals and as a group.

Readers of this book might assume that much of the material contained within it does not apply to the 'well' elderly population, this view can be challenged for the following reason. Although a population, for example many of the elderly, might not have immediate significant health care problems, the role of the nurse will be to *monitor* the overall health of that

Table 1.1 Scottish population by age groups.

Age group (yrs)	1971	1981	1991
0 – 64	4 576 200	4 422 400	4 472 700
65 – 74	424 400	454 100	426 100
75 +	216 800	272 500	306 000
Total population	5 217 400	5 149 000	5 204 800

Adapted from Scottish Home and Health Department (1980) *Scottish Health Authorities Priorities for the Eighties.* Her Majesty's Stationery Office, Edinburgh.

Table 1.2 Scottish population : age groups as a percentage of the whole.

Age group (yrs)	1971	1981	1991
0 – 64	87.7	85.5	86
65 – 74	8.1	8.8	8.2
75 +	4.2	5.3	5.9
Total population	100	99.6	100.1

N.B. Due to 'rounding' figures do not add up to 100%

Adapted from Scottish Home and Health Department (1980) *Scottish Health Authorities Priorities for the Eighties.* Her Majesty's Stationery Office, Edinburgh.

group. Unless you have a very firm notion of the health problems which are likely to be experienced by the elderly, you will be unable to monitor that health status. In short, unless you are fully aware of the problems which *may* exist, and how to identify them, you will be unable to monitor the health of the elderly. The contents of this book, therefore, are equally applicable to nurses who are caring for the sick elderly, and to those, such as health visitors, who are working with the potentially sick elderly. As with other age groups, many elderly people will require nursing care related to acute illnesses, which they experience more frequently than younger age groups. They also require different care and considerations than younger people who are experiencing acute illness.

Approximately 5% of the elderly population, many of whom are permanently resident in facilities which specialize in their care, are frequently referred to as the 'institutionalized' elderly. In the United Kingdom most of them are resident in nursing homes which may be either Government owned, or owned by voluntary organizations, or run for profit. The next largest group are resident in sheltered housing accommodation, and a relatively small group live at home but attend specialist day hospitals. The remainder of the elderly who are institutionalized are either admitted to geriatric hospitals (for the physically infirm elderly) or to mental hospitals which cater for the mentally ill elderly. Table 1.3 summarizes the major facilities for the elderly in Scotland, a country of over five million people which is typical of many countries in terms of how the elderly population that is not living at home is distributed.

Table 1.3   Summary of major facilities for the care of the elderly.

Type of facility	Financed by	No. of places
Beds in mental hospital	NHS	8800 (1975)
		10 000 (1991)
Geriatric hospital beds	NHS	9400 (1978)
Day-hospital places	NHS	1400 (Target)
Nursing home places	Local authority/Voluntary organization	14 000 (1976)
Sheltered housing places	Local authority	13 300 (1978)

The above figures do not include the beds occupied by the elderly in acute specialities such as orthopaedic, medical, surgical, and ophthalmology.

WHO SHOULD NURSE THE ELDERLY?

All elderly people require a regular and structured nursing care input as a preventive, curative or palliative measure. In most cases, particularly relating to the 95% of non-institutionalized elderly, this principally takes the form of monitoring health care status, the early identification of illness, or the provision of a minimal amount of nursing care. For the other 5%, care is obviously more active, directed to actual and specific care needs, and accounts for a large part of available health care facilities and personnel.

In recent years there has been a tendency in some areas towards relegating the care of the elderly to relatively inexperienced and poorly trained nursing personnel. The myth is that the elderly can be cared for *only* by enrolled or licensed practical nurses rather than by registered nurses, or that they can be cared for *only* by nursing assistants or aids rather than by trained nurses. This unfortunate and unjustified position has been systematic, frequently unchallenged, and has been facilitated by the misguided notion that geriatric nursing does not require a high level of skill; *it does*. The following two anecdotes illustrate the low status which the nursing profession has, unfortunately, occasionally given to the care of the elderly in the past; a position which fortunately is changing.

In a hospital in which this author worked some years ago, a very able ward sister made it known to me that she would like to work in one of my psychogeriatric wards. On making this request known to the senior nurse administrator her reply was: 'Sister X is one of the best in this hospital; she is far too good to work in a *geriatric* ward'. The second anecdote relates to a graduate student who had applied for a job as a staff nurse in a division which featured a geriatric unit amongst a number of other specialist areas. During her interview and subsequent discussions with nursing administrators, she made known her very strong preference for working with elderly people. The response of her interviewers was: 'We do not really need nurses with a graduate background to care for the elderly; *anybody* can do that kind of work'. Although these examples may be exceptional, they are important reminders that we have to be alert to the existence of such negative attitudes within nursing.

Another possible reason for this relegation of the care of the elderly to inexperienced and poorly qualified staff may involve the relationship between nursing and medicine. There are some who believe, wrongly, that the extent to which patients need intensive and skilled nursing care is always directly related to their need for intensive and skilled medical care. This is partly true in that, invariably, patients undergoing intensive medical care do require intensive nursing care. However, the reverse is not true, in as much as that patients who do not require intensive skilled medical care frequently *do* require intensive skilled nursing care; for example, many frail and infirm elderly people require no intensive skilled medical care, but will require intensive skilled nursing care. Indeed, there is a very good argument for making nursing the focus of the care which is provided to elderly people, with non-nursing care only being provided at the request of nursing staff and/or their patients.

Finally, a reason for low status being attributed to the care of the elderly relates to a problem which involves nursing generally; that of identifying the role of the nurse. Contemporary nurses are under considerable pressure to identify the unique function of the nurse; a task which is causing some difficulty. An inadequate way of 'resolving' this problem as it relates to the care of the elderly is to describe that nursing role as being 'just routine nursing care', 'just basic nursing care' and 'the use of common sense'. This restricted view of the role of the nurse in caring for the elderly as being menial and without skill does little justice to the elderly or to those who look after them. It is a view which is, unfortunately, widespread, negative and malignant in the extent to which it damages the quality of life of the elderly. It perpetuates the difficult circumstances in which many of our elderly are cared for and in which many of our nurses work. This view militates against the excellent work which is being done by a large number of skilled and highly motivated nurses who are providing an excellent quality of care. The notion that the elderly *only* require routine, basic and unskilled care is one with which this author cannot agree and which this book is intended to dispel. The elderly must be cared for by a nursing staff group which is at least as able, skilled, motivated and professionally trained as those who care for other patient groups. Indeed, as with all patient groups, the providers of professional nursing care must consist mainly of professionally trained (enrolled or registered) nurses.

DEVELOPMENT OF NURSING CARE FOR THE ELDERLY

It has become evident in recent years that the nursing profession is beginning to recognize the complexity and importance of this aspect of nursing. The subject forms a part of most, if not all, nurse training programmes and is increasingly being discussed in professional texts and journal articles. Nursing research relating to the elderly is growing in volume and quality, and is being published in the form of exciting and stimulating articles. The number of eminent nurses who are taking a serious interest in this area of care is undoubtedly multiplying, with important contributions being made in clinical, research and educational areas. This position is to be compared with that of only a few years ago when it would have been difficult to have made these observations.

It is essential that these academic, educational and research changes be reflected in the *delivery* of patient care and that we begin to implement more of what we know can improve the care of this group. If the quality of care is to be unchanged as a result of these important developments, they might as well not have taken place. Much work has still to be done in this profession in order to erase the many negative attitudes which have built up in recent decades. A starting point for continuing this process of change is to recognize and admit that caring for the elderly may well be nursing in its 'purest' form. Indeed, if we abandon the care of the elderly to those who are not nursing professionals, the whole concept of nursing as a profession may well have to be called into question.

Within some health care systems the allocation of resources and personnel to those specialist facilities which care for the elderly, although improving, has been traditionally poor. Within areas such as a hospital which includes a section in which the elderly are cared for, the allocation of resources is frequently similarly inadequate; for example, the allocation of staff and other resources to a psychogeriatric unit within a psychiatric hospital may be relatively bad. The reasons for this are not easy to understand, but may include the sequence of events described in Figure 1.1.

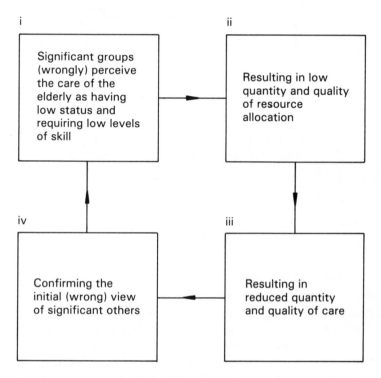

Fig. 1.1   An example of possible reasons for bad allocation of staff and resources.

Figure 1.1 demonstrates a situation in which administrators, those who allocate resources, perceive the care of the elderly as having low status and requiring minimal resources and accordingly allocate limited resources and staff to that area. Consequently, the quality of care provided to the elderly in that situation is, of necessity, of a low quality. This delivery of low quality care confirms the (wrong) assumption made by those who allocate resources.

Figure 1.2 has a different starting point, one in which the elderly, having been allocated adequate resources and personnel, receive a high quality of

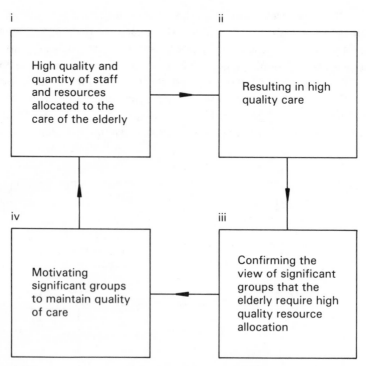

Fig. 1.2   An example illustrating good allocation of resources and consequent high quality of care.

care. Those who provide resources and personnel, and who may well wish to maintain the high standard, continue to provide a quality of personnel and resources designed to maintain this relatively high standard of care. Thus, the quality of care which is provided remains high as does the status of the speciality.

It is not being suggested that either of these two models answers this complex question. However, a new and specific recognition of the complexity of the high quality care required by the elderly will do two things. First, it will provide a starting point from which clinicians can provide specific and goal-directed high quality care to the elderly. If they are presently unable to provide this care, for example because of lack of staff and resources, they will now be in a better position to argue for these resources. Second, those who are in a position to allocate additional materials and staff will be better prepared to evaluate the outcome of that increased allocation. Part of the problem in the past has been that clinicians have had difficulty in specifying exactly why they require extra personnel and resources. Similarly, administrators have been unwilling to allocate these because they have not been convinced that the elderly require them. This book should provide a convincing argument for appropriate facilities and personnel for caring for the elderly person, an argument which may be of equal use to clinicians, administrators and the elderly themselves.

GERIATRIC NURSING

This book relates to the *nursing needs* of the elderly, and to the meeting of those needs. It is not about anatomy, physiology or about diseases of the elderly, these subjects can best be studied by reference to other specialist texts on these subjects. Indeed, the nursing care of the elderly must not be seen in isolation from these other appropriate related subjects. You will find it useful to study these subjects either before, or at the same time as, using this text.

A balance will be maintained throughout this book in relation to the use of community/institutional examples of nursing care. The editor's view is that the nursing care requirements of a person do not change with the context in which he is being nursed; for example, whether a person is living at home or in hospital makes no difference in relation to his needs and potential problems such as elimination or anxiety. Throughout this book, therefore, no real distinction will be made as to whether or not the elderly person being discussed is living at home, in a nursing home, in a sheltered housing facility or in a hospital.

Similarly, in the editor's view the nature of the patient's illness, ranging from being 'well', acutely physically ill, chronically ill or mentally ill, does not change the range of his potential nursing care needs. This book relates to *all* elderly persons irrespective of their health status, the type of illness which they experience or the environment in which they are cared for.

The care of the elderly generally, and the role of the nurse in particular, is one which is currently being given urgent and close examination in many countries (McGilloway 1979, Bryan 1981, Cormack 1981, de Leon 1981, Endo 1981, Golander & Hirschfield 1981, Mantle 1981, Reid 1981), Cormack 1982, Duncan 1982). The unique and highly specialized nature of this field of nursing was highlighted by Mantle (1981) who wrote:

'I believe that Geriatric Nursing is highly specialised and nurses must develop special insights, knowledge and skill for this field of practice' p.670.

That these special insights and skills *are* developing is demonstrated in papers by Department of Health and Social Security (1978), Butler (1980), Help the Aged (1982), Bergman *et al.* (1983), Childs (1983), Knowles (1983), McIntosh (1983) and McLaren (1983). These writers, and others, represent a new and dynamic push towards excellence in the care of the elderly, their writings being typical of a vast literature on the subject which has appeared in recent years.

Some writers recognize that we still have some way to go before achieving our goal of excellence in geriatric nursing. Hockey (1983) posed the question:

'Why do we maintain that there is greater skill in giving an injection than in listening to an anxious, bewildered or confused elderly person?' p.64.

Specific examples of 'problem areas' which remain in this specialist field of nursing were highlighted by Syred (1981) and Richard (1983). The latter writer described instances of care which were disgraceful examples of 'nursing' practice.

In the field of research, geriatric nursing is rapidly reaching a stage of maturity (see Kayser-Jones (1981) for an excellent review of this subject). Academically, the importance of this field is becoming more apparent as can be seen in the work of Doyle (1982), Tollett (1982), Cormack (1983) and Kohuth (1983).

Continued development of the care of elderly persons throughout the world is dependent on those people who make up the readership for whom this book is intended, you and others like you. This area of nursing probably represents one of the most personally and intellectually demanding challenges for professional nurses. With hard work, motivation and a clear understanding of the nature of old age, and of the contributions and needs of the elderly person, you *will* succeed.

REFERENCES

Bergman R., Echerling S., Golander H., Sharon R., Tomer A. (1983) *Nursing The Aged: Institutional and Personal Factors Influencing the Work of Nursing Personnel in Long-Term Care Institutions.* Tel-Aviv University Press, Tel Aviv.

Bryan N. (1981) Nursing Care of the aged in Australia. *Journal of gerontological Nursing* **7**, 664–70.

Butler R.N. (1980) Meeting the challenges of health care for the elderly. *Journal of Allied Health* **9**, 161–8.

Childs E. (1983) Adding life to years. *Nursing Mirror* **157**, 16–18.

Cormack D.F.S. (1981) Nursing care of the elderly in Scotland. *Journal of gerontological Nursing* **7**, 749–58.

Cormack D.F.S. (1982) Nursing in Poland. Caring for the elderly. *Nursing Times* **78**, 334–5.

Cormack, D.F.S. (1983) An educational perspective from Scotland. *Journal of gerontological Nursing* **9**, 596–9, cont. 603.

de Leon S.A.P. (1981) Nursing care of the aged in Mexico. *Journal of gerontological Nursing* **7**, 739–43.

Department of Health and Social Security (1978) *A Happier Old Age.* Her Majesty's Stationery Office, London.

Doyle D. (1982) Nursing education in terminal care. *Nursing Education Today* **2,** 4 – 6.

Duncan L. (1982) Observations of eldercare in the U.S.S.R. *Geriatric Nursing* **3,** 257 – 9.

Endo C. (1981) Nursing care of the aged in Japan. *Journal of gerontological Nursing* **7,** 681 – 8.

Golander H. & Hirschfield M. (1981) Nursing care of the aged in Israel. *Journal of gerontological Nursing* **7,** 677 – 80.

Help the Aged (1982) *An Experience of Caring.* Help the Aged, London.

Hockey L. (1983) What have we achieved? *Nursing Times* **80,** 64.

Kayser-Jones J.S. (1981) Gerontological nursing research revisited. *Journal of gerontological Nursing* **7,** 217 – 23.

Knowles L. (1983) Gerontological nursing 1982. *International Journal of Nursing Studies* **20,** 45 – 54.

Kohuth B.J. (1983) A national first. *Journal of gerontological Nursing* **9,** 236 – 41, cont. 255.

Mantle J. (1981) Nursing care of the aged in Canada. *Journal of gerontological Nursing* **7,** 671 – 6.

McGilloway F.A. (1979) Care of the elderly: a national and international issue. *Journal of advanced Nursing* **4,** 545 – 54.

McIntosh J.B. (1983) Experimental care for the elderly. *Nursing Times* **79,** 56 – 7.

McLaren B. (1983) *Report of a study to make recommendations for a model of care for the elderly in the South West Surrey Health District.* South West Surrey Health District.

Reid E. (1981) Nursing care of the aged: An overview of education, research and practice in England and Wales. *Journal of gerontological Nursing* **7,** 733 – 38.

Richard L. (1983) Time for action. *Nursing Mirror* **156,** 17 – 19.

Scottish Health Service Planning Council (1980) *Scottish Health Authorities Priorities for the Eighties.* Her Majesty's Stationery Office, Edinburgh.

Syred M.E.J. (1981) Changing the face of geriatric care. *Nursing Times (Occasional Papers)* **77,** 5 – 8.

Tollett S.M. (1982) Geriatric and gerontology nursing curricular trends. *Journal of Nursing Education* **21,** 16 – 23.

Chapter 2
Elderly People in Contemporary Society

The assertion that 'old age in our society is held not only in low regard but in contempt' appears to be a harsh statement to make (Elder 1977), but when one examines the images of old age which sometimes crudely and often more subtly influence our perceptions, and identifies the prevailing myths surrounding it, such an observation seems to come very near the truth.

Growing old, like growing up, is both an individual and a social experience. What it is like to be a teenager or an old man is a distinctly individual experience, at either age a happy and exciting one for some and a sad, wearying one for others, but it is also an experience which is fundamentally shaped by the society and culture in which we live.

IMAGES OF OLD AGE

In language and literature we find images of ageing and of the older person which both reflect and influence our view of the 'reality' of growing old. For many children who do not live in close daily contact with grandparents, great-uncles and great-aunts, the picture of old age presented to them is certainly contradictory. In fairy tales the image of the shrewd, authoritarian, magically powerful and occasionally benevolent old king is counteracted by the wicked, frightening and ugly old witch. Childrens books and television advertisements offer a more pallid, sanitized and homely version of grandfathers who tell stories and grandmothers who bake cakes. The older child becomes aware of the image of old age which encompasses helplessness, enfeeblement and impotence while at the same time singing hymns and saying prayers conjuring up the image of God as an old man, white bearded, all powerful and even tyrannical which alternates confusingly with a similarly aged but more benevolent picture of 'God the Father'.

The contradictions in these images give us a clue which might help to explain the contrasts of power and impotence in mythical and religious images of old age.

The image of an impotent old age including its sexual connotations may be a realization of a wish-fantasy of the young. In the histories of most western European peoples, the times when a patriarchal style of family, community and even national life predominated are not far past. Such a position included the widespread experience of the younger man (and sometimes woman) having to wait for the death of the father or the mother until he (or she) could assume full responsibility for their own adult aspirations and actions. Moreover, the 'elders' as superiors at work or leaders in politics and government are powerful and successful figures who are perhaps envied by a younger generation. Thus a mixture of fear and envy may result in a wish to dethrone them leading to an unconscious death wish directed at the old.

The theme of the overthrown king is a frequent and usually dramatic one in the literature which may help the old to understand the need of the young to supplant them; even if older people may not see the freshness and originality in the actions of their successors which the younger people are prone to perceive. Neither may the young always acknowledge that their powers are based on the achievements of past generations. This may be particularly so in our society where desires and fantasies are centred on youth, on the necessity of holding on to youth and its energies and on the commercialization of sexual attractiveness.

In a highly competitive, career-orientated society which is based on the ideology of success through hard work and self-sacrifice and which has developed a concept of medical care as a technical repair service, the almost mechanical image of the old person as a worn-out and tired machine impoverishes the general conception of a human being and belittles the value of human life in all its stages. Life, which as a whole has no meaning, is aptly represented symbolically by its final stage 'sans teeth, sans eyes, sans taste, sans everything'. Shakespeare puts these words into the mouth of a cynic who sees all the stages of life in ugly and ridiculous images from the newborn child 'mewling and puking in the nurse's arms' through affected youth, boastful maturity to final senility.

There are more positive images of old age, some as optimistic as Victor Hugo's: 'When grace is joined with wrinkles, it is adorable. There is an unspeakable dawn in happy old age'.

However, a glance through any book of quotations reveals that the images of ageing tend to be negative.

The words which we use and which are available to us reflect our general values and assumptions about the world around us. Our strenuous efforts to find acceptable euphemisms for describing older people by using such terms as 'senior citizen' or 'members of the third age' are pseudo-liberal and pseudo-tolerant endeavours to camouflage the stigma which we have attached to being old in the first place. It is mildly reassuring that according to Puner (1978) 'perhaps only the British persist in calling them "old people" '. Equally suspect is the use of stereotyping jargon words such as 'OAPs', 'Geriatrics' or the abominable diminutive 'Gerrys' which is unfortunately current in some nursing quarters.

In humour we find another source of the prevailing imagery of old age. A study conducted by Palmore (1971) at Duke University demonstrated that most jokes reflect a negative view of ageing while some are downright hostile. That even in old age sex stereotyping combines with other prejudices is shown by the fact that there are hardly any 'old bachelor' jokes but that those about 'old maids' take only third place after merriment induced by physical feebleness and age concealment. There are also more jokes which reinforce a negative image of old women than those which denigrate old men. This may point to a 'double standard of ageing' which is prevalent in our society.

This double standard is perhaps most clearly seen in the pressures which are exerted on women to keep looking as young as possible for as long as possible. In a man face lines are taken as a sign of character. They indicate emotional strength and maturity, both qualities which are generally far more esteemed in men than in women. Even scars in men's faces are often not felt to be unattractive as they too enhance the image of vigour, strength and action. On the other hand lines of ageing or any scar, however minor, in a woman's face are inevitably regarded as unfortunate blemishes. Contemporary society offers a concept of 'femininity' which places special emphasis on physical attractiveness which is identified with youthfulness; at the same time it discourages the development of qualities and skills which increase with age. 'Masculinity' on the other hand is identified with competence, autonomy and control, qualities which are not threatened to anything like the same degree with advancing age.

In its most extreme manifestation, the double standard of ageing which enhances a man but progressively can destroy a woman erects a clear taboo for a woman while a man is applauded for his vigour and attractiveness. To marry a woman much younger in years enhances an older man's standing and is seen as remarkable and plausible. If an older woman marries a much younger man, both partners will suffer rejection and even condemnation. The woman is certainly not given any credit for her vitality but is likely to be seen as predatory, selfish and even exhibitionist. Her younger partner is considered to be extremely neurotic, in need of a mother figure, suspected of being a secret homosexual and is almost certainly treated with contempt (Puner 1978).

The friendship between a younger man and an older woman is considered odd in our culture whether a sexual component is present or not; odd to the point of being *a priori* evidence of mental incapacity to some people.

Legacies left by older women to younger men friends are not infrequently contested by relatives who maintain that the woman must have been mentally incapable and must have been suffering from delusions when she made her last will. The explanations offered to sustain this allegation are often particularly revealing of the contradictory images which we hold of old people.

It is considered absurd by some that a young man should have genuinely fallen in love with an old woman and utter disbelief is expressed at the notion that there might have been any mutual sexual attraction. If the woman has expressed verbally or in writing any such love or attraction, it is seen as evidence of delusional thought. Declarations of friendship, love or devotion to an older woman from a younger man are dismissed on the assumption that he is only interested in her money. Puner (1978) points out that the myth that marriage is reserved for the young and that sexual intimacy is somehow proscribed in old age has been so powerful and pervasive that it has 'caused millions of older persons to live lives of lone-liness and frustration'.

POPULAR MYTHS ABOUT AGEING

A number of such myths sustain the negative images of old age (Butler & Lewis 1982). Although as at any other stage in life, there are wide variations in physiological, psychological and social functioning between people of the same chronological age, the *dominance of chronological ageing* is a powerful myth. Not since early childhood when the overzealous application of developmental 'milestones' may cause parents serious anxiety if their children seem to be lagging behind, does reaching a certain chronological age have such direct social consequences as for those of 'retirement' age. The myth that at the age of 60 or 65 years a woman or a man has reached the end of a productive life has become a reality with the widespread introduction of compulsory retirement from paid work. There may be compelling political reasons for pursuing a compulsory retirement policy but little other evidence would support compelling people to stop work at a given age. Human ageing studies show clearly that people age at different rates. Physiological indicators show a greater range from the mean in old age than in any other age group. People may become more diverse rather than more similar as they age (Butler & Lewis 1982).

Women may become more acutely aware of the stereotyped perceptions of the influence of chronological ageing than men, and that at an earlier time in their lives when whatever they consider to be amiss in physiological, psychological or social terms is put down with the insistence that it must be due to their 'awkward age'. Even the use of such patronizing language in describing the potential effects of menopausal changes is a forewarning of things to come. Another variation or extension of the myth of chronological ageing is the conviction that all old people are 'senile'. Although far from being a precise medical term, the *myth of senility* has detrimental and dangerous results when used excessively by doctors and lay people alike in explaining the behaviour and conditions of older people. Perfectly justifiable depression, grief or anxiety experienced by old people is labelled as a manifestation of senility and thereby considered to be a chronic, untreatable state. As Butler and Lewis (1982) put it:

> 'Senility is an especially convenient tag put on older women by doctors who do not wish to spend the time and effort necessary to diagnose and treat their complaints'.

The mistaken notion that all ills in old age must be due to the person's increasing senility may be part of a wider *inevitability myth*. No-one should deny that physical and mental decline, isolation and poverty are real and serious problems for many old people, but there is a great danger and injustice in seeing these problems as the inevitable consequence of an ageing process. Not only are isolation and poverty found among other age groups, they do not represent the actual situation of the majority of older people in the United Kingdom. Reinforcing the mistaken idea that advancing age automatically must lead towards loneliness and misery can be a self-fulfilling prophecy. It can also be used as a justification for the lack of social and political action if what is essentially a result of social conditions is represented as the result of a physiological process.

In a society where the economic productivity of the individual assumes primary importance and where the 'creation of wealth' becomes the guiding political principle, all its 'unproductive' members are devalued. Old people suffer this devaluation along with the chronically sick, the unemployed and the poor of all ages. Housewives, artists and students are other examples of undervalued social positions. Whether a society should recognize the invaluable functions which only its economically 'unproductive' members can perform or not, the assumption that older people can no longer be productive is completely unwarranted.

The *myth of unproductivity* presumes that old people are disengaged from life, declining and uninterested. We know, however that in the absence of disease and social adversity older people tend to remain actively concerned about themselves and their communities (Butler & Lewis 1982). Many are still employed in spite of having suffered compulsory retirement. Their work may be on a casual basis, usually part-time and often deliberately concealed from officialdom if the modest income threatens to affect pensions or to attract increased taxation. A considerable amount of voluntary work is undertaken by older people who either do not need to increase their incomes or who are unable to find paid work.

Some elderly people do not experience compulsory retirement: usually those who are self-employed or who work in occupations with a later or no compulsory retirement age. Politicians, judges, ministers of religion, orchestral conductors, academics and doctors are often fully employed well into their seventies. Nor is it unusual for older people who have retired from one kind of occupation to embark on a new career.

The *myth of resistance to change* is as suspect as all the others. Once adult characteristics are established, they tend to remain remarkably stable, usually from late teens or the early twenties onwards. However, the ability to change or to respond to changes depends more on previous and lifelong personality traits than on anything inherent in old age.

When surveying accounts of achievements in old age—Freud, Verdi, Michelangelo, Picasso, Einstein, Tolstoy, Shaw, Toscanini and Stravinsky are common examples—some points are worth noting. It is obvious that the work of already famous people is more likely to be noted and remembered than that of 'ordinary' people. The response of most people that they would not expect to complete an opera at the age of 80 or to conduct an orchestra in their 97th year would seem realistic. In the language of sociology, we would not expect to take any of those mentioned above as 'role models', but we might be able to identify with the postwoman on a remote Hebridian island who pursued her strenuous work well into her seventies or of the boatbuilder who launched his last vessel at the age of 83. The pages of local newspapers provide many examples of achievements in old age which come much closer to the work of 'ordinary' people.

It is also pertinent to make a distinction between sustaining achievements and embarking on new enterprises as old age approaches. The examples of famous and publicly unknown people show the extent to which vitality, intelligence and creativity may be sustained into advanced old age. Puner (1978) suggests that:

'The chances of being creative in old age are immeasurably enhanced if we have been creative in youth and middle age'.

Although popular opinion may reflect the acknowledgement that old people are able to sustain their earlier achievements, the myths about the capacity to learn being reduced by increasing age are very tenacious (Elder 1977). The classical, often inflexible and frequently irrelevant approach to the measurement of intelligence which has dominated psychological research for a long time did not encourage research into the learning capacities of people, and particularly not into the way in which elderly persons learn. Studies like that of Harwood and Naylor are therefore still comparatively rare

(Kastenbaum 1979). Being alert to the recognizable differences in mental decline and survival among different people as they aged, the two researchers took a group of 80 people with an average age of 70 years (the youngest was 63 years and the oldest 91 years old) and taught them German in once-a-week lessons using novel and appropriate instruction materials and methods for people of widely different experience. Although the group's intelligence, as measured by formal testing, was above average (their mean IQ score equalling 118), their experience of formal schooling was well below that common in their community. The members of the group were representative of a wide socio-economic range including former waitresses, telephonists, teachers and civil servants. After only three months more than half of the group passed a formal examination at a level which schoolchildren take normally three years to reach. After another three months (that is, six months after the start of the programme) just under half of the group passed a matriculation standard examination usually taken by 16-year-old secondary school pupils.

Apart from the measurable achievement, Harwood and Naylor (cited in Kastenbaum 1979) comment 'that the attitude of the majority of our students underwent a revolution before a few weeks had passed. So widespread and deep rooted has the 'old age' stereotype become in our society that it has been widely accepted by the elderly themselves. Those of them who had smiled disbelievingly at assurances of their capacity to succeed ... could not escape the impact of their progress'. Even more importantly, they found (Elder 1977) that

'these scholars gained greatly in confidence. Many began to branch out into new fields of skill and knowledge acquisition. Their social life was enriched too, through regular, purposeful meetings with their peers'.

In Britain, many elderly people are starting out on the road towards further education. For a large majority of those who had reached working age before the Second World War, this is the first opportunity for fulfilling longstanding ambitions and interests. Attendance at day or evening classes in local educational institutions seems to be a common choice but there is little doubt that the unique opportunities provided by the Open University have attracted a sizeable number of older people. Under the auspices of a co-ordinating committee for disabled students the Open University provides a range of technological aids to compensate for sensory losses, and it may well be the only institution of higher education which instructs its lecturers to speak slowly and through a microphone! Elderly students are undoubtedly encouraged by such concrete assistance and by the individual interest and concern of committed student counsellors (Elder 1977).

It may be easy to appreciate that perceptions of old age which see this period of life as one of inevitable decline, predictable senility dominated by unproductivity, and a stubborn resistance to any change are indeed negative and are arousing fear and contempt.

The *myth of tranquillity* appears to counteract these predominantly negative images with its vision of old age as a time of idyllic serenity and sweetness when older people enjoy the fruits of their labours in the cosy bosom of their families. It is a picture of neat clichés which assigns to the old person the role of a resigned, gracious, passive dweller in an 'afterlife' in which personal value resides only in the past and in which not complaining about the present is a prerequisite of dignity and pride. Much inspired by children's reading, it reinforces the wishful thinking of the younger generation soothing their fears of growing old. It also allows the denial of substantial stresses which can occur in old age and in particular it ignores those problems related to environmental conditions—low income, bad housing and isolation—which are most probably the more common causes of withdrawal, depression and loss of mental ability. These in turn can then be safely ascribed to the ageing process itself bringing us full circle back to notions of inevitable senility (Butler & Lewis 1982). The stereotypes expressed in the myth of tranquillity which assign seemingly 'positive' virtues to the old person can be equally as restricting as the obviously more negative ones created in other myths by equating serene 'dignity' with passive acceptance and compliance. What all such myths have in common is that they treat the elderly as an undifferentiated, homogeneous group which either by their virtue or by their degradation stands outside humanity (de Beauvoir 1977). Butler and Lewis (1982) observe that:

> 'Medicine and the behavioural sciences have mirrored social attitudes by presenting old age as a grim litany of physical and emotional ills. *Decline* of the individual has been the key concept and *neglect* the major treatment technique'.

How can such an image of old age which reflects, and then only partially, the situation of about 5% of all elderly people be reconciled with or superseded by Albert Schweitzer's 'I still have much to do' approach in his 87th year which may be far more characteristic of the hopes and desires of the other 95%?

THE CONTRIBUTION OF ELDERLY PEOPLE TO THEIR SOCIETY

If, as has already been mentioned, the loss of status and power in old age is to a large extent the result of the small visible and direct contribution made by the elderly to the production of goods and services in a profit and wealth orientated society, the obvious answer might be to allow and encourage them to increase and to make more visible their usefulness in industrialized society (Jones 1976). Although there is undoubtedly personal satisfaction in feeling useful and needed in very specific ways for which elderly people ought to be given the opportunity like those of any other age group, to adopt this as the principal or only argument harbours considerable dangers.

The sole pursuit of this argument would have at least two undesirable consequences for old people. Most obviously, it would simply delay the day when increased frailty or infirmity would force them to cease any productive activity resulting in the low status they have so far strenuously avoided. Less immediately apparent, and particularly in a time of economic recession, may be the insidious pressure that could be exerted on older people to continue working with or without pay to demonstrate their willingness to produce and serve for the good of the community. It is not just accidental that mainly professional, creative and self-employed workers continue in their occupations beyond the statutory retirement ages. This may be partly due to more flexible retirement ages than are common in manual occupations, but it is undoubtedly influenced by the high level of 'psychic gratification and status' that can be derived from such work (Jones 1976). Work for the majority of people is a source of exhaustion, drudgery and alienation and is experienced as dispiriting confinement which most people would leave behind gladly after up to fifty years. Jones (1976) proposes that:

'It seems natural and reasonable that men, creatures of limited strength and endurance, and of numbered days, should both look forward to and enjoy their retirement after years of labour'.

Furthermore, beyond the disadvantages inherent in such a proposal for old people, to measure the worth of a human being solely on his demonstrable usefulness to society would render equally expendable the mentally handicapped or physically impaired child, the chronically ill man or woman and the recidivistic thief. The horrors of the 'euthanasia' programmes of Hitler's Germany in the 1930s and early 1940s are still in the living memory of many. It may seem a long way from an incessant public debate about the immense 'problems' which the rapidly increasing numbers of old people will pose to the industrialized nations by the turn of the coming century, to a programme of state sanctioned murder in a particularly vicious dictatorship. However, both lie, if at different ends, on the same path.

There is one crucial difference between the rejection and even contempt meted out to other powerless and apparently 'unproductive' groups in our society and the elderly. We may have been fortunate to have enjoyed reasonable physical and mental health throughout life, we are not going to change colour overnight, we may not ever become chronically incapacitated and we may not intend to start on a recidivist career but it is almost certain that we shall become old. We shall then also become the victims of our own prejudices and lack of humanity. Albert Schweitzer's plea, 'Please, have a little reverence for *my* life' may become our unfulfilled need.

In offering old people the opportunity to continue contributing to *their* society if they so wish, or to disengage themselves peacefully and comfortably, *their* right to choose must be acknowledged before all else. In their own individual ways, some surely more than others, old people have already made their contributions to a society which often throughout their lives has not given much to them in return. It is usually the disadvantaged child and adult who has to live out an old age of poverty and deprivation, but even should there be some who may not have 'earned' the respite that old age should bring, our need to care, console and forgive is essential if we wish to remain human. Only on that basis should the potential contributions of old people be considered. There is no doubt that older men and women not only can sustain many of their lifelong skills, but that they have knowledge and interests which are less common in younger age groups and from which we can benefit personally and collectively. The unique sense of having lived a long time, of having experienced life in its full cycle from birth to death many times in one's family, of having coped with crises and long drawn out, wearying difficulties, of having done one's best even if it does not amount to great success in the eyes of the world, and simply of having learnt to live with oneself in reasonable equanimity produces even in the more irascible person a feeling of serenity. This, combined with a changing sense of time which allows the older person to abdicate from striving for future gains and achievements, allows the much fuller enjoyment of the moment. This notion was aptly expressed by Butler and Lewis (1982) who wrote:

'The elemental things of life—children, plants, nature, human touching, physically and emotionally, color, shape—assume greater significance as people sort out the more important from the less important. Old age can be a time of emotional and sensory awareness and enjoyment'.

To be able to share moments of such rest and quietude with younger people enhances them for the old person but also provides a powerful stability and security for the young.

An increasing emotional investment in, and attachment to, familiar objects of daily life as well as the common human desire to leave a legacy spring from the older person's growing sense of continuity. Only man is conscious of having a history. The preservation of family objects, heirlooms, keepsakes, photograph albums and old letters does not only provide an identity for all members of the family but often extends into a genuine interest in capturing and enriching local history. The restoration of old things requires patience and often a fairly stubborn tenacity which at a younger age may have appeared out of proportion to the results or gains that one wanted to achieve. Tasks which may appear less attractive to younger people may be more fully appreciated by an older person. Whether one is conscious of a somewhat shorter attention span or not, serial tasks which allow a certain repetition, short breaks and unhurried completion may suit many an older person. However, neither old nor young people want to be patronized by being given 'simple things' to do. Older people enjoy a challenge, if it appears to be within their capabilities. The unpopularity of 'employment schemes' for young people who feel, rightly or wrongly, that they are merely 'filling in time' is reflected in the old person's unwillingness to join in activities which are fairly meaningless in themselves and are thoughtlessly devised in order to 'occupy' the old people. There are not many people who would normally play games first thing in the morning, yet inviting and sometimes even compelling elderly people who attend day centres or live in institutional settings to play cards or dominoes as soon as breakfast is cleared away is a very common approach. Their possibly indignant refusal is not infrequently interpreted as a further sign of increasing senility!

Creativity, curiosity and a delight in surprises do not desert people in old age. If anything, the innocent pleasure of 'playing truant' from routine responsibilities no longer disrupts working and family commitments and is eagerly shared by younger and older children. Real, demonstrable needs of individuals, families and communities engage the interest and commitment of the older person and allow him or her to make a freely chosen positive contribution. Yet to make this possible to a far greater extent and for many more old people, the negative images of old age and the destructive popular myths about ageing need to be abandoned. We shall know that this is happening when we meet someone exclaiming, 'Oh, I'd love to be eighty!'

REFERENCES

de Beauvoir S. (1977) *A Very Easy Death*. Penguin Books, Harmondsworth.

Butler R.M. & Lewis M.I. (1982) *Aging & Mental Health: Positive Psychosocial and Biomedical Approaches*. C.V. Mosby Company, St. Louis.

Elder G. (1977) *The Alienated: Growing Old Today*. Writers and Readers Publishing Co-operative, London.

Jones S. (ed.) (1976) *Liberation of the Elders*. The Beth Johnson Foundation in association with the Department of Adult Education, University of Keele.

Kastenbaum R. (1979) *Growing Old: Years of Fulfilment*. The Life Cycle Series. Harper & Row, London.

Palmore, E (1971) Attitudes toward ageing as shown by humor. *The Gerontologist* Autumn: 1 181–6.

Puner M. (1978) *The Good Long Life: What We Know About Growing Old.* The Macmillan Press, London.

FURTHER READING

Hobman D. (ed.) (1981) *The Impact of Ageing: Strategies For Care.* Croom Helm, London.

Phillipson C. (1981) Women in later life: patterns of control and subordination. In Hutter B. & Williams G. (eds) *Controlling Women: The Normal and the Deviant,* pp.185–202. Croom Helm, London.

Chapter 3
Sexuality and Ageing

Sexuality is a wide-ranging term which encompasses a number of attributes and feelings an individual may possess. It relates to the male or female gender into which the individual was born, the extent to which the individual is comfortable with the sex role, and the ability to demonstrate those behaviours which are collectively referred to as masculinity or femininity.

Healthy and normal sexuality enables us to make choices about the way in which our sexual needs will be met. Providing that these needs are satisfied in a way that is legal, involves other consenting adults, and that is mutually satisfying to those involved, then a whole range of expressions of sexuality may be regarded as healthy and normal.

Although sexual intercourse and other forms of the intimate and physical aspects of sexuality are important, the term has a much wider and much more important meaning. Sexuality relates to the ability to enjoy being with, caring for, relying on, touching, seeing and communicating with other persons who are usually, but not always, of the opposite sex. Many close and intimate interpersonal relationships are sexually satisfying although they may never develop into anything more physical.

The sexually mature adult is happy and comfortable with his or her own sexual identity and finds physical and intellectual contact with other people rewarding. Self-esteem, a subject discussed later in this text (see Chapter 26), is an important part of sexual identity and one which allows the individual to 'feel good' about his own ability to give and take in a sexual exchange.

SEXUALITY AND SOCIETY

As a result of the limited frame of reference which many use in relation to sexuality (it being seen as *only* relating to sexual intercourse) the position of the elderly is often given less attention than it should be. The youth-oriented society into which many Western countries have developed, places a further barrier in the way of fully considering the sexuality of all adult age groups. Since adults, the male in particular, reach a peak in physical sexual activity at a relatively early age, probably between 18 and 30 years, later adulthood and old age are narrowly perceived as being part of a continuous sexual decline.

The subject is undoubtedly something of a taboo one, resulting in very little frank and free exchange about it in most societies. It is not unusual for it to be regarded as something which is 'dirty', something that *we* should do but that our parents should not, and something which is totally abhorrent in relation to old people.

SEXUALITY AND NURSING

Nursing, which is part of the wider society, has the same difficulties and anxieties about the subject as people generally. If one of our patients should have a problem in this area, it is extremely unusual for it to be either life threatening or terribly obvious, resulting in a relatively low key, embarrassed, or confused approach to it. Despite the fact that the subject is fundamental to the happiness of most adults, we are often either unwilling or unable to give it the prominence which it deserves. In fairness, this difficulty is caused by the attitude of society to the subject, our attitude to it, and the attitudes and difficulties which are experienced by our patients.

Some years ago a female nursing colleague of mine and another nurse were bedbathing a partially paralysed long-stay male patient. During the bed bath, and unknown to either the nurses or the patient, the patient became increasingly sexually stimulated and developed an erection. Midway through the bedbath the patient ejaculated and covered one of the nurses with semen. Needless to say, the nurses and the patient were acutely embarrassed by this episode and responded accordingly. The distressed nurse, who was covered with the semen, was replaced by another nurse who then assisted with the rest of the bedbath. The episode was not discussed with the patient, nor was any attempt made to explore means by which the problem may have been minimized or prevented. In order to maximize our undoubtedly great potential in reducing sexual problems in our patients, it is essential that we give some consideration to our personal feelings on this subject. The following questions are offered as discussion topics which will enable you to explore your personal feelings about this sensitive and important subject.

You walk into the room of a young male patient and find him masturbating. What would your short-term and longer-term response be?

An elderly male patient asks if you can ensure his privacy in his room for the duration of his wife's visit that afternoon. How would you respond?

You are a female nurse and an elderly male patient persists in touching the top of your leg each time you are close to him. How would you handle this?

You are in charge of an old folks home which has a number of double rooms used for elderly married couples. A male and female patient, who are not married, ask if they could share a room on a long-term basis. How would you respond?

Two elderly homosexual patients spend a considerable amount of time together and occasionally sit in the ward holding hands. How do you feel about this?

There are obviously no right and wrong answers to these questions which are applicable in all circumstances. However you might find that discussion of these situations promotes a wider and more sympathetic view of them. Additionally, the discussion will offer some preparation for these, or similar, situations which will undoubtedly occur during your professional nursing career. It is not being suggested that we should allow our patients to have a free, unfettered and irresponsible attitude towards sex which takes no account of our feelings or of the feelings of other people in the environment. Rather, it is suggested that we take a sympathetic and understanding view of the need for people to have an intimacy with, and closeness to, other people of their choice, be allowed to express their sexuality in a reasonable and understanding manner, and be able to express their sexuality without fear of ridicule or punishment.

MYTHS AND STEREOTYPES

Many myths and stereotypes regarding the sexual inability of the elderly exist. The most potent of these myths is that old people do not have a need for sexual expression of any kind. This common misbelief, which many elderly persons probably also have, undoubtedly causes many of them to either avoid personal contact of this nature, or feel extremely guilty about it if they either actually express their sexuality, or feel the need to do so.

There is a common belief that any sexual interest which is shown by an older man towards a young woman is either dirty in the extreme, or indicative of some kind of mental illness. Laury (1980) in an excellent article entitled 'Sensual activities of the ageing couple' reports the following example of the age barrier that exists.

'Mr G a seventy year old recently widowed, alert, successful businessman, made some feeble sexual propositions to his new secretary and invited her to go to dinner with him. Disgusted and outraged, the secretary telephoned the boss's daughter in front of him and reported her father's "unbelievable behaviour", adding that he must see a psychiatrist or be admitted to a mental institution. The old man, consequently, felt so depressed that indeed he did see a psychiatrist'.

Another myth is that the decreased sexual activity, in terms of sexual intercourse, of the older person is evidence of the decreased *sexuality* which accompanies the ageing process. In reality, the way in which sexuality is expressed *changes* with age rather than diminishes.

A third common myth is that the physical changes associated with ageing, particularly those which result in disease processes, make sexual activity in the elderly either inadvisable or impossible. In reality, the extent to which physical illness precludes normal sexual activity is an area which has been given far less attention than is necessary for a full understanding of the subject. In those illnesses in which the subject has been studied, acute myocardial infarction for example (see Thompson 1980), the resumption of normal sexual activity is usually indicated at a fairly early stage after the acute symptoms recede. In a discussion of illness and sex Griggs (1978) highlighted the role of the nurse in giving positive advice to elderly people who are suffering from illnesses which interfere with normal sexual activity.

A further myth is that those minorities, homosexuals for example, who have alternative sexual orientations lose these sexual orientations as they become old. In an excellent article on the subject Noyes (1982) discusses the problems experienced by older homosexual men and recommends a positive role for nurses caring for these, and other, minority groups.

BARRIERS TO SEXUAL EXPRESSION

A potent barrier to sexual expression among the elderly is the expectation of society that they be asexual and disinterested in the subject. This expectation, which the elderly have also (wrongly) been conditioned to accept, results in negative attitudes towards the subject.

The increasing isolation which is often associated with the ageing process, *partly* due to the departure or death of children and spouses, may decrease the opportunity to enjoy the company of the opposite sex. This position is particularly pertinent in relation to the large numbers of unmarried or widowed women in most Western societies.

The extent to which the elderly couple are given the same amount of privacy, either in their own home or in an institution, as that afforded to younger people is probably much less. This is particularly so in relation to the elderly institutionalized person who may be perceived as an asexual person who needs little privacy, or as being accustomed to being seen naked or semi-naked by other patients and groups of staff.

The isolating effect of most types of institutionalization delivers a severe blow to the sexual expression of the elderly person. With limited privacy, and possibly even limited visiting arrangements, the extent to which a near-normal sexual relationship can continue after hospitalization may be severely limited.

ROLE OF THE NURSE

Byers (1983) argued that all nursing personnel should become aware of the position of sexuality in relation to the elderly population. There can be no doubt that this subject forms an important part of the care of all patient groups, including the elderly who are particularly disadvantaged in that the subject has a double taboo for them.

As nurses we need to be aware of the normal physical and psychological changes which occur in the elderly population and how these relate to a change in sexual functioning. In order to understand these changes, and utilize this knowledge effectively, we must examine our own attitude towards the subject. Our ability to become open and comfortable with the concept of sexuality will enable our patients to discuss their questions and problems with us. We should never assume that if patients have problems in this area they will take the initiative in mentioning them; our sensitivity, knowledge and understanding must be used to facilitate these discussions.

We must become aware of the specific problems experienced by the elderly in relation to sexual expression, and be able to make specific suggestions which will, we hope, help to eliminate these problems. In recent years the literature has increasingly offered considerable help and advice to the health care professions; all who work with the elderly must make full use of that excellent literature.

Each of us must become familiar with the effect of specific diseases, and the drugs used in their treatment, on the sexual activity of our older patients. This knowledge will enable us confidently to offer help and advice in relation to the problems which have occurred, or which are likely to occur as a result of the disease and/or treatment.

Finally, we must earnestly believe that, as suggested by Aletky (1980):

'Broadly defined, sexuality can be a desire for contact, warmth, tenderness or love. To refuse to address sexual issues of nursing home residents is to ignore a basic part of their existence'.

As Stanford (1977) reminds us, sexual expression varies between individuals;

some may prefer kissing, touching, holding and lying next to each other as an appropriate alternative to sexual intercourse.

It is not being suggested that the health care professions generally, or nursing in particular, have answers to all the questions and problems relating to sexuality and the elderly. Rather, it is being suggested that we need to take a very positive view of the subject, regard it as one which concerns nurses if we are indeed to deliver comprehensive nursing care, and be as concerned about sexuality as other more obvious problems such as anxiety, dehydration, nutrition and trust.

REFERENCES

Aletky P.J. (1980) Sexuality of the nursing home resident. *Topics in clinical Nursing* **1,** 53–60.

Byers J.P. (1983) Sexuality and the elderly. *Geriatric Nursing* **4,** 293–7.

Griggs W. (1978) Staying well while growing old. Sex and the elderly. *American Journal of Nursing* **78,** 1352–54.

Laury G.V. (1980) Sensual activities of the ageing couple. *Medical Aspects of Human Sexuality* **14,** 32–7.

Noyes L.E. (1982) Gray and gay. *Journal of gerontological Nursing* **8,** 636–9.

Stanford D. (1977) All about sex . . . after middle age. *American Journal of Nursing* **77,** 608–12.

Thompson D.R. (1980) Sexual activity following acute myocardial infarction in the male. *Nursing Times* **76** 1965–7.

FURTHER READING

Charatan F.B. (1978) Sexual functions in old age. *Medical Aspects of Human Sexuality* **12,** 151–60.

Falk G. & Falk U.A. (1980) Sexuality and the aged. *Nursing Outlook* **28,** 51–5.

Finkle A. & Finkle P.S. (1977) How counselling may solve sexual problems of ageing men. *Geriatrics* **32,** 84–9.

Kaas M.J. (1978) Sexual expressions of the elderly in nursing homes. *Gerontologist* **18,** 372–8.

Lilliard D.J. (1982) A double-edged sword: Ageism and sexism. *Journal of gerontological Nursing* **8,** 630–4.

Masters W.H. & Johnson V.E. (1981) Sex and the ageing process. *Journal of the American Geriatric Society* **29,** 385–90.

McCarthy P. (1979) Geriatric sexuality: Capacity interest and opportunity. *Journal of gerontological Nursing* **5,** 20–4.

McCary J.L. & Hammet V.L. (1978) Quiz. Prevalent sexual myths. *Medical Aspects of Human Sexuality* **12,** 109–16.

Nelson S.E. (1977) All about sex education for students. *American Journal of Nursing* **77,** 611–12.

Schmall V. (1982) Sex and ageing—a game people play. *Geriatric Nursing* **4,** 263–4.

Shoemaker D.M. (1980) Integration of physiological and sociocultural factors as a basis for sex education to the elderly. *Journal of gerontological Nursing* **6**, 311–18.

Spennrath S. (1982) Understanding the sexual needs of the older patient. *Canadian Nurse* **78**, 25–9.

Chapter 4
Ageism

Ageism, a term used by Butler (1975) to describe the prejudices and stereotypes that are applied to older people *simply* because they are old, might be regarded as a problem of 'civilized' societies, of the nursing profession and of many nurses who care for the elderly. This chapter will discuss ageism, the extent to which it exists in society *and* in nursing, explore some of its possible causes and look at ways in whch it might be reduced.

Ageism is a negative phenomenon which results in viewing the elderly in a stereotyped and prejudiced manner. They are seen as lacking in individuality, having less worth than younger people, having more negative aspects of personality, and being less attractive to work with. Ageism will result in the use of such derogatory terms (which may be wrongly used as 'endearments') as geriatrics, gerrys, grannies, grandma and grandpa. It also takes the form of an inability to enjoy working with older people, or to allocate to them the quantity and quality of nursing care which they deserve.

Although nurses are widely regarded as being all-loving, all-caring and incapable of having prejudices such as those associated with ageism, it *must* be recognized that ageism does exist in nursing. It is only by recognizing it that we can begin to try and understand its causes and (hopefully) begin to look for remedies to it. Indeed, we should be encouraging each other to verbalize our feelings about the elderly as individuals and groups in order to better understand our attitudes towards them. It is important to realize that nurses were not the inventors or initiators of ageism, merely the perpetuators of it. The guilt of the individual nurse, therefore, need be no more or no less than that of the nursing profession as a whole, and of society generally. That ageism is not inevitable is evidenced by those societies in which it does not exist, and by those individuals who live in ageist societies but who do not practice ageism. There can be no doubt that there are many excellent, committed professional nurses who are not tainted with ageism and from whom we have much to learn.

EXPRESSIONS OF AGEISM

Ageism can take many forms which range from those relating to society as a whole, to the nursing profession generally, to institutions which care for the elderly, and to individual nurses and other care givers. It can range from the compulsory retirement of fit, healthy and productive 65-year-old men, to the *occasional* expectation that an elderly hospitalized person should eat her breakfast whilst seated on a commode. Remember, the purpose of this chapter is *not* to apportion blame, to punish, or to produce guilt, its purpose is to help recognize the problem of ageism and explore some ways in which it might be minimized.

This discussion will be based on the premise that the elderly deserve *and* require a higher (rather than lower) quality and quantity of professional nursing care. More than any other age group, people who are over 65 years of age are at greater risk of ill health, experience more frequent (and longer) episodes of ill health, and will frequently require intensive nursing care during the process of dying.

SOCIETY

In an increasingly materialistic society, the elderly can be viewed as an unproductive burden on others who are, or will be, productive. They may also be seen as worn out and broken down machines who have outlived their usefulness and are now ready for the 'scrapheap'. The previous achievements of the old person, which have resulted in the prosperity and development of today, may be given little value by a society which is generally unconcerned with acknowledging past contributions.

Contemporary youth-oriented societies value being young, looking young and being economically productive and independent; a value which fails to take account of different forms of success and achievement which belong to the elderly; wisdom, experience and past contributions having little value in such societies.

Ageism also takes the form of using the old as the subject of jokes, particularly as they relate to their alleged lack of sexual ability and interest. Palmore (1971) presented a collection of jokes which, in many ways, reflect the negative views held by society; some examples are as follows.

On death: The funeral of a comedian in London was attended by many old-time comedians. During the ceremony, one said to his neighbour, 'Ow old are you, Charlie?' 'Ninety' replied the old timer. ''Ardly worth going 'ome, eh?'

On diminishing mental ability: 'Four stages of memory loss: (1) Forget names; (2) forget faces; (3) forget to zip up fly; (4) forget to zip down fly'.

Many of the jokes reported by Palmore were of a sexual nature.

The sexual life of a man, 'Triweekly. Try weekly. Try weakly'.

Oscar Wilde said, 'Young men want to be faithful and are not; old men want to be faithless and cannot'.

Of old age, 'The time of life when a man flirts with girls but can't remember why'.

Ageism could result from an unconscious denial of death, a subject which is very difficult for a youth-oriented society to come to terms with. This denial of eventual death, and of the elderly because of their association with it, is more a feature of Western societies. Oriental societies tend to accept both death and the elderly person as *important* parts of the life cycle.

Despite the fact that society tries to ensure that its members live to a 'ripe old age', it can do more to ensure that the additional years are of a quality which will make them something to be enjoyed by the individual. Although *some* additional money, buildings and other resources are being made available, the underlying problem of ageism is still not being given appropriate attention. Perhaps society is waiting for the initiative to be taken by one part of it; it would be rather sad if the nursing profession missed this opportunity.

THE NURSING PROFESSION

As with society generally, a significant part of nursing is prejudiced against the elderly (with a minority of important exceptions). The form which the prejudice takes depends on the level at which it occurs; the following are representative examples.

First, the tendency to relegate the care of the elderly to relatively unskilled and untrained staff; for example, a Government report (Scottish Home and Health Department 1979) suggested that confused elderly patients should be cared for by nursing assistants (aides) with qualified nurse supervision. One has only to look at 'nursing' homes and other geriatric care facilities, and compare their poor staffing arrangements with those of other short-stay/acute facilities to conclude that a deliberate and systematic policy apparently exists which discriminates against the quantity and quality of nursing staff given to the elderly. This discrimination is not universal in that some societies, or parts of societies, *do* allocate to the elderly a fair and reasonable share of the available resources. It may be that those who discriminate in this way do so unconsciously, or that they may (wrongly) equate the need for less intensive medical care, which the elderly are known to require, with less intensive *nursing* care.

Second, the quantity and quality of nursing education which is offered to many nurses as part of their basic training is often inadequate. Although there has been some recognition of the need for a specific theory and practical component in recent years, and an increasing number of post-basic diploma, masters and doctoral programmes, it continues to be an area in which much needs to be done. As important as the duration and content of a specialist geriatric nursing input into basic nurse education, is the attitudinal change which occurs in students as a result of the experience. Green (1981) expressed this notion as follows:

'It is often true in the teaching of nursing that the crux of a particular content area does not lie in the inherent theories and facts, but more in the attitudes and feelings that students hold about that particular content area' p.169.

The role of the nurse teacher, clinician and administrator in engendering positive attitudes in nurse learners is of considerable importance, as is their need to understand why negative attitudes occur. Elliot and Hyberston (1982) in a survey of factors in the elderly which elicit a negative response found the following to be important; socially unacceptable behaviour, abusiveness and incontinence. If we regard these factors as the *very* reason why some elderly people require our assistance, then we will value the elderly rather than, as reported by Nuttall (1983), regard caring for them as being beneath our dignity. Similarly, an understanding of the ageing process, chronicity and multiple pathology will help us to appreciate that caring for the elderly (if the job is to be done properly) is the most demanding of any nursing role.

The third example of prejudice in nursing is the relegation of the care of the elderly who occupy part of an institution to the least experienced and qualified staff. Although there are important exceptions, the acute/short-term wards in both psychiatric and general hospitals tend to be given priority in terms of staff and resources and are frequently more attractive to staff. The following anecdote illustrates this point.

A trained nurse was reprimanded for professional incompetence while working in an acute/short-stay ward. As part of her 'punishment' the nurse was moved to a geriatric ward where she allegedly could do the patients 'no harm'.

Fourth, the many examples of care provided to the elderly being of a very much lower quality than they deserve. These examples come from well-documented sources, from personal experience, and from the experience of almost all nurses and learners who have worked with elderly people. Typical of the many examples is the one described by Kayser-Jones (p.46, 1981) in which patients were made to wait in 'shower chairs' (similar to a commode with the bed-pan removed) for hours before being taken to the shower room. Many patients could not distinguish between the shower chair and the commode and '. . . had bowel movements while waiting for their bath, and the odour or urine and faeces pervaded the hallways . . . . Men and women were bathed simultaneously in the same shower room'.

Although there are very many important exceptions, both in terms of individuals and institutions, we are still some way from eradicating the insidious causes and results of ageism in nursing. The issue is being increasingly raised by such writers as Kimsey *et al.* (1981), Benson (1982), Lillard (1982), Settin (1982), Tatham (1982), Thompson (1982), and Jones and Gilliard (1983). Clearly, there is no easy solution to this problem which must be tackled from personal administrative and educational viewpoints. A number of personal and general strategies may be used in order to raise the status of, and interest in, this most challenging of *nursing* specialities.

Personal Strategies

As individual nurses we need to view the elderly as requiring high quality *nursing* care, and as being a group who experience unique problems. This group often requires long-term care which may or *may not* result in 'improvement' or 'success'. At the one extreme, dehydration may be reversed in a matter of hours, at the other extreme irreversible incontinence may have to be dealt with symptomatically for a number of years. The chronic nature of the nursing needs of the elderly is often also acute, thus we have the need for acute nursing intervention over a prolonged period of time (long-term *acute* care).

Care, rather than cure, is of fundamental importance from a nursing viewpoint. The best example of this unique function relates to caring for the dying patient, a nursing function which can only be performed well by the *crême-de-la-crême* of the nursing profession. We must resist any suggestion or misguided notion that 'anyone' can nurse the elderly person.

The excellent literature relating to the care of the elderly should be found and used, particularly the increasing number of articles contained in specialist journals such as *Geriatric Nursing* and the *Journal of gerontological Nursing*. Contributing to the literature on the subject can only serve to improve its status and help combat ageism. Making use of the literature convinces us that the care of the elderly is not *just* 'basic' or 'routine'; it demonstrates the complexity of the subject and the professionalism required to deliver high-quality care.

Individual nurses, including those in training, have a right to expect that they be given an appropriate theoretical and practical education relating to the elderly. If the training is not comprehensive in terms of physical/psychological/social aspects of care, then the cycle of ageism—low quality care–low status–ageism—will continue.

Similarly, individual nurses should expect to form part of a ward team which is appropriately trained *and* staffed and working in reasonable environmental conditions. Nothing is better designed to dampen the enthusiasm and destroy morale more than having to face a continuous struggle in which the quality and quantity of staff are not of the required levels, and in which the environment militates against the provision of good care.

Finally, individual nurses should look for inspiration and leadership in the many developments which are taking place in terms of institutions, methods of care and general recognition of the importance of the speciality. Kohuth (1983) in a discussion of the first endowed chair of gerontological nursing in the United States of America was in no doubt that the nursing speciality was 'coming of age'.

General Strategies

The combined efforts of educators and nurse administrators provide an effective weapon against ageism in nursing. Their efforts, combined with those of clinicians, could effectively lead the way towards reducing ageism in society by providing high-quality care as evidence of an increased status for the elderly.

Nurse educators, in common with nursing generally, can devise means of projecting their own rejection of ageism by providing meaningful and innovative gerontological training programmes (see Gunter & Estes (1979) for an overview of geriatric nursing education). Nurse administrators also have an important role to play in ensuring that the quantity and quality of care which we are capable of providing for the elderly *actually* reaches them. Despite the continuous overdemand on staff and resources in the health care system, administrators can play a major role in combating ageism by:

1   recognizing the need of the elderly to be given a quality and quantity of care which is at least equal to that of any other group, thus, ensuring that the elderly obtain a *fair share* of the available resources;

2   by resisting any suggestion by non-nurses that 'good' nurses should be concentrated in acute/short-stay specialities, and so doing much to increase the status of geriatric nursing.

Conclusion

There can be no doubt that, just as it exists in society, ageism exists in the nursing profession and in individual nurses. The first step in overcoming this serious problem is to identify and discuss it, rather than to deny it exists. Although *nothing* can excuse the delivery of low-quality care, abuse of the elderly or any form of ageism, it is imperative that we work hard at understanding why these problems exist and what can be done to reduce them. While it still remains important for individual examples of abuse or neglect to be reported immediately to the nurse in charge or some other appropriate person, the long-term solution lies in eliminating ageism.

Having set our own house in order, perhaps we can help society to make the elderly feel less guilty about being old. This guilt was described by an elderly woman during the 1983 general election campaign in the United Kingdom, she said:

'Far more important than the additional pension increase is the need to give old people back their dignity. In this country it is a "crime" to be old'.

REFERENCES

Benson E.R. (1982) Attitudes toward the elderly: A survey of recent nursing literature. *Journal of gerontological Nursing* 8, 279–81.

Butler N. (1975) *Why Survive? Being Old in America.* Harper and Row, New York.

Elliott B. & Hyberston D. (1982) What is it about the elderly that elicits a negative response? *Journal of gerontological Nursing* 8, 568–71.

Green C.P. (1981) Fostering positive attitudes toward the elderly. A teaching strategy for attitude change. *Journal of gerontological Nursing* 7, 169–74.

Gunter L. & Estes C. (1979) *Education for Gerontic Nursing.* Springer Publishing Company, New York.

Jones R.G. & Galliard P.G. (1983) Exploratory study to evaluate staff attitudes towards geriatric psychiatry. *Journal of Advanced Nursing* 8, 47–57.

Kayser-Jones J. (1981) A comparison of care in a Scottish and a United States facility. *Geriatric Nursing* 2, 44–50.

Kohuth B. (1983) A national first: The endowment of a professorship in gerontological nursing makes history. *Journal of gerontological Nursing* 9, 237–41 (cont. 255).

Kimsey L.R., Tarbox A.R. & Bragg D. (1981) Abuse of the elderly—the hidden agenda. *Journal of the American Geriatrics Society* 29, 465–72.

Lillard J. (1982) A double-edged sword: Ageism and sexism. *Journal of gerontological Nursing* 8, 630–4.

Nuttall P. (1983) News Item. *Nursing Times* **79**, 64.

Palmore E. (1971) Attitudes toward ageing as shown by humor. *The Gerontologist* Autumn 1, 181–6.

Scottish Home and Health Department (1979) *Services for the Elderly with Mental Disability in Scotland.* Her Majesty's Stationery Office, Edinburgh.

Settin J.M. (1982) Overcoming ageism in long-term care: A solution in group therapy. *Journal of gerontological Nursing* **8**, 565–7.

Tatham S.A. (1982) Factors which affect learners attitudes to the elderly. *British Journal of Geriatric Nursing* **1**(5), 12–13.

Thompson M.K. (1982) Why not better care for the elderly? *Journal of the Royal College of General Practitioners* **32**(235), 113.

FURTHER READING

Anderson C.L. (1981) Abuse and neglect among the elderly. *Journal of gerontological Nursing* **7**, 77–85.

Beck C.M. & Phillips L.R. (1983) Abuse of the elderly. *Journal of gerontological Nursing* **9**, 97–101.

Campbell M.E. (1971) Study of the attitudes of nursing personnel toward the geriatric patient. *Nursing Research* **20**(2), 147–51.

Dimond M. (1980) Caring: Nursing's promise to the elderly. *Geriatric Nursing* **1**, 196–8.

Hickey T. & Douglass R.L. (1981) Mistreatment of the elderly in the domestic setting: An exploratory study. *American Journal of Public Health* **71**, 500–7.

Plawecki H. & Plawecki J. (1980) Act your age. *Geriatric Nursing* **1**, 179–81.

Chapter 5
Theories of Ageing

The human being, in common with all other living things, undergoes a process of ageing which ultimately leads to death. One of the unique features of man is his ability to understand and appreciate his mortality and to attempt to establish the cause of becoming old. In the attempt to understand *and* explain the factors which cause this, a number of theories of ageing have been developed. These theories are many and include biological theories, psychological theories and those which relate to the individual's environment and social circumstances.

None of the major theories of ageing are accepted as being the sole cause of the phenomenon, it may be that all play a part in causing each and every one of us to age and die. Although some of the major theories are presented below in isolation from each other, remember that they are interrelated and might be collectively responsible for the consequences of ageing.

While the causes are not yet known, only *theories* exist, we need to recognize that present theoretical knowledge can go some way towards either delaying the ageing process or, more importantly, enhancing the life experience of the individual for a longer period than is possible at the moment. Thus, although an understanding of the process might not increase the average lifespan, it may enable the health care system to improve the quality of life of individuals during their latter years. It is also necessary to appreciate that not all individuals in the same species age at the same rate; we are all familiar with the very 'old' fifty-five year old and with the 'young' seventy-five-year-old person. Similarly, we are also aware of the extent to which different parts of the person might age at different speeds; for example, one person may have a musculoskeletal system which has aged prematurely, another may have a brain which is prematurely ageing, and yet another may have a respiratory system which has aged prematurely.

FACTORS INFLUENCING AGEING

In addition to the existing theories of ageing, it is known that other factors will influence the speed with which a given person will age. Although it is inevitable that an individual will age and die, the following circumstances will modify the speed with which the process takes place.

The process is often hastened because of the additional burden of chronic illness such as chronic bronchitis, physical deformity, congenital defects, recurring mental illness, or any of a number of other conditions. It is recognized, of course, that the existence of many chronic illnesses may well be as a *result* of a premature ageing process rather than the *cause* of it.

Environmental conditions which are harsh, lacking in stimulation, which offer poor social support systems, and which do not offer the person security and self-esteem will add to the rate at which deterioration takes place. Similarly, a work environment which places excessive and unnecessary physical and emotional stress on the individual, without the necessary support systems, results in physical and psychological 'burnout'. One is increasingly familiar with colleagues who are occupationally 'old' because of a harsh working environment, this syndrome being frequently documented in relation to the nursing and other professions.

Nutritional excesses and shortages undoubtedly have a major role to play in the general health status, and therefore ageing pattern, of the individual. It is ironic that a very large portion of the population of this planet is poorly nourished, and therefore ages quickly, whilst another major part of the population is shortening its lifespan because of excesses in nutrition.

Self-abuse in the form of excessive intake of potentially toxic material is a further factor which influences ageing. Examples of these substances are locally grown stimulants which are widely used and abused in many third world countries, alcohol, tobacco, and the increasing use of 'hard' drugs throughout the 'Western' world.

Genetic factors clearly play a part in the speed with which an individual ages, this being evidenced by the existence of many generations of a family who have a known long lifespan, and the existence of many families who have a known short lifespan. It would seem that, to some extent, we are born with a genetic blueprint which plays a part in determining how long each of us will live.

Exercise, both physical and psychological, appears to have a role to play in relation to the ageing process. In general terms it would seem that an optimum amount of physical and psychological exercise will result in a healthier old age, if not a healthier *and* longer old age.

Finally, the individual must be free to choose the extent to which he positively or negatively influences his personal ageing process. Some of us choose to avoid potentially harmful situations or circumstances, whilst others apparently invite serious or less serious personal threat. Some choose a life style which, because of personal excesses, will undoubtedly hasten the ageing process; others choose to pursue a less adventurous and 'healthier' life style and undoubtedly have a healthier old age because of it. The Sumo wrestlers of Japan, who are invariably grossly overweight, sacrifice an average twenty years of the normal seventy-three-year Japanese lifespan in order to maximize their success in their chosen career. The importance of understanding the factors that influence ageing is to present individuals with a choice; a choice which must always be made *by* the individual rather than *for* him.

THEORIES OF AGEING

The existing theories of ageing can be conveniently categorized into two major groups: the personality theories and the biological theories.

Personality Theories

The personality theories of ageing focus primarily on the personality of the individual and on his psychological make-up. They are also concerned with the manner in which the individual responds to and interacts with other *people* in his environment. These theories are relatively unconcerned with the physical make-up of the individual or with his genetic background. The three major personality theories are: exchange theory; disengagement theory, and activity theory.

EXCHANGE THEORY

The exchange theory is based on the notion that interactions between individuals and groups exist and flourish because they are rewarding to the individuals. These interactions will continue for as long as both 'sides' continue to profit from the interaction. When one individual, or group, becomes unable to provide the other with a reward then the continued existence of the relationship is threatened.

Dowd (1975) in his paper entitled 'Aging as exchange: A preface to theory' describes social exchange in terms of profits, rewards and costs. As the power and status of the elderly diminish with age, resulting from reduced health and reduced social contact, economic hardship and increasing dependence the old become less able to play a full and equal part in exchange relationships. As the balance of power, and therefore relationship control, increasingly shifts in favour of the young members of society, so the older person becomes more isolated, more dependent and less powerful.

In seeking to apply this theory, we must provide the elderly with opportunities for increasing their power, status and involvement. Such an approach will include maximizing the old person's self-esteem, seeing his age as a positive rather than negative factor, providing opportunities for increasing involvement and decision making, and taking the lead in helping society to understand more fully the positive aspects of and potential contributions from its elderly members.

DISENGAGEMENT THEORY

The disengagement theory, described by Cummings and Henry (1955), views ageing as a reciprocal disengagement involving the individual and society. The resulting decrease in interaction between the ageing person and society generally is seen as releasing the elderly person from the norms and roles of society, thus freeing him to adopt a relatively self-centred and reflective existence. The value of this arrangement to society is that its younger members have power and control passed to them, making it possible for society to continue to function after the death of its elderly members.

There are many obvious individual exceptions to the disengagement theory which are not easily explained by it. Many older persons continue to be involved in society, hold powerful positions in it, and continue to do so for many years after becoming 'old'. It could be that some elements of our society, many academics, artists, politicians and other professionals for example, either refuse to disengage or are encouraged by society not to do so.

An understanding of the disengagement theory can help us to understand the behaviour of older people who have decreased social interaction, and are relatively self-centred. Indeed, an appreciation of the disengagement theory may explain and possibly prevent many of the negative attitudes which are held regarding the elderly person.

ACTIVITY THEORY

The activity theory views the elderly as being essentially the same as middle-aged people apart from the inevitable physical changes. According to this theory those who stay active and involved in old age will achieve a satisfying and successful ageing process. The social and psychological needs of the elderly are, according to Havighurst et al. (1968), different from those of younger age groups. However, the increasing isolation of the elderly results from society's withdrawal from them, resulting in an isolation which is not of the elderly person's choosing.

The application of the activity theory in nursing relates to the extent to which the elderly are offered opportunities to continue to be actively involved in events and decision making. As nurses, we must be careful not to expect our elderly patients to be unnecessarily dependent on us, nor should we expect them to take on a full and complete 'sick role' in circumstances where they may be not sick at all, or only marginally sick.

It is evident that none of the personality theories of ageing can fully explain the ageing process, nor can they explain the large numbers of exceptions which do not appear to be explained by a given theory. The short-comings of existing theories and their failure to take into account individual personality differences was recognized by Havighurst *et al.* (1968) who reported that:

> '. . . as men and women move beyond age seventy in a modern, industrialised community like Kansas City, they regret the drop in role activity that occurs in their lives. At the same time, most older persons accept this drop as an inevitable accompaniment of growing old; and they succeed in maintaining a sense of self worth and a sense of satisfaction with past and present life as a whole. Others are less successful in resolving these conflicting elements—not only do they have strong negative affect regarding loss in activity; but the present losses weigh heavily, and are accompanied by a dissatisfaction with past and present life.' p.171.

Biological Theories

Biological theories focus on the physiological and structural changes which take place in the individual, causing the person to age and die. Although this process is relatively species specific, some species have a much longer life-span than others, there also exist considerable differences within species. As with the personality theories, it is likely that no single biological theory can explain the ageing process. The following theories of ageing have been selected from a large number of examples as being representative of them: self-destruct theory; genetic error theory; stress theory, and the immuno-logical theory.

SELF-DESTRUCT THEORY

It has been postulated that human cells have a 'self-destruct' programme which is contained within the DNA in each species. The operation of this programme causes a series of ageing events, resulting in the death of the individual. Strehler *et al.* (1971) describe this programme of ageing and cell death as being the result of the activity of 'on/off switches' found in the genetic material of the cell.

GENETIC ERROR THEORY

Szilard (1959) suggested that random somatic mutations which were caused by normal low-level background radiation resulted in further mutations which interfered with the proper function of DNA. Subsequent accumulation of these mutations could cause chromosomal interference and cell death.

STRESS THEORY

Shock (1957, 1970) expressed the view that the decrease in functional reserve of organs was a major feature of the ageing process. The body of the elderly person could, Shock suggested, no longer cope with the stress of the environmental change as rapidly as it could at an earlier stage. He also suggested that the problem lay not in the inability of the body to adapt to change, but rather in its inability to adapt rapidly enough.

IMMUNOLOGICAL THEORY

This theory, as described by Burnet (1970) and others, suggests that the ageing body may produce antibodies against the healthy tissues within that body. These so-called 'autoantibodies' may play an important part in a range of autoimmune diseases.

CONCLUSION

It is possible that none, or all, of the above theories of ageing are responsible for the ageing process. However, although much still needs to be discovered about it, much more is known than is applied by nurses and other health care professionals. As additional evidence becomes available it may be possible to construct a single well-defined theory of ageing which will enable health care professionals to maximize the quality of later life. The importance of understanding the ageing process can be that it will enable life to be added to years rather than years to be added to life.

REFERENCES

Burnet F.M. (1970) An immunological approach to aging. *Lancet* **2**, 358–60.
Cummings E. & Henry W.E. (1955) *Growing Old*. Basic Books, New York.
Dowd J.J. (1975) Aging as exchange: A preface to theory. *Journal of Gerontology* **30**(5), 584–94.

Havighurst R.J., Neugarten B.L. & Tobin S.S. (1968) Disengagement and patterns of aging. In Neugarten B.L. (ed.) *Middle Age and Aging.* University of Chicago Press, Chicago.

Shock N.W. (1957) Age changes in some physiologic process. *Geriatrics* **12**, 40–8.

Shock N.W. (1970) Physiologic aspects of aging. *Journal of the American Dietary Association* **56**, 491–6.

Strehler B., Hirsch D., Gusseck R., Johnson R. & Bick M. (1971) Codon-restriction theory of aging and development. *Journal of theoretical Biology* **33**, 429–74.

Szilard L. (1959) On the nature of the aging process. *Proceedings of the National Academy of Science U.S.A.* **45**, 30–45.

Chapter 6
Psychological and Social Changes in Ageing

As important as the physical changes associated with ageing are the psychological and social changes, and the accompanying loss which inevitably occurs. Although a number of selected changes are presented in separate 'compartments' throughout this chapter*, it is recognized that all of these items are strongly interlinked. An understanding of these changes is only relevant if they are remembered and taken into account during our contacts with elderly people. In applying this understanding we become more able to help our patients achieve a better quality of life, and better able to appreciate the reasons for different behaviours in the elderly.

PSYCHOLOGICAL CHANGES

Psychological changes are those which primarily affect the way in which the *individual* reacts to and influences his immediate environment. These are changes which primarily occur within the *emotional* make-up of the person, and which can be influenced by gaining an understanding of the way in which the individual thinks and responds to specific situations.

Dependence

The many physical and psychosocial changes which are experienced by the elderly result in an increasing dependence on others in society. This dependence increases throughout the ageing process and reaches a peak when the individual approaches death and eventually dies. Although the level of dependence will vary between individuals, it is inevitable. Thus, age-associated dependence is a gradual and variable phenomenon, as nurses we sometimes make the mistake of assuming that a person must either be independent *or* dependent. Consequently, when we admit an old person to hospital or some other facility, we often (wrongly) assume that he must automatically become totally dependent on us. What must be borne in mind

*The reader should also consult specific chapters elsewhere in the book.

is that dependence exists on a continuum and may be very slight or very great, or more often, somewhere in between. As nurses we should respond accordingly. Similarly, we sometimes make the error of assuming that a person's level of dependence can change in only one direction; it can only get worse. In reality the level of dependence can change quite dramatically over periods of time, thus requiring frequent evaluation and changes in the direction and nature of nursing care.

I am reminded of the staff nurse who wiped a patient's nose for her while commenting 'she hasn't been able to blow her nose for years'. Ten minutes later a student and I were with the patient in her bedroom when her nose began to run. The student offered the patient a tissue, the patient wiped her nose with the tissue and disposed of the tissue in a nearby bin.

Trust

Two major changes in relation to trust occur in many older people; either they have a naive trust in all they meet, or they have a natural reservation and distrust in relation to those they meet for the first time. In the former case, because of their perceived relative social disadvantage and lack of power, the elderly may feel sufficiently dependent on others to always trust them. This presents obvious dangers in relation to the person encountering others who have less than good intentions. In the latter case, low trust levels present less of a problem for the old person than for those whom he encounters; indeed, it may be regarded as a desirable self-protective mechanism. Nurses, care givers and other acquaintances must accept the fact that many elderly people are slow to 'warm up' and trust people they meet for the first time. It is natural for them to be cautious and have reservations during their initial encounters with people whom they meet casually. This has important consequences for those who care for the hospitalized elderly, bearing in mind that the hospitalized person may be 'expected' to fully and completely trust each and every one of a large number of people with whom he comes into contact during a short time period.

The very close relationship between physical and psychological changes in ageing can be well illustrated by reference to the fact that the hard of hearing, a large percentage of whom are elderly, are more likely to experience trust problems than those who hear well.

Intelligence

Earlier research studies suggested that a considerable decline in intelligence accompanies ageing. In recent years these research-based assumptions have been criticized on the grounds that the intelligence tests used may have been more suited to younger rather than older persons, that the relevance of the test material has been dubious in relation to the elderly, and that the tests may have taken little account of the environmental circumstances of the elderly. The criticisms are based on the considerable reaction speed which some tests require and which is diminished in the elderly, on the increased incidence of ill health in the elderly, and the increased anxiety which they may experience whilst being tested.

Although there appears to be a decline in some aspects of intelligence which is associated with age, one should more properly view the elderly as having *changes* in intelligence rather than a global decrease in it. Undoubtedly those aspects of intelligence which are related to experience, 'wisdom', and long-term memory may be more easily handled by the older person. Conversely, elderly persons who have been inactive, unoccupied, poorly educated or who have lacked recent mental stimulation may perform badly in intelligence tests.

The relationship between intellectual changes and short-term memory deficits should not be underestimated however. Although long-term memory may remain relatively unimpaired until old age, short-term impairment is a frequent occurrence. Difficulty with storing and recalling recent information is often related to its lack of relevance, decreased motivation to remember it, and to increased anxiety levels during both the learning and recall processes.

Given time, encouragement and motivation, short-term memory can be dramatically improved in the older person. Although some problems with memory and 'intelligence' frequently occur during extreme old age, there is much that can be done in order to minimize the accompanying problems.

Hostility

Whilst hostility may not of itself be a feature of the ageing process, it often results from the existence of other changes such as low self-esteem, anxiety and dependence. The stereotype view of the elderly as being 'awkward', 'cantankerous' and 'generally difficult' can result from a sense of frustration caused by a temporary inability to adjust to the ageing process.

It is not difficult to understand the hostility which results from the frustration experienced by a person who finds it impossible to communicate verbally following a cerebrovascular accident. Nor is it difficult to appreciate the hostility which follows from the guilt and loss of self-esteem after an episode of incontinence in an older adult.

Affect (Mood)

In principle, two variations in affect may occur with increasing age; elation and depression of mood. In practice, however, depressed affect is much more common and much more problematical than elated affect. The incidence of low-level non-pathological depression in the elderly is thought to be quite considerable. This may be partly due to a decline in physical health, general loss of such things as friends, income and social position, inadequate support systems and a gradual loss of self-esteem which is partly imposed by society. Because of the frequent denial by elderly persons of the existence of diminished affect, this area of assessment and intervention is crucial for nurses and other care givers. Remember, the incidence of *successful* suicide in the elderly population is high, often predictable, and often preventable.

Anxiety

A strong free-floating anxiety is a common experience which is compounded by many other features of the ageing process such as short-term memory loss and increasing dependence. At a time when the physical, psychological and social status of the elderly person is changing rapidly, he is becoming less able to adapt to this change. The resultant anxiety can be severe and disabling if appropriate steps are not taken to minimize it. One factor which tends to increase anxiety is lack of information about one's environment, and about present and future health status. Consequently, older people will seek much more information about these events (occasionally to the extreme annoyance of staff).

Older people take more time to learn, therefore having to learn makes them anxious, and because anxiety causes people to learn less effectively, they find it more difficult to learn. Similarly, the pre-existing rigidity of some elderly persons will result in anxiety in new circumstances, and the resulting increase in anxiety will tend to reinforce the rigidity. We must bear in mind that our patients are emotionally 'fragile' and require much additional explanation, time, reassurance and opportunity to adjust.

Self-esteem

There can be no doubt that we exist in a society in which youth, physical beauty and social and economic independence are considered to be of high status. We live in a society where to be old, toothless, balding, poor, dependent, wrinkled, and economically unproductive carries a very low status. We also live in a society in which ageism is rife, a society in which systematic stereotyping of and discrimination against the elderly person (simply because he is old) is commonplace (see also Chapter 4).

If any single thing has caused the elderly to be worse off physically, economically, socially and occupationally than they *need* be, it is the prevalence of a level of self-esteem which is unnecessarily and unjustifiably low. Successful ageing is dependent on maintaining an appropriate level of self-esteem. To do so the individual must be aware of his own self-worth, must have hope, an identity, be valued and loved by other individuals and by society generally. It is probable that if the self-esteem of members of our elderly population was raised to its appropriate level, most, if not all, of their other problems which could be resolved, would be resolved.

Social Skills

The changes in social skill functioning which take place are in two areas; psychomotor and interpersonal skills.

PSYCHOMOTOR SKILLS

A decline in psychomotor skill functioning results, in large part, from musculoskeletal changes, tactile deterioration, loss of fine muscle co-ordination, less flexible joints, and any of a range of illnesses such as cerebrovascular accidents and osteoarthritis which interfere with psycho-motor activities.

Successful ageing may depend on the development of alternative psychomotor strategies and techniques in order to overcome the constraints imposed by the ageing process. Care givers must be particularly alert both to the psychomotor skill problems of the elderly person, and equally aware of the means of overcoming them.

INTERPERSONAL SKILLS

Loneliness, solitude, introversion and social isolation are possible causes of decreased interpersonal skills. Any form of interference with communication abilities also imposes serious constraints. Equally important is the fact that there is an obvious and sometimes negative generation gap between the elderly as a group, and others in the population. This generation gap is of special importance when one considers the great age difference of professional staff such as nurses, and of the elderly for whom they care.

We must be continually alert to the need of our elderly patients to be given every opportunity to maintain and practice their interpersonal skills.

This will mean attention to such detail as ensuring that dentures fit well, attending to hearing deficits, adjusting seating arrangements in order to maximize communication, providing an environment which stimulates the use of interpersonal skills, and fully recognizing that many aspects of the ageing process will interfere with the use and development of these skills.

Reality

The extent to which a person becomes orientated to a changing environment, and the extent to which he correctly perceives the structure and content of a new environment diminishes with age. Both of these changes are related to the many other normal features of ageing and to the need of the elderly to be given more time to adapt to change.

REALITY (ORIENTATION)

Although disorientation is a common feature of many of the psychotic conditions associated with old age, senile dementia for example, it is also a feature of the 'normal' ageing process for many elderly individuals. Because of a decline in short-term memory, increased anxiety, rigidity, and the need for change to be slower rather than quicker, the older person can become quite disorientated when exposed to a rapidly changing new environment. The best example of this relates to the transfer of a mentally healthy person from home to hospital and the inevitable exposure to a totally new and often confusing environment and to a large number of new people. The resulting short-term disorientation may well be 'normal' and disappear in a few hours or in one or two days.

REALITY (PERCEPTION)

In order to perceive the environment correctly it is necessary that all of the senses are functioning well. That the senses, hearing and vision for example, diminish in acuity in old age is a clear pointer to the possibility of perceptual deficits occurring. The distrust resulting from partial deafness, the illusions resulting from visual deficits, and the drug-induced hallucinations are examples. Additionally, the high incidence of acute confusional states in the physically ill elderly person is a major cause of perception difficulties.

All those who work with the elderly soon come to know that they are not the same, either physically or psychologically, as younger people. They require a new understanding, different nursing techniques, greater allowances, and a high quality of care which will compensate for the considerable pathological and 'normal' disadvantages which they experience.

SOCIAL CHANGES

A number of social changes, many associated with loss, occur with increasing age. Many elderly people compensate for these losses and changes, others succumb to them with tragic results. It is important that we not only appreciate these changes, take account of them, but also that we assist the elderly in developing alternative coping strategies.

Loss of Dependants (the 'Empty Nest' Syndrome)

At a time when families are increasingly mobile it is likely that children who leave home will move to another city or country, and distance the elderly person from their children and grandchildren. Additionally, this usually leads to the loss of continued contact with the friends and acquaintances of children and grandchildren.

Occupational and Economic Loss

Once the normal retirement age, 60 or 65 years of age, is reached there is significant loss in terms of one's occupation, the acquaintances and friendships which result from that occupation, and the economic security which it gives. Despite the existence of a widespread social security network in many countries, the elderly person is still seriously disadvantaged from an economic point of view. Economic and occupational loss both bring with them a considerable diminution in personal and social status.

Health Loss

The elderly are undoubtedly at greater risk of both acute and chronic illness episodes, a fact which increases with age. Normal changes in appearance which are associated with old age invariably have a negative connotation which result in the 'loss' of a youthful attractiveness and appearance.

Mobility and Independence

Mobility, and the independence which it brings, is limited both from a personal and public viewpoint. The individual may have difficulty not only in relation to personal movement such as sitting down, standing up and walking, but also in relation to the use of private and public transport. As age increases, a car driver will be more likely to stop driving his own car and rely more on public transport. In due course, the frequency of using public transport is usually also decreased.

Loss of Friendships

The circle of friends and contemporaries undoubtedly diminishes as age increases and friends and acquaintances die. A person might remark 'there were fifteen of us in my class at school, eight of them have died, I wonder who will be next'. The social isolation and loneliness of many old persons is a tragic consequence of an increasing withdrawal from society, and of rejection by it.

Loss of Spouse

Bereavement, which can have a traumatic and depressing effect on the surviving partner, is an inevitable experience amongst the elderly married population. Almost half of widowed and single persons over the age of 65 live alone, more importantly they are often lonely. There is little doubt that the high incidence of depression in bereaved elderly persons is strongly related to the grieving process and the effects of isolation and loneliness, with the risk of suicide being particularly high in this group.

Loss of Life

All individuals know they will die, the elderly are aware that it is likely to occur sooner rather than later. The withdrawal and isolation which is part of the ageing process may be regarded as a 'rehearsal' for death but it is undoubtedly a painful and uncomfortable experience for many. Furthermore, it is a process which only the old can help us to understand. It is something for which not all persons are as well prepared as the 91-year-old very fit Polish lady who said to me, 'I can't understand why I am still here when all of my friends have gone. I think death has forgotten about me; death has passed me by'.

CONCLUSION

Although nobody *dies* of 'old age', it is a time when specific diseases are more likely to attack and kill. There are exceptions to the general rule that men and women in industrialized societies can (at birth) reasonably expect to live to about 70 and 75 years old respectively. One often reads of extraordinary old people who are considerably older than the average 70–75 years and who are held up as shining examples of a 'good' old age. However one must remember that people like Albert Schweitzer, Charlie Chaplin, Bertrand Russell, Albert Einstein, Pablo Picasso and Winston Churchill were all 'exceptional' old people. Any suggestion that they should be regarded as the *norm* only serves to increase the guilt, low self-esteem and alienation of the 'average' elderly person. The reality is that the elderly must be assisted to adapt to and accept the ageing process as a 'normal' feature of life, rather than be encouraged to seek everlasting and unnatural youth.

The reality of old age is that it is accompanied by many losses which often occur one after the other. The person may not have enough time to recover from one loss before another happens. This experience of multiple loss, with little time for recovery, can lead to isolation, helplessness, depression and suicide. Much can be done by health care professionals generally, and nurses in particular. This responsibility is a heavy one. However, skilled work by dedicated professionals can do much to help those individuals who have difficulty in coping with the changes and losses which inevitably accompany the ageing process.

FURTHER READING

Barrowclough F. (1981) The process of ageing. *Journal of Advanced Nursing* **6**, 319–25.

Brock A.M. (1984) From wife to widow: A changing lifestyle. *Journal of gerontological Nursing* **10**, 8–15.

Diekelmann N. (1978) Pre-retirement counselling. *American Journal of Nursing* **78**, 1337–8.

Dresen S.E. (1978) Autonomy: A continuing developmental task. *American Journal of Nursing* **78**, 1344–6.

Griggs W. (1978) Sex and the elderly. *American Journal of Nursing* **78**, 1353–4.

Helper M. (1982) Facing death together. *gerontological Nursing* **3**, 394–5.

Hirst S.P. (1984) Promoting self esteem. *Journal of gerontological Nursing* **10**, 72–7.

Hogstel M.O. (1978) How do the elderly view their world? *American Journal of Nursing* **78**, 1335–6.

Horn J. & Donaldson G. (1976) On the myth of intellectual decline in adulthood. *American Physiologist* **31**, 701–19.

Marshall D. (1981) Toward a stimulating retirement. *Geriatric Nursing* **2**, 143–5.
Schwartz D. (1982) Catastrophic illness: How it feels. *Geriatric Nursing* **3**, 302–6.

Chapter 7
Physical Changes in Ageing

Although the ageing process varies in rate and intensity between individuals, there are a variety of aspects of that process which are inevitably experienced by all of us as we become 'old'. Apart from being important factors in the development of those diseases which are commonly experienced by the elderly (see Chapter 8 for a review of these), they have important implications for the type of health care we deliver, and for the manner in which we deliver it; for example, a person with reduced muscle volume and strength, reduced height and stiff joints will need special consideration in relation to the distance of the top of the bed and bath from the floor. The items selected for inclusion in this chapter all have a particular relevance to *nursing* care. In reading this section you should ask yourself: 'How does it relate to bathing, admitting, feeding and mobilizing a person? How does the change affect the person's relationship with his environment, ability to communicate and his independence, and so forth?'

The relationship between different types of physical and psychological changes adds to the complexity of this subject; for example, those which reduce activity may result in dependence, dehydration, poor communication and inadequate nutrition. Similarly, those which reduce hearing acuity, affect interpersonal relationships, trust and self-esteem. Because virtually all the changes mentioned here will be dealt with more fully in the appropriate 'concept' chapter*, they will only be reviewed here.

ACTIVITY

One of the most obvious changes seen in the elderly person relates to reduction in activity levels. Apart from a general reduction in activity, a number of more specific alterations also occur.

---

*See specific chapters in Part 2.

Muscle

A general decrease in muscle mass, strength and tone is common. The loss of strength is clearly demonstrated by comparing the hand grip power of younger and older people. A number of studies of this subject have shown a decline from approximately 45 kg of pressure at age 35 years to 20–25 kg of pressure at 85 years and over. In both sexes the hand grip of the dominant hand remains greater, although reduced, in later years.

The reduction in hand grip power with increasing age is typical of *all* major muscles in the ageing person, and must be fully accounted for in nursing care activities which depend on the use of our patients' muscles.

Skeletal System

An obvious change relates to the general posture of the person either when standing 'normally' or when attempting to stand erect. Typically, particularly with extreme old age, one sees flexion, inevitable kyphosis of the dorsal spine, knees, elbows and wrists slightly bent, 7–10 cm loss in height and reduced joint mobility.

Bones become lighter and more brittle in association with and as a result of *osteoporosis,* a common skeletal disorder, occurring at least twice as often in women as in men. The increased fragility of bone tissue in the elderly accounts for much of the increased incidence of fractures, particularly those of long bones such as the femur.

Joints, especially the articulating surfaces, become 'roughened' with age and generally are reduced in their ability to move freely and comfortably. Restricted movement and painful joints are a feature of the lives of many elderly persons who inevitably adapt by restricting their activity.

CARDIOVASCULAR SYSTEM

Unless disease processes such as hypertension or congestive cardiac failure occur, heart size may be unaffected by ageing. Indeed, the size may well be reduced due to decreased physical activity and, therefore, less demand for cardiac output results. Valves may become rigid and thickened because of fibrosis and sclerosis, with the myocardium using oxygen less efficiently as age increases. Myocardial degeneration and neural deterioration add to general reduction in the ability of the heart to function.

Blood pressure increases in both sexes, with the systolic increasing more than the diastolic, and the increase being greater in women than in men; for example, a typical systolic increase might be from 153 mmHg for a 60-year-old man, to 166 mmHg for an 89-year-old man. For a woman, a typical systolic increase might be from 155 mmHg aged 60 years to 179 mmHg for an 89-year-old woman.

Atherosclerosis and arteriosclerosis are significantly increased in old age and are major contributors to illness and death in this age group.

SLEEP

Problems such as difficulty in falling asleep, early wakening, insomnia and falling asleep during the daytime are often experienced by elderly people. These problems may, in some part, result from a diminished activity during the daylight hours, and from the tendency of older people to fall asleep during the daytime because 'there is nothing else to do'. Alternatively, it may be that problematical sleep patterns result from underlying problems such as anxiety or depression.

It is important that we assist older people to establish a healthy and 'normal' sleep pattern which provides them with the amount of sleep that they personally require. This may involve taking additional exercise, reducing daytime cat naps to perhaps one of fifteen to forty five minutes, and not going to bed much earlier than he or she did during middle age.

Schrimer (1983) in an excellent discussion of sleep and the elderly presents a number of nursing strategies which can be used in order to improve patients' sleep patterns. Bahr (1983) provides an informative literature review of sleep–wake patterns in the aged and firmly places the nurse in the position of 'facilitator' in helping patients improve the quantity and quality of their sleep. A number of implications of the subject for nursing research were included in an excellent paper by Lerner (1982).

Nursing care must take full account of the elderly person's reduced activity levels, diminished strength, reduced height and reduced ability to undertake psychomotor tasks which require a rapid neuromuscular response or the fine control of small joints. One must recognize that the elderly person will be less skilled in all areas of physical activity compared with a younger person.

Patients should be given the opportunity to maintain their activity levels for as long as they wish to do so. de Vries (1970) found that age-related inactivity was partly due to the ageing process *and* partly due to a functional decline resulting from a general loss of physical fitness. de Vries offered a controlled exercise programme to a volunteer sample of old men and found that a general increase in activity and in physical fitness resulted. It is not being proposed that nurses should subject older patients to an enforced exercise or activity programme, rather, it is suggested that meaningful and realistic activity programmes be made available to those older patients who wish to participate in them.

RENAL TRACT

A well-documented reduction in renal mass occurs in old age and results in a declining renal function which may be exacerbated by the effects of chronic disease of the kidney. A widely accepted calculation for the number of glomeruli in the human kidney is 800 000 to 1 000 000 at the age of 40 years, with reduction of up to one half by the age of 80 years. The resulting reduction in the filtration rate of the kidney has important implications for the hydration status of the person, and his ability to eliminate drugs which are excreted by the renal system.

Urinary Elimination

Bladder muscles become weakened with age resulting in decreased bladder capacity. Hypersensitivity of the urinary expulsion mechanism may be caused by increased irritability of the bladder muscle, the normal desire to urinate becoming considerably more urgent. Bladder capacity invariably diminishes leading to increased frequency of micturition.

Prostatic enlargement occurs in most elderly men although the extent will vary considerably from individual to individual. Problems with either urinary retention or 'dribbling' become increasingly frequent as the years advance and constitute a serious embarrassment and inconvenience to those who experience either.

Elderly women, especially those who have had children, are more likely to experience relaxed muscles of the pelvic floor. Stress incontinence, the involuntary passing of urine upon coughing or laughing, is quite frequent.

Dehydration

Elderly people, particularly if they are hospitalized, are prone to dehydration from one or more of a number of causes including a diminished thirst response, lack of access to fluids, deliberate reduction in fluid intake to avoid incontinence, use of diuretics, and exposure to heating and ventilation systems which increase sweat loss.

The physiology of the elderly person is particularly sensitive to changes in his hydration status which may result in the onset of an acute confusional state. This diminution of the ability of the elderly person to cope with even minor changes in his fluid position presents us with a situation in which an acute medical emergency can be relatively easy to prevent by ensuring that appropriate fluids are taken.

RESPIRATORY SYSTEM

There are several changes in the structure and function of the respiratory system which can give rise to problems for the ageing person, and which play an important part in the increased respiratory pathology in this group.

Respiratory System Structure

The ageing lung tends to enlarge due to loss of elasticity, resulting in an increase of residual capacity of up to 45 to 55% by the age of 90 years. The number of alveoli are reduced and are increased in size. These factors, along with the increased residual capacity, dramatically reduce the breathing efficiency of the older person.

The almost inevitable kyphosis reduces the mobility of the rib cage and inhibits the contraction power of the respiratory muscles, increasing the incidence of respiratory infection.

Respiratory Function

There is a progressive lowering in the vital capacity of the lung, resulting in a relative lack of ventilation of lung tissue even at rest, causing high incidence of hypostatic pneumonia. The elderly need to exert more effort in breathing deeply in order to achieve full expansion of the lung. Although immunity to viral infections almost certainly increases with age, there is a greater tendency to suffer from bacterial infections.

'Normal' respiratory difficulty is a common feature, and one which requires that the elderly be given additional time in which to undertake activities requiring moderate exertion. Much can and should be done in order to maximize respiratory function by the use of exercise generally, and respiratory exercise in particular. Although the dangers of respiratory infections are particularly evident during bed rest, they should be regarded as a real threat at all times.

GASTROINTESTINAL SYSTEM

The stomach decreases in motility, hunger contractions decrease, gastric secretions decrease and the emptying time of the stomach also decreases. Gastric atrophy and accompanying gastritis increase in frequency and may be a result of ageing or of a pathological process.

Intestinal absorption may be decreased due to decreased digestive juice secretions, decreased motility, degradation of the absorbing surface and reduced intestinal blood flows. Constipation, commonly experienced by the elderly, may result from reduced large bowel peristalsis.

The efficiency of the digestive system undoubtedly diminishes with age, giving rise to frequent digestive complaints by the elderly. Particular attention must be paid to the nutritional consequences of growing old, and to the fact that many emotional disturbances such as anxiety and depression seriously affect nutritional status.

Teeth and Gums

Although it is virtually inevitable that gums will recede and some loss of teeth will occur, a good oral hygiene and dental programme can do much to minimize these problems. Well-fitting dentures, rather than those which are ill-fitting and uncomfortable, will reduce embarrassment and also cause the person to enjoy food and communicate better.

Taste and Smell

Taste and smell, both important factors in the enjoyment of food, deteriorate significantly with age. These, and other factors, may cause the older person to complain of 'loss of appetite' therefore highlighting the need for food to be offered and presented in an attractive, appetizing and appealing manner.

Saliva

The volume of saliva can be reduced by as much as 60% in the elderly resulting in a dry tongue and mouth, and in chewing difficulties. There is also a marked decrease in salivary ptyalin causing difficulties with the digestion of starch.

Nutrition

A number of changes take place which, cumulatively, effectively reduce the nutritional status of the elderly person. Although these changes may result in an insidious, rather than acute, nutritional problem occurring they are nevertheless sufficiently serious to cause many people to be acutely mal-nourished, *even* in institutional settings.

Faecal Elimination

Faecal incontinence increases with advancing years and may occur in as many as 20% of hospitalized elderly patients. The awareness of a full rectum diminishes with age as does the muscle tone of the rectal sphincter. Although the internal sphincter may well be normal, the external sphincter is frequently over-relaxed. In younger people the two sphincters operate in such a way that flatus can be passed without allowing the passage of faecal matter, this ability is diminished in the elderly and often adds to the incidence of faecal incontinence.

Constipation is relatively common and, although partially due to the decreased motility of the large bowel, may be made considerably worse by a low-roughage diet, lack of exercise, deliberate withholding of the stool, and the accumulative effects of faulty bowel habits.

As nurses we must be particularly aware of, and sensitive to the needs of the elderly in relation to faecal elimination, because the outcome of faulty elimination mechanisms is an acute source of irritation and embarrassment to our patients. We must take full account of the changes which are due to the ageing process.

All aspects of elimination are the source of considerable concern to the elderly person. Elimination, regarded as a particularly private function, is regarded as something which the adult ought to be fully able to control. Elimination problems such as incontinence of urine and faeces are often (wrongly) regarded as forms of infantile or totally unacceptable behaviour. It is worth noting that it is very often the onset of faecal and/or urinary incontinence which causes the relatives of elderly people who are being cared for at home to seek their admission to a nursing home or other type of facility.

SEXUALITY

Although sexual intercourse does not, and need not, cease with old age it is undoubtedly modified because of the physical changes which take place. Nurses have an important role to play in relation to minimizing the extent to which the normal physiological and physical processes of ageing interfere with sexual activity.

The walls of the vagina become considerably drier, itchy and thinner. Vaginitis is a frequent complaint made by elderly women, a condition made worse by sexual intercourse. Temporary relief may be obtained by the use of lubricants such as KY jelly, a substance which can be used during sexual intercourse to reduce any actual or potential discomfort resulting from increased friction.

Although impotence in the male after the onset of extreme old age is very likely, many instances of impotence in the 'younger' old man may be psychogenic rather than physical in nature. Sexual performance probably begins to decline after the age of 25 years and is related to the decline in both frequency and duration of erection.

Both sexes experience a whole range of other changes relating to the ageing process (musculoskeletal weakness, respiratory deficiency and elimination problems) which interfere with normal sexual activity. The role of the nurse is to appreciate that continuing sexual activity during old age is normal and natural for most individuals who will need considerable assistance in overcoming the physical barriers to a successful sex life in old age. For those couples who find 'normal' intercourse impossible because of changes which have seriously limited physical activity, alternatives such as oral intercourse or mutual masturbation should be considered.

PAIN

As with all individuals, the existence of pain in the elderly is something which requires urgent attention; until it is relieved the person cannot realize his full potential. Although the elderly person can feel pain with the same degree of intensity as someone younger, it is something which he is more likely to endure for one of a number of possible reasons. Pain might be perceived as something about which one needs to feel stoic, or which should not be reported in case it is found to be indicative of something sinister and which requires vigorous medical intervention. I have personal experience of an 80-year-old lady who endured pain for ten years, forbidding her husband or others to report it in case she should be hospitalized and submitted to vigorous invasive surgery. In the event, the pain was found to have been caused by a minor medical condition which was resolved relatively easily.

A major feature of pain, even minor pain, is that it increases in intensity as anxiety, loss of control, and increased accompanying emotional experiences such as grief, fear, guilt and depression occur. In recognizing the often limited personal emotional resources of some elderly people, particularly those who are hospitalized or who are ill in some other situation, we must not be altogether surprised by over-reaction to relatively minor pain experiences.

COMMUNICATION

A range of changes take place in the lifestyle, anatomy, physiology and motivation of the elderly which reduce the effectiveness by which they can communicate with others. Selected changes will be presented which are representative of the general alteration in the functioning of the elderly person which interferes with communication skills.

Hearing

Some degree of hearing loss occurs due to a decreased efficiency of the actual hearing mechanism or (more commonly) to excess ear wax which is relatively easy to remove. Other causes include prolonged exposure to high level noise, recurring ear infections, and drug-induced ear damage. The high incidence of deafness in the elderly due to causes other than excess wax, about 3% aged 70 years and over 8% aged 85 years, constitutes a major challenge for nurses working in this area of care.

The extent to which impaired hearing reduces the ability of the elderly to interact and socialize cannot be over-estimated. The role of the nurse in maximizing hearing ability and in minimizing the consequences of bad hearing is an extremely important one. These consequences include communication and interpersonal difficulties, reduced trust, depression, anxiety, immobility, dependence and reality-perceptual deficits.

Vision

Visual acuity which is the ability to discriminate fine detail of an object, undergoes a marked deterioration beyond the age of about 65 years. This deterioration probably results from the lens and vitreous humor becoming less effective. Fozard *et al.* (1977) suggest that blurred vision may also result from a change in the curvature of the cornea which tends to flatten as the person's age increases. There is also a diminution in the ability of the eye to react to increases and decreases in light, posing particular problems when the person moves between rooms with different light intensities.

Touch

There is a diminished ability of the touch receptors resulting in a decreased ability to recognize fine, and even rough, texture and in relation to those psychomotor skills which demand the sensitive use of touch. Although changes in touch sensitivity in the elderly have not been researched as well as changes in relation to other senses, there are indications that there is probably a particular decrease in the sensitivity of the skin on the palm of the hand (Kenshalo 1977).

Decreased acuteness in the sense of touch can cause problems in relation to such activities as identification of different coins, sewing fastening buttons or clips, and obtaining pleasure from the 'feel' of objects.

Taste

Taste buds diminish in quantity and quality as the person ages. Although taste buds can regenerate, their loss exceeds the rate at which they can multiply. Other factors which result in a deterioration of taste are smoking, the general state and dryness of the mouth, and the overall quality of the food that is being tasted. Because food has a great psychological importance for all individuals, particularly the elderly person with diminished taste, it is of great importance that the quality, taste, colour and smell of food offered, be of the highest quality. It may also be that the older person requires 'special' flavours such as garlic, spices, alcohol, hot sauces, or any of a number of aperitifs which will enable him to compensate for diminished taste ability.

Smell

Smell is caused by a chemical reaction in which molecules of volatile materials initiate activity when they come into contact with olfactory receptor cells in the nose. It would appear that, although the sense of smell is not significantly affected by the ageing process alone, other factors associated with age may affect it (Engen 1977). A general decrease in the health status of the person results in a defective smell mechanism, as will long-term exposure to strong smells, tobacco smoke or any substance which will irritate the nasal cavity.

Many of the potentially unpleasant smells associated with the care of hospitalized, or non-hospitalized, incontinent patients can be minimized by using appropriate ventilation, odour control machines, and by preventing the causes of such odours. The pleasant smell of food, soap, cologne or freshly cut flowers is something which the elderly are entitled to enjoy.

SKIN AND HAIR

A major and obvious change takes places in the 'outer covering' of the ageing person. A decrease in subcutaneous tissue, coupled with thinning and drying of skin, results in severe inelasticity and a greater tendency to break or tear. These changes, and others relating to muscle tissue, place the person at high risk in relation to the development of pressure sores. The nursing implications of changes in the wound healing process include pressure sore formation and healing, and need to be accounted for when dealing with such circumstances. Bruno and Craven (1982) point out that these changes include vascular insufficiency, immune system decrease in antibody and neutrophil production, decreased rate of mitotic activity of epithelial cells, and decreased responsiveness of homeostatic mechanisms.

Atrophy of sweat glands and a decreased blood supply to the skin add to the general deterioration in its condition with the resulting texture (including wrinkles) being 'typical' of old age.

Nails grow more slowly and in a thick and irregular way.

Hair loss and/or greying is common, as is the development of excess facial hair on the ageing female, a potential source of considerable embarrassment and threat to self-esteem.

The ability of the skin to measure external temperature, and regulate internal temperature, decreases dramatically with increased age. Hypothermia in the elderly (see Collins *et al.* 1977 and Millard 1977) is well documented, and a paper by Kolanowski and Gunter (1983) presents a number of approaches for preventing hypothermia. The variation in 'normal' temperature in the elderly is the important subject of an article by Thatcher (1983) entitled '98.6°F. What is normal?'

THE BRAIN

It has been estimated, from a combination of weight loss, surface area changes and cell counts, that every day of our adult life 100 000 of our neurones (which are non-renewable) die. The brain changes are both regionalized and generalized with an example of the latter being the accumulation of Lipofuscin age pigments in the neurones. Another important generalized change is the progressive arteriosclerotic change which affects the cerebral arterial system.

The microscopic and macroscopic brain changes whch occur have an important relationship with many of the pathological and 'normal' differences which may exist between young and old people. Examples of these differences include senile and arteriosclerotic dementia, short-term memory problems, resistance to change, inability to respond rapidly, and difficulty in coping with multiple stimuli.

As nurses we need to be acutely aware of the anxiety which these actual or anticipated changes in the brain cause for people who are old, or who are becoming old. In many respects, these changes are reflected in the negative use of the ageist descriptive label 'senile', thus adding to the pain of growing old.

DYING

Almost all deaths occur over the age of 70 years of age, and all old people will die sooner rather than later. The inevitability of death is a certain result of the cumulative effects of changes which occur with age.

The fact that the process of dying is a potential problem for many elderly persons makes it an area in which nurses must move freely and with considerable confidence and sensitivity. It is often (wrongly) assumed that the inevitability of death is something which the elderly population all become increasingly comfortable with as they age. This assumption can be easily challenged on the basis that at least a small, but significant, number of elderly people fear the process of dying or death itself.

It is not being suggested that all old people are 'ill' or that the selected changes outlined in this chapter are pathological, therefore indicative of a disease process, or that they represent illnesses. Rather, it is suggested that these changes are a normal and natural part of the ageing process which must be taken into account by nursing staff and others who care for elderly people. These changes do, however, result in a tendency for the elderly to experience multiple disease process (multiple pathology) and disease processes which tend to be chronic rather than acute (chronicity).

MULTIPLE PATHOLOGY

Because of the degenerative nature of the ageing process, and because of the cumulative effect of chronic disease experiences, elderly persons tend to suffer from a number of disease processes at any given time; for example a person may suffer from a combination of osteoarthritis, congestive cardiac failure, late onset diabetes and varicose veins. The concept of multiple pathology also applies in relation to the nursing needs of patients who, irrespective of the specific disease processes involved, may require nursing care in relation to incontinence, deafness, immobility, respiratory distress and disorientation simultaneously.

CHRONICITY

Although the elderly are just as likely to experience illnesses of an acute nature such as pneumonia, fractures and illnesses requiring immediate surgical intervention, they are much more likely additionally to experience illnesses and more general problems which are of a chronic nature. Chronicity is due in part to the general physical decline associated with old age, with the cumulative effects of diseases such as repeated attacks of acute bronchitis resulting in chronic bronchitis, and to the extended timespan in which they are 'at risk' in relation to suffering diseases which are of an irreversible and chronic nature.

CONCLUSION

Beyond maturity all of us suffer a decrease in our ability to repair the normal wear and tear to which we are exposed. The changes that inevitably come with ageing are well documented and should be understood by nurses and other care givers in order that they can take account of them when caring for the elderly. Indeed, the whole point of achieving an understanding of the ageing process is in order that it be taken into account during our relationship with, the delivery of care to, and during our everyday contacts with elderly people.

REFERENCES

Bahr R.T. (1983) Sleep-wake patterns in the aged. *Journal of gerontological Nursing* **9**, 534–7, cont. 540.

Bruno P. & Craven R.F. (1982) Age challenges to wound healing *Journal of gerontological Nursing* **8**, 686–91, cont. 715.

Collins K.J., Dore C. & Exton-Smith A.N. (1977) Accidental hypothermia and impaired temperature homeostasis in the elderly. *British medical Journal* **1**, 353–6.

de Vries H.A. (1970) Physiological effects of an exercise training regimen upon men aged 52–88. *Journal of Gerontology* **25**, 325–36.

Engen T. (1977) Taste and smell. In Birren J.E. & Schaie K.W. (eds) *Handbook of the Psychology of Aging*. Van Nostrand, New York.

Fozard J.L., Wolf E., Bell B., McFarland R. & Pubolsky S. (1977) Visual perception and communication. In Birren J.E. & Schaie K.W. (eds) *Handbook of the Psychology of Aging* Van Nostrand, New York.

Kenshalo D.D. (1977) Age changes in touch, vibration, temperature, kinesthesis and pain sensitivity. In Birren J.E. & Schaie K.W. (eds) *Handbook of the Psychology of Aging*. Van Nostrand, New York.

Kolanowski A. & Gunter L. (1983) Thermal stress and the aged. *Geriatric Nursing* **9**, 12–15.

Lerner R. (1982) Sleep loss in the aged: Implications for nursing research. *Journal of gerontological Nursing* **8**, 323–6.

Millard P.H. (1977) Hypothermia in the elderly. *Nursing Mirror* **145**, 23–5.

Schrimer M.S. (1983) When sleep won't come. *Journal of gerontological Nursing* **9**, 16–21.
Thatcher R.M. (1983) 98.6°F. What is normal? *Geriatric Nursing* **9**, 22–27.

Chapter 8
Diseases Commonly Experienced by the Elderly
(A Review)

To make full use of this book, and obtain an appropriate understanding of the diseases reviewed in this chapter, you will have to study selected texts dealing with geriatric medicine and geropsychiatry. A number of excellent books on the subject are available including the five described in the Further Reading list at the end of this chapter. In order to indicate the width of material contained in these five typical examples, a note of the contents of each is included.

Although virtually all diseases experienced by the young can be experienced by the elderly, the reverse being *almost* as true, there are a range of illnesses which are much more likely to affect the older population. The diseases which are reviewed in this chapter are *examples* of that range and do not constitute an exhaustive review.

The diseases selected for inclusion are, for the sake of convenience, generally separated into physical and non-physical sections. It is recognized that this division is somewhat arbitrary in that all diseases have both physical and non-physical components. An excellent example of this 'overlap' are the *acute confusional states* which have a physical cause and a consequence which is both physical and non-physical.

In order to care for the elderly as a group, you will need to have a detailed knowledge and understanding of the causes, signs, symptoms, course, prognosis, treatment and general presentation of all diseases (physical and non-physical) which are commonly experienced by that group. (See texts in Further Reading list at the end of this chapter.)

THE DEMENTIAS

In their various forms, the dementias constitute one of the most common and serious groups of illnesses of old age. Ten per cent of people aged over 65 years are moderately/severely demented, with the incidence increasing rapidly with age to as high as 25% above the age of 80 years. As medical science increases longevity, the incidence of dementia (often referred to as the 'quiet epidemic') will continue to rise and present a great challenge to nursing and other health care staff, as well as to the relatives of sufferers.

The major features of dementia (of which there are a number of types) are: a picture of chronic and extensive brain disease, late onset, intellectual deterioration, severe memory impairment (particularly for recent events), disorientation for time, person and place, all occurring *without* clouding of consciousness. Additionally, the dementing process is one of slow insidious onset, a gradual deterioration and irreversibility. The progressive nature of dementia means that the person will only be mildly demented, with his 'normal functioning' being largely retained during the early phase, for part of the period of illness. Thus, the severity of the disease is very much on a continuum, resulting in different care requirements at different stages of the illness.

Not all elderly people suffer from dementia, although many who do not may experience *some* short-term memory impairment. The normal changes associated with the ageing process should *not* be equated with dementia. This problem of *benign senile forgetfulness* (or benign 'dementia') was recognized and described by Kral (1965) who clearly documented the differences between the memory dysfunction of dementia and that due to the 'normal' ageing process. See Table 8.1 for a comparison of the features of benign senile forgetfulness, senile dementia (Alzheimer's disease) and multi-infarct dementia.

Senile Dementia (Alzheimer's Disease)

The current view held by the majority of workers in the field of gero-psychiatry is that Alzheimer's disease and senile dementia are one and the same, and this view is reflected by the increasing use of the term 'senile dementia of Alzheimer type'.

Senile dementia has a slow and gradual onset which can be rather difficult to recognize at an early stage. Intellectual impairment may be preceded by restlessness, agitation, irritability, egocentricity and suspiciousness. Consciousness is not affected. Short-term memory, and latterly long-term memory, becomes increasingly impaired resulting in gross disorientation for time, person and place. Hallucinations and delusions of various types are not uncommon and add considerably to the difficulty presented in 'managing' these patients.

Judgement, in terms of ability to make decisions requiring insight and intellectual ability, declines and often results in the person endangering his

Table 8.1 Differences and similarities between benign senile forgetfulness, senile dementia (Alzheimer's type) and multi-infarct dementia.

	Benign senile forgetfulness	Senile dementia (Alzheimer's type)	Multi-infarct dementia
Age of onset	75 years +	45 years +	45 years +
Sex affected	Most frequently found in women	Most frequently found in women	Most frequently found in men
Course	Very slow, mainly affects memory	Progressive/ global	'Step-wise' progression. Focal
Dysphasia (time of occurrence)	Absent	Early	Earlier or later
Impaired: insight, personality, intellect (time of occurrence)	Late	Early	Late
Physical signs and symptoms	None	Limited/late	Dizziness, headache, tremors, etc.
Lifespan	Unaffected	Longer than multi-infarct dementia	Shortened

life, or the lives of others (for example by pouring paraffin on an electric or coal fire to make it burn well). *Affect* (mood) may be disturbed in terms of either depression or elation, or a mixture of both. *Memory* is impaired, resulting in considerable anxiety early on, and in virtual total memory loss in later stages. *Comprehension* and communication problems increase with the demented person losing much of his ability to comprehend the sensory input from his environment, and experiencing increasing difficulty in communicating with others.

The life-expectancy of persons suffering from senile dementia need not be shortened as a result of the illness. With good nursing care (which demands the highest possible level of excellence in relation to both physical *and* non-physical problems) there is no reason why a near to normal lifespan should not be achieved. In the latter stages of senile dementia the patient will become almost totally dependent on others in a wide range of areas such as feeding, drinking, dressing, bathing, using the toilet, movement and so on.

Multi-infarct Dementia

The term 'multi-infarct dementia' has now largely replaced the long-used term 'arteriosclerotic dementia'. While post-mortem examinations show the presence of multiple cerebral infarcts in persons with this illness, not all persons who suffer from cerebro-arteriosclerosis will develop multi-infarct dementia. The relationship between this illness and raised systemic blood pressure (a feature of the ageing process, see pp. 59–60) is well documented.

The physical origins of the disease result in it most often being initially seen by geriatricians rather than by psychiatrists. Early changes in the health of the person include weight loss, general physical decline, headaches, falling, fainting, drowsiness and strokes. The continued occurrence of minor strokes (multi-infarctions) is accompanied by periods of general confusion, agitation, anxiety or emotional lability.

Continued episodes of cerebral infarction result in a gradual deterioration in the patient in a classic 'step-wise progression'. Thus, the person deteriorates slightly after the first infarction and remains at that level for some time. A further episode makes the illness more serious, and so on until the dementia is gross and all-pervasive in terms of deterioration in memory, intellect, personality, communication ability, orientation and dependence. (See Table 8.1 for a summary of major features of this type of dementia relative to others.)

Life-expectancy is considerably shorter than for senile dementia, with the probability that the person will die of a major stroke a relatively short time after the onset of the illness. Multi-infarct dementia is less common than senile dementia and accounts for about 20% of all dementia sufferers.

DEPRESSIONS

Depression, of various types, is a major feature of the group of illnesses experienced by the elderly. In general, the incidence of neurotic depression is greatest in the 35- to 45-year-old age group, and psychotic depression is manifested most frequently in the 55- to 65-year-old age group. However, in surveys carried out by people who are not necessarily psychiatrists, the highest prevalence of depression has been in persons aged more than 65 years (Levy & Post 1982). In a study of the management and nature of depressive illness in later life Post (1972) examined a sample of 100 persons aged over 60 years who were admitted to a psychiatric unit after a diagnosis of depression. He found that of this sample 37% had severe and psychotic depression, 24% were labelled as 'intermediate psychotics' and 39% were labelled as neurotic depressives.

Suicide and the Elderly

While more younger people attempt suicide (parasuicide) than actually commit it, a ratio of about 10 to 1, the reverse is true in the elderly population. That the elderly population have a higher *actual* suicide rate is evidenced by the generally accepted estimate of 25% – 30% of all suicides being performed by elderly persons who constitute only 10 – 15% of the population. (See Schulman (1978) for an excellent discussion of suicide and parasuicide in old age.)

Depressive Pseudomentia

There are instances when depression may be confused with, or present as an apparent, dementia. An important work on this subject was written by Kiloh (1961) and is well worth reading. Pseudomentia is frequently encountered in elderly patients who, in fact, have a severe depressive illness; because many agitated or severely retarded depressed elderly patients may appear 'confused' or 'disoriented', they can be wrongly diagnosed as being demented. This condition is usually differentiated from true dementia by a more precise date of onset as obtained from informants, rapid deterioration from the date of onset to the time of referral to a psychiatrist, some awareness of memory deficit, ability to give some account of the progression of the illness and responsiveness to treatment of the depression.

PARANOID DISEASES

Paranoia, which is an extreme form of pathological suspiciousness, can occur as a feature of some illnesses such as dementia, or represent a distinct disease entity. As with many disease processes, paranoia can exist on any part of a continuum ranging from mild chronic suspiciousness to severe paranoia in which delusions of persecution are a prominent feature.

In old age, paranoia, if present, is likely to be a feature of a disease such as dementia, or a recurrence of an illness such as chronic and long-standing paranoid psychosis.

Levy and Post (1982) report that persistent persecutory states are relatively rarely encountered in psychogeriatric practice, although they cite other writers as calculating that 10% of elderly persons admitted to mental hospitals were paraphrenic. In the author's experience, paranoid diseases, or illnesses in which paranoia may be a prominent feature, are sufficiently common for nurses to be made aware of them. Furthermore, working with a paranoid person is particularly difficult and requires a nursing approach of considerable sophistication.

ACUTE CONFUSIONAL STATE
(DELIRIUM)

All age groups are at risk from this illness, which almost always has a physical illness precursor, but it is far more likely to affect the elderly as compared with the young adult population.

Acute confusional states have a *sudden onset* leading to gross confusion/delirium in a few hours or a day or two. Confusion is always present, with considerable fluctuation in severity. The confusion symptoms include memory impairment, disorientation, hyperactivity, alteration in consciousness levels (clouding of consciousness), disturbed sleep patterns, hallucinations, delusions, hostility, misinterpretation of environmental stimuli (illusions) and limited concentration.

The physical manifestations of this condition are those of an acute general physical deterioration and may include tachycardia, fever, dehydration, tremor, dry tongue and sunken eyes. Additionally the specific signs and symptoms of the illness/cause of the delirium are present. In the elderly, acute confusional states are more easily precipitated and usually last longer than in younger persons. In both age groups, however, delirium is usually a short-term syndrome, lasting for a few days or one to four weeks, with treatment being the treatment of the underlying cause. On occasions, in all age groups, the physical stress of the delirium, or the underlying illness, will result in death.

Acute confusional states result from any illness process which interferes with the activity of the brain in any of a number of ways. Examples of common causes include: malnutrition; cerebral hypoxia; infection (local or general); dehydration; metabolic and endocrine disorders; trauma; blood loss; intoxication by alcohol or other chemical agents, including drugs; severe pain; hypo- or hyper-thermia; and psychological stress (see Lipowski 1980). Table 8.2 outlines the important differences between acute confusional states and chronic confusional states (the dementias).

PARKINSON'S DISEASE (PARKINSONISM)

Parkinson's disease constitutes the cause of about 10% of all admissions to geriatric wards. At one extreme this disease may present as a very treatable and mild syndrome, at the other as a rapidly progressive illness with a considerable dementia component.

Typically, an obvious tremor presents although it can, in some cases, be difficult to detect. A fixed, staring expression with infrequent blinking is present as may be a 'small-step' gait, reduced arm swing and a bent posture.

The illness, particularly if untreated, can lead to increasing inactivity,

Table 8.2 The major differences between acute and chronic confusional states.

Details	Acute confusional states	Chronic confusional states
Age of onset	Can affect all age groups	45 years +
Rapidity of onset	Very rapid	Slow and insidious
Clouding of consciousness	Yes, marked alteration in levels of consciousness	No
Treatment	Of the underlying cause	Symptomatic
Duration	Acute/short term	Chronic/long term
Prognosis	Good, providing underlying cause is successfully treated	Poor, long-term deterioration

difficulty in rising from a chair, clumsy movements, impaired fine movement and general susceptibility to falls and accidents.

Despite their problematical side-effects, a number of drugs are effective in controlling the rigidity and weakness associated with parkinsonism, although they may have less effect on the tremor.

HUNTINGTON'S CHOREA

Huntington's chorea, an inherited disease transmitted by a single autosomal dominant gene, usually develops in the fourth or fifth decade of life. The physical aspects of the illness are frequently accompanied by non-physical symptoms including depression, agitation, hostility, hallucinations, delusions and paranoia. Dementia usually develops during some stage of the disease, which is a progressive and fatal one.

Huntington's chorea is differentiated from other types of dementia and choreaform diseases by its hereditary character, involuntary jerking movements and snake-like writhing of the body. There is a *relatively* good preservation of memory, even during the advanced stage of the illness.

Although fairly uncommon, this disease is important because of the intensive nursing care required by sufferers, and also because of the important hereditary implication for the families of sufferers. *On average,* half of the children of a person who suffers from Huntington's chorea will develop the disease, none of the children of non-sufferers will develop it.

Unfortunately, it is only after passing the normal child-bearing age that the child of a sufferer will know whether or not he/she has inherited the illness.

SKELETAL DISEASES

Diseases of joints and bone tissue are extremely common in old age. Although they result partly *from* reduced mobility, they are also a major *cause* of reduced mobility and are an often painful and obvious reminder of the ageing process.

Bone Diseases

Paget's disease, a bone disease of unknown aetiology, affects some 5% of elderly patients. The localized nature of Paget's disease results in bones becoming expanded, softer and deformed. Although all bones may be affected, those most frequently involved are the clavicles, femora, skull, pelvis, lumbar spine and tibiae. Medical intervention may be required to treat pain and fractures.

Osteoporosis results in bone tissue becoming generally less dense and therefore more susceptible to fracture and collapse. Either type of damage may occur as a result of trauma such as a fall, or may result from minimal stress such as that caused by walking or being turned in bed. The high frequency of fractures in old age is largely attributed to the elevated incidence of osteoporosis in both sexes, but particularly in women. Vertebral collapse, resulting in *kyphosis* (Dowager's hump) is common, especially in elderly women.

Treatment in the form of drug therapy, including calcium supplements, is of value. More important from the nursing viewpoint is the central and effective role of the nurse in relation to prevention, by health education, which includes the use of appropriate diet and exercise prior to and during the period of old age.

Osteomalacia is a generalized disease of bone in which the osteoid matrix is formed normally, but fails to calcify properly. The resulting 'soft bone', pain, muscle weakness and biochemical testing can result in the diagnosis of this very treatable disease. The major types of osteomalacia include those due to lack of vitamin D, drug side-effects, renal failure and inappropriate absorption of calcium.

The treatment of this illness in the form of vitamin D therapy can result in dramatic improvement.

Joint Diseases

Septic arthritis, a pyogenic infection of individual joints, occurs rather infrequently, with joints affected by rheumatoid arthritis and osteoarthritis being particularly vulnerable.

Rheumatoid arthritis usually begins in middle age. This chronic condition is, however, an important cause of secondary degenerative joint disease in old age. Potent analgesics, even those which are known to cause addiction, may be necessary to control the pain frequently experienced by elderly sufferers. In general, steroid therapy is avoided in elderly patients with this illness.

Osteoarthritis, a degenerative joint disease, is the major type of arthritis found in the elderly population. The major change caused by osteoarthritis is the loss of articular cartilage in the joints in which increased friction and crepitus result. Pain and restricted movement are the principal features with all joints being at risk.

CHEST DISEASES

Almost all forms of chest diseases are experienced by the elderly with some being particularly common. These diseases must be seen in the context of the gradual and general deterioration which takes place in the respiratory system as part of the ageing process.

Infections

Bronchitis (acute and chronic), *lobar pneumonia, bronchopneumonia* and *empyema* are all important causes of morbidity and mortality in older people. Chest infections frequently precipitate heart failure and result in a combination of both illnesses. The respiratory changes in old age, in addition to the 'normal' respiratory limitations imposed by the ageing process, can make medical diagnosis more difficult in this age group.

Pulmonary tuberculosis, although comparatively rare, can easily be over-looked, and may be effectively treated.

Cancer

Cancer of the lung, particularly the bronchus, is one of the most common cancers affecting the older person. Treatment is not very satisfactory, with surgical intervention carrying a fairly high operative mortality rate. Secondary lung cancer, and metastasis resulting from the primary bronchial tumor are common.

ENDOCRINE DISEASES

Diabetes mellitus is often mild and of late onset. Although symptoms may be minor and only found during routine blood/urine sugar testing, diabetes can be more serious. In many instances the illness may be associated with obesity, occasionally with pancreatic disease, including carcinoma of the pancreas.

Hyperparathyroidism, which is more common in elderly women than in men, is associated with a consistently raised serum calcium level and a normal or elevated level of serum parathormone. Progressive mental deterioration and renal failure may result if the disease is left untreated.

Thyrotoxicosis often presents in an atypical fashion in the elderly with cardiac complications of heart failure being common. 'Apathetic' thyrotoxicosis in the form of apathy, weight loss and depression may occur with general muscle weakness and fatigue.

Myxoedema presents in the elderly in a way which is usually similar to the onset in younger adults with mental and physical slowing, apathy, puffiness of the face, a croaky voice, cold intolerance, occasionally deafness, and constipation. Apparent dementia, or a depressive-type psychosis, is not unusual. Therapy in the form of lifelong L-thyroxine replacement is often effective.

GASTROINTESTINAL DISEASES

In addition to the age-related changes which take place, a number of gastro-intestinal diseases often affect the elderly.

Parotitis (inflammation of the parotid glands) results from a number of primary causes which include local and general bacterial infection, febrile illnesses and dehydration.

Hiatus hernia, which may be asymptomatic, most frequently affects women and is usually associated with obesity. In the most common type of hiatus hernia, the 'sliding' type, the upper part of the stomach and the cardio-oesophageal junction rise up through the diaphragm. Although treatment is usually conservative, surgery may be required despite its relatively high mortality rate in the elderly.

Peptic ulcer, with a peak incidence in middle life, presents in the elderly in the same way as in the younger adult. Pain, in any of a number of abdominal areas, although most common in the left side of the lower chest, weight loss, vomiting, anaemia and general debility are common symptoms. At one time it was thought that very large peptic ulcers were often malignant, this is now known to be untrue. Drug therapy is the treatment of choice, with surgery being required in some cases.

Malabsorption, caused by a combination of disease and age-related deterioration of the gastrointestinal tract, can result in a variety of nutrition-deficiency-related diseases, including general malnutrition and a range of vitamin deficiencies.

Carcinoma of the gastrointestinal tract, with cancer of the stomach being one of the most common malignancies in the elderly, can occur in various parts of the system. The pancreas, oesophagus and rectum are commonly affected. Radical treatment, in the form of surgery, does not have a high success rate and may be inappropriate because of late diagnosis, resulting metastasis and general physical frailty.

Gall-stones, which are often asymptomatic and not detected until post-mortem examination, give rise to symptoms such as intolerance of fat, dyspepsia, cholecystic attacks and episodes of obstructive jaundice. Cholecystectomy may be the treatment of choice if the symptoms are severe. Otherwise, conservative treatment is more usual.

Jaundice, often of the obstructive type with malignant diseases being a major cause, is common. Pancreatic carcinoma and others such as carcinoma of the stomach and resultant metastasis are major causes of obstructive jaundice. Gall-stones, which will result in fluctuating levels of jaundice, are another common cause.

Diverticular disease, most frequently affecting the sigmoid colon, has been found in almost half the post-mortem examinations of the elderly. The role of diet, particularly the lack of dietary fibre, is well documented in relation to diverticular disease. A high-fibre diet, such as that achieved by adding bran, is a simple and effective means of reducing the symptoms of diarrhoea, abdominal pain and bleeding.

Haemorrhoids, internal and external, result in painful dilated veins covered with a film of mucous membrane. Internal haemorrhoids originate inside the bowel and become thicker and more painful as they develop. Bright red blood is present in the stools and, in long-standing cases, anaemia occurs. External haemorrhoids occur at the external margin of the anus and consist of small, dilated, painful veins.

While surgery is an effective form of treatment, local applications (cream or suppositories), phenol injections and/or control of constipation are also used to reduce haemorrhoidal tissue. The role of constipation control in preventing this disease is very important.

KIDNEY AND UROGENITAL DISEASES

Kidney size reduces in old age, with the nephrons becoming smaller in size and number. The general reduction in renal capacity and efficiency means that the elderly have much less 'reserve' and are more vulnerable to the risks of disease.

Uraemia of the pre-renal, post-renal and renal types results from substantial renal impairment commonly found in the elderly. This condition requires prompt recognition with treatment usually being conservative, with renal transplant or dialysis rarely being considered. The role of the nurse in encouraging appropriate fluid intake, compliance with medication regimen and diet control is of obvious importance.

Urinary tract infections generally, polynephritis and cystitis in particular, have a high incidence rate. Additionally, asymptomatic bacteriuria may be associated with mild dysuria or frequency of micturition, particularly in women.

Prostatic disease of the benign prostatic hypertrophic type is often found in old men and leads to the troublesome symptoms of urinary dribbling, nocturia, frequency and dysuria. Acute retention of urine, or chronic retention with overflow present serious problems. Prostatectomy carries a low risk, permanent and indwelling catheters may be used in some instances. Carcinoma of the prostate is one of the most frequent cancers found in elderly men.

Gynaecological disorders of many types are found in elderly women, ranging from mild 'senile' vaginitis to more serious diseases such as carcinoma of the uterus and cervix. The latter develops in approximately 1.5% of women at some point in their lives, and occurs twice as often in older women compared with those aged less than 65 years.

NUTRITIONAL DISEASES

Recent surveys reveal an alarmingly high incidence of nutritional deficits in the elderly, with general malnutrition existing despite the ageing process having little impact on the ability to eat and digest food.

Dehydration, which is usually secondary to some other more specific disease process, can have serious, if not fatal, consequences. The role of the nurse in preventing dehydration, or treating the 'uncomplicated' form which is simply due to an inadequate fluid intake, is crucial.

Malnutrition, resulting in a range of specific nutritional deficiencies, is often secondary to other disease processes; for example, a dementing or depressed person may be incapable of preparing and/or eating food properly. Vitamin A,B,C and D, calcium, iron, magnesium and potassium deficiencies result in their own specific pathology.

Gout, caused by the accumulation of excess uric acid which is deposited in the joints, results in recurring episodes of acute arthritis. Up to 3% of elderly men and 0.5% of elderly women suffer from gout.

Obesity, particularly in the elderly female, gives rise to a great deal of secondary morbidity in the form of arthritis, diabetes, respiratory and cardiovascular problems and general inactivity. Excessive calorie intake (particularly if the person's budget encourages them to buy high-calorie, inexpensive foods) and reduced activity are the major causes of obesity.

DISEASES OF THE CARDIOVASCULAR SYSTEM

Heart disease of a variety of types is experienced, with some 15% of all persons admitted to geriatric units suffering from cardiac failure. A selection of the more common diseases are outlined below.

Valvular diseases of the mitral and aortic valves may require intensive medical intervention but are, more commonly, of the chronic, degenerative and (occasionally) asymptomatic types.

Cardiac arrhythmias increase in incidence with old age with atrial fibrillation being related to the gradual increase in fibrous tissue within the conducting system of the heart. Complete heart block, with a typically slow but regular pulse, is not uncommon, nor are both right and left bundle branch blocks.

Ischaemic heart disease is possibly one of the most important classes of cardiac disease in the old person, with the highest incidence occurring in men. Myocardial infarction, although acute, often presents in a less dramatic/critical form in the elderly as compared with the younger person. While some infarcts may result in sudden death, others are 'silent' and symptom free. Angina pectoris, less often found in the elderly bearing in mind the high incidence of other heart diseases, can often be controlled by chemotherapy when symptoms are troublesome.

Bacterial endocarditis of the subacute type in those aged 60 years or more, represents one-third of all diagnosed cases. Although carrying a serious prognosis if untreated, the outlook with treatment is relatively good.

Heart failure, which may be secondary to any of a variety of other diseases, is a major feature of cardiac pathology in old age. Although the presentation, treatment and prognosis are similar to that in a younger age group, cardiac failure frequently results in acute confusional states in the elderly. Where the cause is due to an irreversible condition, treatment will have to be permanent. In some instances, short-term medical treatment will cure the underlying cause and, subsequently, alleviate the cardiac failure.

Cardiac arrest, and its medical and nursing management, requires careful consideration and, when possible, planning. Where a good prognosis is present, and if prompt and efficient resuscitation is possible, active and intensive intervention may well be appropriate. However, if resuscitation following cardiac arrest only represents a means of postponing a patient's inevitable and imminent death, and suffering, it may be felt to be inappropriate in some instances.

Hypotension, including *postural hypotension,* and *hypertension* are both common in old age. Pathological increases or decreases in blood pressure can, for the most part, be fairly effectively controlled by appropriate chemotherapy. Patient education, particularly as it relates to the causes and consequences of postural hypotension, can do much to alleviate these conditions and their consequences.

Atherosclerosis and associated *arteriosclerosis* are major causes of pathology in old age, carrying serious consequences for health status. Resultant conditions include hypertension, arteriosclerotic dementia, peripheral vascular disease and strokes.

Thromboembolic diseases, including *venous thrombosis* and *pulmonary embolism,* are commonplace, with post-mortem studies demonstrating the presence of recent pulmonary emboli in about 30% of routine examinations of the elderly.

Anaemia, although not rare in the population generally, is found among the elderly in the form of *iron-deficiency anaemia* or *pernicious anaemia.*

DISEASES OF THE CENTRAL NERVOUS SYSTEM

A number of diseases of this system occur, in addition to those such as dementia and parkinsonism mentioned earlier (see pp. 72–8). Additionally, a wide range of illnesses such as cardiac failure, anaemia, hypotension and toxaemia have a noticeable effect on the functioning of the central nervous system.

Cerebrovascular accidents, commonly referred to as 'stroke' or CVA, may take the form of cerebral thrombosis, cerebral haemorrhage or cerebral embolism. Although the mortality rate is high, and the prognosis is poor if the patient is comatose for 24 hours or more, many elderly people recover either partially or totally.

Rehabilitation, in the form of immediate and intensive physiotherapy accompanied by nursing actions to maximize independence, is crucial. The long-term consequences of a cerebrovascular accident are, for many patients, serious and very difficult to accept. Dysphasia, which may well be mistaken for confusion, is particularly stressful for patients and those who care for them.

Transient ischaemic attacks, believed to result from arterial disease in either the carotid or vertebro-basilar systems, cause a number of disturbances of cerebral functions as evidenced by such problems as vertigo, temporary speech disturbance, visual difficulties and giddiness.

Herpes zoster (shingles), a painful condition distributed along the affected nerve root, can result in considerable general disablement. Treatment is rather difficult, neural complications such as those affecting the eye may result in hospitalization.

DISEASES OF THE EYE

Cataracts, a lens opacity causing blurring of vision, may affect one or both eyes. Treatment of cataract, the most common eye disease of old age, is by surgical removal of the lens.

Glaucoma, which can be either of the acute or chronic type, may result in loss of vision and is usually responsive to treatment with chemotherapy.

Macular degeneration causes a loss of central vision so that the part which is sharpest and clearest deteriorates, resulting in difficulty with 'fine vision' such as that required to sew or read fine print. Treatment is usually supportive and conservative with the use of spectacles.

Ectropian and *entropian* are common and can cause corneal damage and/or extreme personal irritation.

Retinal detachment, a condition by no means confined to the elderly, is often treated with bed rest or by surgery if the elderly person is physically fit.

DISEASES OF THE EAR

Deafness, a symptom of disease, is a serious and debilitating condition frequently experienced by old people. Wax in the outer ear can result in *conductive deafness,* infections in the form of *otitis media* may result in hearing loss and ear drum perforation. *Perceptive deafness* can follow obstruction of the blood supply to, or nerve damage to, the inner ear.

Presbycusis, a naturally occurring diminution in hearing acuity which accompanies old age, begins around the age of 30 years, becomes noticeable after age 35–45 years, and becomes gradually worse. High-frequency sounds become difficult to hear, affecting the quality of the person's speech, particularly that of women.

Both ears are normally affected, with men more at risk probably because of their increased exposure to high levels of occupational noise. When deterioration is severe enough to cause inconvenience, a hearing aid may be necessary.

SKIN DISEASES

Pruritus, a troublesome complaint taking the form of a localized or more generalized itch, is either idiopathic or has a known cause. It may also be secondary to some other primary disease process including that of diabetes mellitus or renal disease.

Intertrigo, a condition affecting touching skin folds, is more common in the obese elderly and is often associated with lack of personal cleanliness.

Scabies, an easily treated disease cause by a burrowing mite, is recognised by the presence of 'burrows' in the skin and by severe itching and scratch marks.

Psoriasis, which presents with sharply defined reddened skin areas with abnormal scaling, increases and decreases in severity over time.

Chilblains, resulting in tenderness, burning sensations and itching on the affected areas, are often, but not exclusively, found on the feet.

Eczema, which can occur at any age, may be in the acute or chronic form in the old person. The itch associated with eczema can be a source of considerable irritation and distress.

Pressure sores may be of the superficial or deep type and are associated with immobility and a general deterioration in the physical/mental condition of the elderly person. The role of the nurse, and of those working under her direction, is of paramount importance both in terms of preventing and treating pressure sores.

CONCLUSION

The purpose of this chapter is to present an *overview* of diseases commonly experienced by the elderly. All nurses who work with old people, irrespective of whether they work in a 'general', 'psychiatric' or 'community' setting can only work effectively if they have an adequate knowledge of all such diseases.

It is not being suggested that all old people will have one or more of these diseases at any given time, although the majority of old people will undoubtedly suffer from a clinical or sub-clinical form of one of these. However, virtually all individuals will suffer from, if not die as a result of, one of these diseases during their old age.

REFERENCES

Kiloh L. G. (1961) Pseudo-dementia. *Acta Psychiatrica Scandinavica* **37**, 336 – 51.

Kral A. V. (1965) The senile amnesic syndrome. In *Psychiatric Disorders in the Aged.* Manchester W.P.A. Symposium, Ciba Geigy, Manchester.

Levy R. & Post F. (Eds) (1982) *The Psychiatry of Late Life.* Blackwell Scientific Publications, Oxford.

Lipowski Z. J. (1980) Delirium updated. *Comprehensive Psychiatry* **21**, 190.

Post F. (1972) The management and nature of depressive illness in late life: A follow through study. *British Journal of Psychiatry* **121**, 393 – 404.

Post F. (1982) Affective disorders in old age. In Patkell E.S.(ed.) *Handbook Of Affective Disorders.* Churchill Livingstone, London.

Schulman K. (1978) Suicide and parasuicide in old age: A review. *Age and Ageing* **7**, 201 – 9.

FURTHER READING

Anderson F. (1976) *Practical Management of the Elderly,* 3rd edn. Blackwell Scientific Publications, Oxford. A 452 page book which focuses on the *management* of the patient, rather than the signs and symptoms of the illness. The emphasis is on physical diseases, with one chapter on mental disorders.

Coakley D. (Ed.) (1981) *Acute Geriatric Medicine.* Croom Helm, London. A 290 page book dealing, as the title suggests, with *acute* geriatric *medicine,* contains a readable chapter on acute confusional states.

Coni N., Davidson W. & Webster S. (1977) *Lecture Notes on Geriatrics.* Blackwell Scientific Publications, Oxford. A 332 page book covering most aspects of geriatric medicine and including one chapter on mental illness.

Hodkinson H. M. (1981) *An Outline of Geriatrics*, 2nd edn. Academic Press, London. A 166 page book covering most aspects of geriatric medicine and including one chapter on mental disturbance in old age.

Levy R. & Post F. (Eds) (1982) *The Psychiatry of Late Life.* Blackwell Scientific Publications, Oxford. A 297-page book which examines all aspects of mental illness and the elderly. The psychiatric illnesses associated with old age are particularly well presented.

Chapter 9
Models of Care

A model of care relates to the way in which you see the cause of the problem, and to the choice of nursing care which you subsequently make. To illustrate the different ways in which an identical problem can be seen, and subsequently dealt with in terms of nursing care models, consider the following imaginary situations.

Situation 1

Mr Jones is recovering from surgery and should now be fully mobilized and up and about all day. He should be virtually independent of nursing staff and be using the toilet and bathroom facilities without assistance or supervision. However, he is continuing to spend all day in bed, insists on being taken to the bathroom in a wheelchair, and will not use a tub bath unless assisted and given full supervision.

This information might indicate the existence of one of a number of problems, that relating to 'activity' for example. In dealing with the activity problem one could adopt the *medical* model of care and organize an activity programme designed to increase Mr Jones' level of activity. Another approach would be to adopt the *psychotherapeutic* model and spend time in private conversation with Mr Jones in an attempt to understand his reasons for remaining inactive, and to help him gain a level of self-understanding and motivation which will cause him to wish to become more active.

Situation 2

Mrs Smith is about to undergo a minor surgical procedure and informs you that she is very 'anxious' about the procedure and is concerned about the prospect of experiencing pain afterwards.

Nursing care relating to this situation could also take a number of forms including the use of the medical model or the use of the psychotherapeutic model. In using the medical model, you would seek, and possibly obtain, the prescription of appropriate tranquillizers from the medical staff.

Alternatively, in using the psychotherapeutic model, you would utilize your interpersonal skills and discuss the outcome of this minor surgical procedure as it related to pain. If, as is often the case, the level of pain can be described to the patient, her anxiety may decrease as her level of knowledge about the expected pain increases.

It is not being suggested that any given approach is always useful in all situations. Rather, it is proposed that you should be familiar with a variety of models of care and, in a given situation, use one or more of these in relation to that individual situation.

The following example goes further in that it demonstrates how four commonly used models might be used in an identical situation.

Situation 3

Mrs Brown lives at home, her husband died three months previously and she describes herself as feeling very 'anxious'. She frequently phones her son and daughter who live in a nearby village and asks them to come over and comfort her. They respond to this telephone call by visiting her, bringing over her grandchildren and by spending a considerable amount of time with her.

The four possible solutions to this situation reflect four models of care.

SOLUTION 1 (MEDICAL MODEL)

You could report the anxiety to the family doctor who might prescribe minor tranquillizers to control it. This approach, which is based on the medical model of care, assumes that the cause of the anxiety is *physical* in terms of its cause and solution. It can be seen that you play a *relatively* minor and inactive part in this form of therapy, the major responsibility for treatment being that of the medical staff. Your role is largely concerned with identifying and reporting symptoms.

SOLUTION 2 (PSYCHOTHERAPEUTIC MODEL)

In adopting the psychotherapeutic model you would assume that the problem (anxiety) was an intrapersonal one, in that it had much to do with Mrs Brown's personal emotional make-up. In trying to resolve the problem using the psychotherapeutic model, you would use your *interpersonal skills* with Mrs Brown and try to enable her to identify and resolve the cause of her anxiety. In so doing you would play a very active part in resolving the anxiety, and would be using yourself as a therapeutic tool.

SOLUTION 3 (SOCIOTHERAPEUTIC MODEL)

In using the sociotherapeutic model you would arrange a meeting between Mrs Brown, other members of her family and yourself. An attempt would be made to identify the cause, and possible cure, of Mrs Brown's anxiety in terms of its *social cause and consequences*. In using this model, it is assumed that other important people in Mrs Browns's life feature in the cause of her anxiety, and have a role to play in minimizing it. It can be seen that, as was the case in the psychotherapeutic model, you have a very active part to play in this form of therapy.

SOLUTION 4 (BEHAVIOURAL MODEL)

You might view Mrs Brown's anxiety as a 'lever' which she uses in order to obtain more attention and comfort from her family. Thus, in the absence of what she regards as being sufficient attention from her family, Mrs Brown subconsciously develops the 'anxiety' which she reports to them. As a result of this information her family give her the attention and comfort which she feels she needs. In short, the 'anxiety' is being *rewarded and reinforced* by the attention of her family.

In taking this behavioural view of the cause and possible treatment of the anxiety, you will arrange with Mrs Brown and her family that she be reinforced for *not* being anxious and that rewards in the form of family visits will be made as a result of Mrs Brown not being anxious. As with the psychotherapeutic and sociotherapeutic models, the behavioural model enables you to play a very positive part in patient care.

It is not the purpose of this text to provide a detailed discussion or description of the major nursing care models. Rather, it is intended to convince you of the need to use all four models in relation to the care of the elderly, if you have been previously introduced to them. Alternatively, it is intended to convince you of the need to learn about, and use, all four nursing care models.

Identifying four *separate* models of nursing care is rather artificial in that it implies that no more than one model can be used at any given time. The reality is that, in the tradition of good-quality nursing, more than one model may be used simultaneously. Indeed, it would not be unusual to find a circumstance in which all four models were being used at the same time; for example, in relation to a person who was dehydrated because he was unwilling, rather than unable, to drink, the following approaches might be used. First, all reasonable physical means of encouraging him to drink fluids may be used, *the medical model*. Second, he may be encouraged to participate in group activities which will increase his access to fluids, and in which other people, patients for example, will act as role models for him in that they drink appropriate quantities of fluids, *the sociotherapeutic model*. Third, he may be given systematic encouragement and compliments when he consumes fluids, *the behavioural model*. Fourth, an individual nurse may develop a sufficiently strong relationship with this man so that the relationship is used to explore his difficulty in consuming fluids, *the psychotherapeutic model*. It may reasonably be argued that there is only one model of nursing, that which includes all four approaches and that these are parts of *a single* model of nursing care rather than four individual models.

PSYCHOTHERAPEUTIC MODEL

Many nurses on being asked whether they use a psychotherapeutic approach with their patients or if they use relationship therapy, will answer in the negative. This rather hasty response is often prompted by the misunderstanding that psychotherapeutic approaches to patient care can only occur in a psychiatric nursing setting, and that it can only be used by those who have a formal training in the subject. It is the author's firm view that psychotherapeutic techniques are presently being used by most, if not all, nurses in all disciplines. The psychotherapeutic approach, which is based on nurse–patient relationships, is one in which the nurse uses her warmth, personality, understanding of human behaviour, empathy and communication skills in order to help individuals overcome specific problems. In a now classic article on the subject Peplau (1962) described interpersonal techniques as being 'the crux of *psychiatric* nursing' (my italics). This rather limited vision of the role of the nurse generally, and non-psychiatric nurses in particular, implies that the use of interpersonal techniques is confined to a relatively narrow group of nurses. This view, if interpreted literally, may lead to the use and recognition of interpersonal and psychotherapeutic skills as only relating to persons with mental illness, and relating largely to one small group of nurses, psychiatric nurses. The reality of the matter, in the author's view, is that *all* nurses in *all* circumstances do and should make considerable use of their interpersonal skills as psychotherapeutic tools.

The point at which interpersonal skills become therapeutic, rather than social, is not easy to identify. However, it is true to say that psychotherapeutic techniques are used in a specific and goal-directed way, relate to specific problems which are being experienced by a person, and are firmly structured in terms of where, when and how they will be used. The following example demonstrates how a psychotherapeutic approach can be used in relation to a patient who has become pathologically dependent on nursing staff. The example includes the principles involved in this technique and the means by which they might be used in relation to this particular problem.

Relationship Formation

The formation of a positive relationship with a patient is an important prerequisite in relation to the use of psychotherapeutic skills. You will deliberately spend time with the patient in order that you can get to know each other. In most instances it is possible, if not desirable, that the patient be made aware that a specific relationship is being developed in order to reach a therapeutic goal. At this point, the interactions which take place may well be social and directed by the patient in terms of choice of subject matter. The therapeutic value of nurse—patient social interactions is of considerable importance in relation to all models of nursing care. During this time you will undoubtedly begin to collect information which will enable you to identify specific nursing care needs. The duration of this phase will vary considerably between patients; six months in relation to some patients with trust problems, and a few hours in relation to more 'accessible' patients.

Assessment Phase

You will begin to take firmer control of the content of the nurse—patient interactions and manipulate it to the extent of causing the patient to discuss potential problem areas. The word 'control' has been carefully used in this context, and should be taken to mean an 'organized' control; for example, the purpose is to prevent the patient spending all of the interaction time discussing totally irrelevant material, the most desirable new model of car for example. The interaction is controlled to the extent that you ensure that areas of actual or potential problem are discussed. In relation to this particular patient who has a dependence problem, you might steer the interaction towards discussing how much the patient does for himself, what he feels about being given help by nurses, whether or not he feels 'dependent' and whether or not he feels he could do more for himself. In short, you are making a nursing diagnosis based on a nursing assessment.

Clarification Phase

As the assessment phase progresses you become more aware of the specific problem areas being experienced by the patient. The 'dependence' problem which has been identified in the assessment phase will now be further explored with him. Indeed, you should clarify that this is really the problem which is being experienced by him, and explore related aspects of it. In this clarification phase the nurse and patient will attempt to find the full meaning of the patient's thoughts and communications, ensuring that each has a full understanding of the problem. The existence of many problems, and dependence is no exception, is difficult for some people to admit, let alone describe. Your task at this stage is to move closer towards achieving a mutual understanding with the patient and open fluent communication.

Exploration

As the patient becomes increasingly willing to recognize and discuss the problem, dependence, encourage him to express his feelings about himself, his relationship with others, and his dependence. A very important part of your role at this stage is to *listen* and *empathize,* deliberately increasing the warmth, understanding and empathy which you convey to the patient. Indeed, many patients feel this type of activity to be therapeutic although the nurse is 'only' listening. As these positive feelings between you and the patient increase, the ability of the patient to communicate and his willingness to focus on the problem will increase.

Focusing

The relatively general nature of exploration will give way to a more pointed focusing on the patient's problem, and he will be encouraged to identify and describe thoughts and feelings relating to it. At this stage, identify specific feelings which are expressed by the patient and focus on them; for example, he might hint that his dependence is a means of controlling others, indeed it may be the principal reason for the existence of the problem. You must be able to pick up these clues and act upon them, encourage the patient to continue on this particular theme, and know how far he can be 'pushed' in any given direction. With experience, you will not only be able to identify those topics which should be pursued, but will also recognize when to 'push' a patient towards discussing them, and when (temporarily) to allow a patient to avoid discussion.

Informing and Reflecting

Although it is highly desirable that a mutual understanding of the problem be made, and a mutual identification of possible solutions, you will often have to play a major part in interpreting the feelings of the patient. This can be achieved by reflecting, and often clarifying, information which is provided by him; for example, you will observe, 'I have the feeling that talking about your dependence makes you angry', or, 'You seem to avoid talking about your dependence, how does it make you feel?' Another approach is to inform the patient, using a form of reality confrontation, which will help to see his behaviour through the eyes of another person; for example, you might say, 'I noticed you asked Mr Smith to make your bed for you this morning; can you tell me more about that, please?', or, 'When we met here a few minutes ago you asked me which chair you should sit on; could we talk about that, please?'

Using Silence

Many nurses, particularly beginners, feel under considerable pressure to avoid periods of silence during a therapeutic interaction. Those who make this mistake find themselves playing an increasingly dominant part in the interaction, with minimal input from the patient, and introducing a large and varied number of topics which may or may not be of relevance to the particular patient and his problems. Silence can and should be used in a positive, therapeutic and constructive manner, providing it is identified as part of the therapeutic process.

An important non-verbal message can be conveyed during silent periods, you are 'telling' the patient that you care enough about him to give him *time*. By allowing the patient to end the period of silence you are indicating to him that *he* can choose the next topic, and that you value his choice. Silence can also be used, in some instances, to raise the patient's anxiety level and encourage him to talk about 'relevant' topics; for example, you may remain silent in response to a patient's social talk, but contribute to the interaction if he should focus on the problem under discussion. Thus, behaviouralist techniques can be used in the psychotherapeutic process.

Validating Your Understanding of the Problem/s

As you develop a clearer idea of the patient's problem, its possible causes and related factors, it is necessary that these assumptions be validated by sharing them with him. In other words, you begin to arrive at conclusions in the form of untested assumptions. These must be made known to the patient in order that he can accept or reject them. If they are correct, but rejected by the patient, then more work needs to be done with him. If the assumptions are correct and are accepted by the patient, considerable progress has been made. During this stage, indeed during every stage of the relationship, both patient and nurse must feel free to validate and clarify in order to avoid misunderstandings.

Identifying Alternative Behaviour

Once a thorough understanding of the dependence problem has been established and fully explored, the next phase will be to discuss alternative means of behaviour. If the patient recognizes that his dependent behaviour is pathological and needs to be modified in some way, then considerable progress has been made. One strategy might be for you and the patient to discuss the sense of achievement which might be experienced by him if he were to contribute more toward his own care. An agreement might be reached whereby he would make his own bed, with the help of a nurse, and discuss progress with this activity during his next meeting with the therapist.

The whole purpose of the psychotherapeutic relationship is to enable the patient *personally* to overcome problems which can be resolved. The success of this approach depends very much on mutual understanding and the belief that he has a considerable part to play in achieving his independence.

Summarizing the Therapeutic Sessions

Each psychotherapeutic session, and the sessions collectively, should end with a summary in which you present a synopsis of the interaction to the patient. This should include a brief description of the topics covered, problems raised, progress made, possible solutions and plans for the future.

This psychotherapeutic process can take weeks, months or even years; it is not being suggested that it is a quick and easy means of delivering nursing care. The psychotherapeutic sessions should occur on a regular basis, one hour per day for example, operate on a structured and therapeutic (as opposed to social) basis, and be seen as a very important part of nursing care delivery in *all* fields of nursing.

BEHAVIOURAL MODEL

The behavioural model of nursing care is different from the psychotherapeutic model in that it is less concerned with the 'psychological make-up' of the patient and more concerned with the actual 'problem'. Behavioural techniques are many and varied and, although they have previously been used largely in relation to the mentally ill and the mentally handicapped person, are equally effective in relation to other patient groups, including the physically ill elderly. An excellent account of behavioural therapy nursing can be found in Barker (1982). Although Barker directs his excellent discussion of the behavioural approaches almost exclusively to the mentally ill and mentally handicapped, all of the material contained in his book can be used in relation to the mentally *and* physically ill elderly person.

A patient who is experiencing an anxiety problem will be used to illustrate the application of the behavioural model.

Assessment

The process of assessment, which is a collective endeavour involving a number of people, and takes place over a period of time, consists of a number of related parts.

GENERAL PROBLEM IDENTIFICATION

Initially, the problem may be identified in a vague and rather general manner. The patient, or others such as nurses or relatives, may report that, 'Something is wrong', or that, 'He is not himself; I think something is wrong'. These general statements are indicative of two things: first, that *something* is wrong with the patient; second, that the 'problem' is sufficiently serious to cause concern. At this point, whether the patient is hospitalized or living in the community, you might become involved in seeking a solution. Having identified the fact that something is wrong with the patient's health status, the next phase is to move from the general to the specific.

SPECIFIC PROBLEM IDENTIFICATION

You and the patient (and perhaps others) now begin to identify the exact nature of the problem which may relate to mood, anxiety, trust or a number of other areas. In this instance you identify 'anxiety' as being the problem, this nursing diagnosis will, of course, be supported by subjective and objective evidence. *Subjective evidence* can take the form of the patient complaining of, 'feeling anxious', or, 'having butterflies in my tummy', or 'feeling on edge all the time', or, 'feeling worried'. *Objective evidence* can result from observations that the patient is experiencing frequency of micturition, pacing the ward floor continuously, wringing his hands frequently, chain smoking or having difficulty in concentrating.

PROBLEM ANALYSIS

Even at this stage of assessment the *precise* nature of the problem is often unclear. It has not yet been established whether the patient is always anxious, occasionally anxious, or is only anxious in particular circumstances. During this phase of the assessment process the patient and nurse describe the problem in very precise terms, describe circumstances which make it worse, circumstances which make it better, and quantify the problem in terms of its frequency and/or intensity.

The importance of 'measuring' the problem cannot be overemphasized, this measurement results from making a very *specific* examination and description of the problem. It can take a number of forms which include a statement of the frequency with which behaviours occur, and a measurement of their intensity. It is important that a detailed writtten record be kept of these measurements.

Having completed the assessment phase, the next step is to identify required changes in behaviour, then design and implement appropriate nursing care.

Identification of Required Changes in Behaviour

Decisions must now be made regarding the required changes in behaviour which will indicate a reduction in, or elimination of, the problem. In other words, decisions must be made about treatment goals. Identifying required behavioural changes will not be difficult providing that the problem, and evidence of it, has been specifically described, analysed, measured and recorded. Of course, the required changes in behaviour should be attainable in the relatively short term. If the goals are too large, both you and the patient will become disheartened and give up before they are reached. Examples of required changes in behaviour are: smoking reduced from 40 to 30 cigarettes per day; floor pacing reduced from 3 hours to 2½ hours per day; complaints of 'feeling anxious' reduced from half-hourly to hourly intervals; frequency of micturition reduced from twenty to fifteen times per day. By identifying and quantifying required changes in behaviour, there can be no doubt about when 'success' has been achieved in relation to the nursing care plan.

Devising the Nursing Care Plan

A nursing care plan is devised, with the help of the patient, which will decrease the amount of time that he is 'anxious', and will increase the amount of time that he is 'not anxious'. One way to achieve this is by using an operant conditioning technique which relies on positive reinforcement. Operant conditioning is a type of learning in which behaviour is changed by altering the consequences which it produces. Let us imagine that in this case the anxious behaviour is reinforced by the attention received from nursing staff and others, the anxiety is being reinforced and rewarded. If, on the other hand, the patient's anxious behaviour were not being 'rewarded', it could be seen that it might diminish in its intensity.

Positive reinforcement may also be used to increase the frequency when he is 'not anxious'. Positive reinforcement is any result of a behaviour which will increase the likelihood of that behaviour recurring in the future. In this case suitable rewards in the form of staff time, attention or some other tangible reward, will be given to this man when he is 'not anxious'. Conversely these rewards will not be made available to him during the times when he *is* anxious.

Implementation of the Care Plan

In implementing the nursing care plan using the behavioural method, it is important that all staff and others such as relatives be fully informed of the strategies to be used. All must deal with the patient in exactly the same way, giving and withholding reinforcement under identical circumstances; for example, it could have been decided to positively reinforce non-anxiety behaviour by giving the patient verbal praise when he has stopped pacing for at least two minutes. Full documentation of the nursing care plan and of subsequent behavioural changes will enable evaluation to be undertaken.

Evaluating the Outcome of the Nursing Care Plan

The previously identified required changes in behaviour are used as the basis of an evaluation of the outcome of the nursing care plan. Although this evaluation is a continuous process, it is more common for a predetermined time to have elapsed between implementation of the nursing care plan and evaluation of its outcome. The form which the nursing care will take beyond the point of evaluation will depend on the outcome of that evaluation.

SOCIOTHERAPEUTIC MODEL

The sociotherapeutic model, which often uses group therapy as an important focus of treatment, is usually, although not exclusively, used in an institutional setting. However, it should be borne in mind that the sociotherapeutic model can be used in any environment, including the patient's home. In that environment, structured group therapy can be organized and include the patient, the relatives, visiting nurse and others. The major features of the sociotherapeutic approach, which make it different from other treatment approaches are threefold.

First, the entire environment is considered to have therapeutic potential. This includes the physical environment, *all* the people in it, and the people who visit it. It also includes those people and places which are visited by the patient when he leaves his immediate environment.

Second, *all* experiences and activities to whch the patient is exposed are considered potentially therapeutic.

Third, it is recognized that *all* persons with whom the patient comes into contact have a potentially *equal* therapeutic contribution to make. It is not the case that nurses, doctors and other professionals are automatically recognized as being the ultimate therapeutic experts. Indeed, the contribution by the professional 'experts' is often overshadowed by the patient himself and other non-professionals in the environment. The unique role of the nurse in terms of the sociotherapeutic approach is to structure and organize this type of care, to recognize and harness the therapeutic potential of the environment, and to ensure that it works in a positive way for the patient.

The potentially therapeutic forces which exist need to be given focus and direction, they must also be closely monitored and evaluated. One way of doing this is to organize a means by which the individuals from the environment meet on a regular and organized basis to maximize available therapeutic potential. This form of meeting, often referred to as 'group therapy' has two major purposes. It can be used to harness the therapeutic potential of the environment and to provide an additional therapeutic experience for its members. In other words, group therapy may be seen as an environment within an environment, as a specialized form of therapy which exists within the context of the person's total milieu.

To illustrate the use of the sociotherapeutic model, a patient with a specific problem (obesity) due solely to overeating will be used. It will be assumed that the problem has a social basis, is influenced by his social circumstances, and is one which can be influenced by the physical and interpersonal structure within which he lives.

In organizing group therapy, full consideration has to be given to who should participate in the group, how often it should meet, and to the purpose of the meetings. This particular group may consist of all patients in the ward who are experiencing a variety of problems. Alternatively, it could consist of a smaller number of patients, each of whom has a problem relating to some aspect of nutrition. The process by which this particular patient might have his problem minimized or resolved in group therapy can take a number of forms including the outline that follows.

Settling in

During the initial meetings, of 1½ hours duration and occurring daily, the patient will spend his time getting to know other members, developing a mutual trust and becoming familiar with the function of the members of the group, particularly the nurse member. You will play a 'leadership' role in terms of introducing new members, reminding the group of its problem-solving function, ensuring that the therapeutic goals of the group are pursued, and providing a summary of the group discussion at the end of each meeting.

Identifying Problems

Having settled in, the patient will be encouraged and expected to identify his problem or problems. Ideally he should identify the fact that he is over-weight and fully recognize that this is a problem. If, on the other hand, he states that he has no problem, that he does not overeat, or that his weight is as it should be, others in the group will be expected to confront him with the reality of the situation. Clearly, being confronted with an unacceptable reality may well be a painful experience. An important part of your role at this time will be to give sufficient support, to help him accept this reality. Alternatively, in some instances, you might have to protect the patient from this type of reality confrontation if he is unable to cope with it at that particular time.

Problem Exploration

Having identified and accepted the existence of the eating problem, the patient will be encouraged to discuss it more fully, as well as its possible causes; for example, he may recognize that he overeats because of boredom, to attract attention, or because it is part of a lifelong eating pattern. In other words, the problem is analysed and its possible causes identified.

Identifying Alternative Behaviour

With the help of others in the group the patient will be encouraged to examine alternatives to overeating. This will be facilitated by the contributions of other group members who have, or have had, similar problems. These potential solutions to the problem will be tried out with the full support and encouragement of others in his environment.

Evaluation of Progress

During a subsequent group session he will be encouraged to talk about his success and/or problems relating to the alternative behaviours which were discussed in previous meetings. He will be expected honestly and realistically to evalute progress and discuss it with others in the group. If his perception of progress is valid, then others may do no more than congratulate him on the progress and continue to give positive encouragement. If progress has been considerable, but he fails to recognize it, then others will have to convince him of it. Alternatively, if he reports considerable progress but, in reality, has made none, then the group will have to confront him with the reality of this.

Summary of the Sociotherapeutic Model

As with other forms of nursing interventions, it is not being implied that the sociotherapeutic model is either quick or easy. Neither is it being suggested that the brief description which has just been provided will enable nurses unfamiliar with this type of treatment to practise it. However, it is hoped that this example will encourage you to believe that the sociotherapeutic model is a real and possible addition to other forms of intervention, and that it will encourage you to read texts on this form of nursing care.

MEDICAL MODEL

The medical model has two distinct parts; one in which you act as an extension of the physician in providing medical care, another in which you see your *nursing* role as extending only to ensuring the physical safety and comfort of the patient.

In relation to problems of disorientation and overactivity which are experienced by a patient, you will need to report to the appropriate medical staff. This information will be used by the doctor to assist him in arriving at an appropriate medical diagnosis and the subsequent prescription of medical treatment. Usually, although not always, the medical treatment will take the form of medication. You will then ensure that the prescribed medications are taken by the patient and that observed effects and side-effects are recorded and reported to the medical staff; this information will then be used by the medical staff to determine the type, if any, of subsequent medical treatment.

Custodial care will take the form of ensuring the safety of the patient, preventing him from wandering outside the ward for example, and generally providing nursing care. This nursing care will include the provision of nutrition, toilet facilities, clothing, warmth and a secure environment. However, if the patient experienced problems in his ability to use any of these items and/or facilities, this would be seen as a medical rather than a nursing problem and would be referred to the medical staff.

CONCLUSION

The conceptual framework which is used in this text deliberately includes problems which are susceptible to *nursing* influence. Indeed, in the vast majority of cases these problems can be best influenced by nursing staff. As nurses we need to realize that there is very little that others, including medical staff, can do with regard to a patient with an anxiety problem, a demented patient who is disoriented, an elderly person who is unwilling to drink, who has a self-esteem problem, or who has difficulty in eating. These problems are primarily *nursing* problems which can be resolved by nursing staff with the assistance of others who include the patient, relatives, medical staff, occupational therapists and fellow patients.

The view taken in this text is that all models of care have a role to play in the provision of care in all contexts in which the elderly are provided with nursing care.

REFERENCES

Barker P. (1982) *Behaviour Therapy Nursing*. Croom Helm, London.
Peplau H. (1962) Interpersonal skills. The crux of psychiatric nursing. *American Journal of Nursing* **62**, 50–4.

FURTHER READING

Alagaratnam W. J. (1981) Pain and the nature of the placebo effect. *Nursing Times* **77**, 1883–4.
Birchmore T. & Clague S. (1983) A behavioural approach to reduce shouting. *Nursing Times* **79**, 37–9.
Campbell W. (1979) The therapeutic community. Problems encountered by nurses. *Nursing Times* **75**, 2038–40.
Davies A. (1983) Back on their feet. Behaviour techniques for elderly patients — 1. *Nursing Times* **79**, 49–51.
Davies A. & Crisp A. (1980) Setting performance goals in geriatric nursing. *Journal of advanced Nursing* **5**, 381–8.
Davies A. D. M. & Snaith P. A. (1980) The social behaviour of geriatric patients at mealtimes. An observational and intervention study. *Age and Ageing* **9**, 93–9.

Davies B. & Holdworth V. (1981) Time for talking. *Nursing Mirror* **153**, 20−1.

Ehrman J. (1983) Use of biofeedback to treat incontinence. *Journal of the American Geriatrics Society* **31**, 182−4.

Finkle A. L. & Finkle P. S. (1977) How counseling may solve sexual problems in aging men. *Geriatrics* **32**, 84−8.

Nigl A. J. (1981) A behaviour management programme to increase social responses in psychogeriatric patients. *Journal of the American Geriatrics Society* **29**, 92−5.

Settin J. M. (1982) Overcoming ageism in long term care: A solution in group therapy. *Journal of gerontological Nursing* **8**, 565−7.

Simpson S. D. (1982) Treatment of sexual dysfunction by behavioural psycho-therapy. *Nursing Times* **78**, 53−5.

Woodhams P. (1984) Nurses and psychologists — the first-hand experience. *Nursing Times* **80**, 34−5.

Chapter 10
Nursing Concepts

One means of viewing patients' nursing care is to relate it to a range of disease processes or medical diagnoses. From such a viewpoint, the diseases commonly experienced by that specific patient group are first of all identified. Having considered a particular disease or disease process, the care relating to a person suffering from that particular disease is then discussed; for example, having described bone fractures generally, and the fracture of the neck of femur in particular, you then discuss the related medical treatment and nursing care. Such an approach includes discussion of related anatomy, physiology, disease, medical treatment, surgical treatment, pharmacology and nursing care.

Although a thorough understanding of many 'non-nursing' subjects is required, an increasingly held view is that it is desirable, if not necessary, to separate a discussion of nursing care from these other subjects.

One problem with linking nursing care to each of the many possible medical diagnoses relates to repetitiveness, since patients with any of a number of diagnoses may be wrongly thought to have similar, or identical, nursing needs. Such a linking of medical with nursing care might imply that the nursing care required by a patient with a given medical diagnosis was unique to that diagnosis, and shared few features with patients from other diagnostic groups. In reality, of course, this is not the case and many patients with different medical diagnoses may require similar nursing care, while many patients with the same diagnosis may require different nursing care. Take, for example, the case of an elderly person who is bedridden because of a fractured neck of femur, one who is suffering from senile dementia and another who is depressed; they are all very much at risk in relation to de-hydration. The medical diagnostic system suggests that all patients with an identical medical diagnosis have identical nursing needs; for example, if one reads about the nursing care relating to a person with a fractured neck of femur, one might assume that all patients with a fractured neck of femur require identical nursing care. This assumption is wrong, the truth being that the person's medical diagnosis will only partly influence his nursing care. Indeed, many patients who are being provided with nursing care have a medical diagnosis which is out of date and no longer applies to them, or have no medical diagnosis at all.

In order to take a rather more dynamic and positive view of nursing care, this text will identify and describe that care in terms of nursing *concepts*. Features of these concepts are that they relate less to patients' medical diagnoses and more to patients' nursing diagnoses and *individual nursing needs*. They relate to potential problems which can be identified by nursing staff and which can, in large part, be positively influenced by nursing intervention. Of course it is not being suggested that we work in isolation from other professional groups, doctors for example, or that we think about these concepts only in terms of nursing care. The importance of our contribution to medical care, and to care provided in support to the contribution made by other disciplines, is fully recognized. One way in which this relationship between medical diagnosis and care, and nursing diagnosis and care can be illustrated is as follows. If an 80-year-old lady has been hospitalized following a fractured neck of femur, the major role of the medical staff will be to diagnose that problem and initiate appropriate medical intervention which will result in the fracture being reduced and reunited. It is probable that a number of nursing needs can be identified, following the fracture and medical intervention, which can be resolved by nursing, rather than medical, intervention. These needs could relate to activity, elimination, anxiety and dependence. In many instances nursing staff will be able to provide care which will minimize or resolve these problems, with or without the assistance of other professional groups, although they will invariably be informed of nursing decisions and actions.

In many circumstances your role will be to prevent these problems occurring, in order to do so you must be aware that the patient is at risk in relation to these particular problems; examples include ensuring that enough fluids are consumed in order to prevent dehydration, developing a positive and meaningful relationship in order to maximize trust, ensuring that patients do as much for themselves as possible in order to minimize dependence, and giving advice on diet and nutrition in order to prevent nutrition problems.

In other situations you may diagnose and treat *nursing* problems without any reference to other members of the team other than informing them; examples include identifying dehydration and initiating appropriate nursing care, recognizing the development of psychomotor social skill deficits and implementing appropriate nursing care, and recognizing a person's anxiety and acting accordingly.

WHAT ARE CONCEPTS?

A concept is an understanding of the relationships between a group of ideas which have something in common. Concepts are less concerned about the facts relating to a particular subject and more concerned with a knowledge *and* understanding of it. The difference between knowing the facts relating to a subject, *and* understanding the concept might be illustrated as follows. Students may be taught that there are three different types of disorientation: disorientation for time, place and person. Features of the disorientation are that the individual is partially or totally unable to: identify himself or other persons (disorientation for person); identify and recognize the place in which he is (disorientation for place); identify and respond to the time in which he exists (disorientation for time). Disorientation is described as an unwelcome symptom of a number of illnesses, particularly the dementias. The role of the nurse in relation to recognizing, and occasionally influencing, disorientation may form part of the facts made available to nursing staff. The traditional manner in which nursing care was taught could be likened to knowledge and facts, in that nurses were taught to recognize the signs and symptoms of an illness and to be able to describe its related medical and nursing treatment.

The difference between knowing the facts related to a subject, and having a well developed concept of it is considerable. In large part this difference relates to the width and depth of *understanding* (as opposed to knowledge) of the subject, an understanding which invariably begins with an introduction to the facts.

In developing a concept of disorientation a much wider appreciation of it will be required. The concept will include an understanding of the cause of disorientation, features of disorientation, levels of disorientation, means of minimizing disorientation and how the disorientation affects the person. The extent to which disorientation influences other aspects of the person's life must also be understood; for example, its effect on hydration, nutrition, communication, activity, pain, hostility, anxiety and self-esteem will be understood. The extent to which the disorientation will affect those who are caring for the person will also be understood, this includes professional nursing staff and the person's relatives. The fact that disorientation is viewed by society as being an important part of 'madness' should also be recognized.

The development of orientation during childhood should be fully appreciated, as must the extent to which it relates to intellectual skills and memory. A degree of insight into how disorientation is experienced by an individual patient will enable you to *empathize* with him rather better than if only the facts about this phenomenon are known.

Differences Between Facts and Concepts

Facts are taught to and remembered by students, the ability to remember and repeat these facts is often an indication of educational 'success'. Concepts are introduced in a way which is similar to planting a seed; the seed is expected to grow.

Students may limit their knowledge of facts to that which they have been taught, assuming (wrongly) that what they have been taught is all that they are required to know. Conversely, they will continue to develop their concept of a subject indefinitely, indeed they will soon realize that what they have been taught and know is relatively limited.

Learners may have difficulty in identifying the relationship between different groups of facts, treating each set of facts as a separate entity. Conceptual thinking implies an ability to see the relationship between issues and items which are obviously, and less obviously, related to the basic concept.

Knowledge of facts remains relatively unchanged over time, as may well be the case in a teacher who has operated on a 'factual' rather than on a 'conceptual' basis. Concepts are dynamic, growing and changing; they develop as the individual develops in experience and maturity.

Facts relating to a specific subject can be perceived in an almost identical manner by a group of individuals who have been taught them, resulting in near-identical answers being provided under examination conditions. Although there will be some similarity between members of a group in their concept of a specific subject, there will also be considerable variation which reflects the uniqueness of each individual's understanding, experience and ability to conceptualize.

Facts are often difficult to relate to situations other than those which form the context in which they were taught. A major strength of concepts is that the principles which they embody can be generalized to many other appropriate situations.

Factual materials are relatively non-threatening to the learner providing that she can remember them. Concepts require the learner to work much harder, requiring a specific personal and unique input from her in order to develop her own concept of the subject being taught.

Teaching facts is relatively easy for the teacher, providing that she can prepare a suitable set of lecture notes or use an appropriate textbook. Concepts are more difficult and more demanding to teach in that they are much more likely to identify gaps in the teacher's knowledge. In using this text it is important to note that *concepts* are being presented, rather than a series of facts about each of the topics. To this extent each presented concept is limited; it is no more than a starting point from which you can develop a wider and more personal understanding of the topic.

DEVELOPING CONCEPTS

Before developing a concept, it should be recognized that a variety of subjects or ideas have something in common; for example, the notion of pain may not be conceptualized in the mind of a child, who regards it as no more than an unpleasant experience. However, the child soon begins to appreciate that there are different types of pain, pains of different intensity and many different causes of, and reactions to, pain. Later still the maturing adult recognizes that different individuals and different cultural groups react differently to the same type of pain. Similarly, it is recognized that pain can fulfil different functions; for example, it can be used as a punishment, be a warning of a disease process, give pleasure to masochists; the individual is thereby *conceptualizing* pain.

The four major steps in developing a concept are:
1   identifying features of the concept;
2   organizing the features of the concept;
3   applying or using the concept;
4   examining the responses to the concept.

1 Identifying Features of the Concept

Having previously concluded that a variety of subjects or ideas have something in common, the next stage is to identify those specific features which may be included within the concept, and be able to identify those which may not. At this stage you should be able to describe a number of features of a concept, anxiety or dehydration for example. In relation to anxiety, or any other concept for that matter, you should be able to identify features which it always has. Nurses should also be able to identify the range of 'normal' as opposed to 'pathological' aspects of the concept, and to identify those characteristics which have no influence on or relationship to it.

2 Organizing the Features of the Concept

The second stage in developing a concept is to organize the previously identified features of it into some meaningful form. In doing so one tries to arrange these features, as far as possible, in a cause and effect sequence; for example, you might describe enforced immobility, lack of access to fluids, reduced fluid intake, thirst and reduced urine output as a series of events in which enforced immobility results in dehydration.

3 Applying or Using the Concept

In nursing it is necessary that concepts have an application which will improve the quality of nursing care. In the previous description of dehydration, resulting in large part from enforced immobility, the practical consequences of understanding these related features of the concept can be easily seen. Indeed, it now becomes more possible to prevent the dehydration by allowing the immobilized person greater access to fluids or by decreasing the enforced immobility.

4 Examining Responses to the Concept

The final phase of conceptual development is in considering the responses of individuals when presented with features of the concept; for example, if the features of the concept 'anxiety' have been properly identified, organized and have some nursing application, then those who have been taught to understand this concept will respond in a similar way in similar circumstances such as when asked to discuss 'anxiety'. The word 'similar' is used rather than the word 'identical' because each individual will respond to the stimulus rather differently because her concept of the presented item will undoubtedly differ somewhat from the concept of all others.

NURSING CONCEPTS AS A TOOL IN NURSING DIAGNOSIS

Part 2 of this book will present selected nursing concepts and discuss them as they relate to the care of the elderly. There are a number of important points which must be borne in mind in relation to these concepts. Each is a normal part of the natural and healthy existence of all individuals, it need not necessarily be 'a problem' or pathological; for example, hydration, dependence, trust, hostility and death and dying are all features of a normal healthy existence.

The importance of these concepts, in terms of nursing care, is twofold; first, to enable you to identify features of healthy elderly people, and to give you a focal point for determining those aspects of the elderly person's existence which *may* be problematical or pathological. Second, the concepts chosen for inclusion in Part 2 also relate, to a greater or lesser extent, to other patient groups. Some concepts such as hydration and anxiety apply to virtually all patient groups. Others such as activity, death and dying, and elimination are potential problems which are more related to the care of the elderly inasmuch as they occur more frequently. It can be seen, therefore, that the concepts relating to the care of the elderly are not, in themselves, unique to that patient group. However, the way in which they are experienced by the elderly person as problems, the evidence which makes the nurse conclude that these items are problematical, and the resulting nursing intervention are likely to be different in relation to this particular patient group. In other words, although the concept is not fundamentally different in relation to the elderly, its presentation, identification, nursing intervention and evaluation have their own special characteristics.

DEVELOPMENT OF NURSING CONCEPTS IN NURSING STAFF

The majority, if not all, of the concepts discussed in Part 2 of this text are known to nurses, even before they start training. Most people know that the consumption of fluids is important to human existence, for example; they know something about the meaning and nature of pain; they know something about the meaning and nature of anxiety; and, whether or not they use the term, they have some notion of what is meant by 'self-esteem'. However, an understanding of these concepts may be confined to personal (young adult) experience, or to people generally in a very loose sort of way. In focusing attention on the elderly person, you are encouraged to extend your understanding of the concept to elderly people, and to identify those 'special' aspects of the concept which relate to that patient group.

TEACHING AND LEARNING GERIATRIC NURSING CONCEPTS

Strictly speaking, concepts cannot be 'taught', they have to be developed by you in a very personal way. However, the purpose of this book is to construct a learning experience which will maximize the extent to which you will develop appropriate geriatric nursing concepts. It should be realized that a selected number of appropriate concepts must be understood as they relate to the elderly, and that a learning experience has been designed which will *introduce* you to these concepts. The author finds it best to provide his students with only enough information to enable them to become started on what will be a lifelong learning process, the use of lecture material having some value, but being limited in many respects. Discussions, particularly student-led discussions, are an extremely useful tool in concept development. Coursework, particularly patient-centred work, can be stimulating, especially if it is undertaken along with the appropriate reading. The teacher should expect that students will develop different concepts, and that this will be reflected in coursework, discussion papers, and examination answers. This form of teaching does encourage a diverse and, sometimes conflicting, range of views which reflect the individuality and personal nature of conceptual development. Although this style of teaching is more difficult for the teacher than, for example, the uniform teaching and repetition of facts, it is necessary in terms of conceptual development. Learning the subject also presents a number of different problems to students.

Some nurses perceive their training as a situation in which they are taught a number of facts, required to remember them, and are expected to repeat them in order to pass examinations. This kind of learning should be regarded only as a basic starting point in conceptual development and as a means of introduction to the subject. Beyond that beginning point you will be expected to go and develop your own concepts, under appropriate guidance of course, and to develop new and useful insights into the subject. Initially you will find it very difficult to accept that *the* concept of a particular subject does not exist, this realization placing a great responsibility on you. You have to develop *your* concept. Initially the realization that the concept development is never ending worries some students, in the longer term, however, it results in a much more meaningful education.

The following chapter will discuss means by which an understanding of geriatric nursing concepts can be applied to the organization of nursing care via the nursing process. It might be argued that conceptualization generally, including the development of nursing concepts, is an art rather than a science. The relatively loose boundaries of concept formation, their highly individual nature and the extent to which they must be personally developed rather than taught, support the view that they constitute an art rather than a science. However, the practical use to which nursing concepts can be put in the organization of nursing care using the nursing process is the point at which nursing science becomes more important than the art. This change of emphasis from art to science, resulting in a balance between the two, is of fundamental importance to the delivery of high-quality care.

The geriatric nursing concepts selected for inclusion in this book, and discussed in Chapters 12 to 29, are those which form a central feature of nursing care for the elderly. This particular selection of concepts should not inhibit the identification of additional ones. You are encouraged to add further items to this list of concepts, providing that the item is relevant to the nursing care of the elderly person. Chapter 11 includes a conceptual framework which can be used, in conjunction with the geriatric nursing process, to make a systematic assessment of the nursing needs of an elderly person.

FURTHER READING

Benner P. (1982) From novice to expert. *American Journal of Nursing* **82**, 402–7.
Gange R. (1977) The Conditions of Learning, 3rd edn. Holt, Rinehard and Winston, New York.

Hardy E. (1983) The diagnostic wheel. *Canadian Nurse* **79**, 38–40.

Henderson V. (1978) The concept of nursing. *Journal of advanced Nursing* **3**, 113–30.

Hoo A.S. (1979) A study into the concept of mobilization of patients post operatively. MSc Thesis, University of Manchester.

Meleis A.I. (1979) The development of a conceptually based nursing curriculum: an international experiment. *Journal of advanced Nursing* **4**, 659–71.

Wilson J. (1963) *Thinking With Concepts*. Cambridge University Press, Cambridge.

Chapter 11
The Geriatric Nursing Process

Although an understanding of concept formation generally, and of geriatric nursing concepts in particular, is a prerequisite for the provision of high-quality care, it does not guarantee that you will be able to provide that care. The means of utilizing concept formation and of applying these concepts in terms of actually *delivering* nursing care is currently referred to as 'the nursing process'. Thus, knowledge and experience of the nursing process allows full use to be made of an understanding of nursing concepts.

THE NURSING PROCESS

The nursing process is a vehicle which enables nursing care to be organized and delivered in a structured and documented fashion. It facilitates, indeed demands, the use of scientific principles in terms of nursing care delivery being systematic, specific, documented and formally evaluated. Although all methods used for implementing the nursing process have the same basic features (assessment, planning, nursing intervention and evaluation), variations do exist in the models which are used to implement it. All models have the same basic features, those which do not contain at least these should be regarded with some suspicion.

The principles of the nursing process are relatively easy to understand although more difficult to implement. The development of appropriate concepts and a conceptual framework which are necessary in order to implement the nursing process are more difficult to grasp. The most important aspect of the development of good nursing care skill relates to the ability to use the appropriate concepts in order to *apply* the nursing process. This section aims to try and demonstrate the important link between conceptual development and the implementation of the nursing process. It also aims to try and illustrate that the nursing process, although different from conceptualization, is very dependent on it.

Nursing History and Assessment

A nursing history is the collection of information which will enable you to examine the present health status of the person who may or may not have current health *problems*. Obtaining a nursing history is dependent on using and referring to a *framework* of potential problem areas; such an assessment framework can be seen in Figure 11.1. The items contained within this assessment framework include those examples such as anxiety and hydration which were used earlier in this book when discussing nursing concepts. Indeed, the assessment (or conceptual) framework contains a range of 'concepts' which *may* present as problems to individual patients. It is not being suggested that a nursing concept and a nursing problem are the same.

However, an understanding of the concept 'anxiety' is necessary if you are to establish whether or not a person has 'a problem' relating to anxiety. Thus, problems relating to all of the items contained within the assessment framework can only be identified if you have a well-developed concept of that item. Furthermore, you will only be able to design appropriate nursing interventions if you have a full understanding of the subject. The relationship between each of the items in the assessment framework must also be borne in mind and never be seen in isolation; for example, it is easy to appreciate that 'anxiety' can be influenced by, and itself influence, every other item in the framework. Indeed, one of the important aspects of conceptualizing, opposed to remembering a series of facts about a subject, is that the interrelatedness of concepts is appreciated more fully. This interrelationship between items also illustrates the complexity of each individual item.

It would be foolish and inappropriate to imagine that because the concept is used to identify a problem using a single word, hydration for example, that the word relates to anything other than a highly complex system of ideas, objects and experiences. This complexity can be seen in the suggested format for assessing patients in each of the concept areas dealt with in Chapters 12 to 29. The use of an assessment framework should be regarded as a starting point from which to develop a wider and more personal ability to make a nursing diagnosis. There can be no doubt that any framework, including the one used in this text, may have limitations for some individual patients. Thus, as is the case in the development of an individual concept, those who use this framework must always ask, 'Are there any other important health care areas in which I must interest myself in relation to this particular individual?'

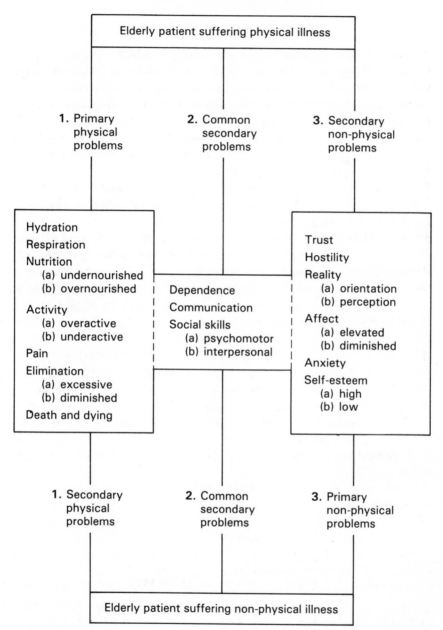

Fig. 11.1 A conceptual framework for the identification of patients' needs and problems. The broken lines between 1, 2 and 3 demonstrate interrelatedness of all problem areas, showing that the division is mainly one of emphasis.

THE ASSESSMENT FRAMEWORK

The assessment framework in Figure 11.1 was developed by the author from a largely physical one which had been developed by other writers (Cormack 1980, 1981). In producing this framework the author was conscious of the need to include items which would be of equal relevance to the physically and non-physically ill elderly person, which would encompass a wide range of physical and non-physical needs, and which contained *nursing* concepts. The criterion for including an item was, 'Is the concept, if it constitutes a "problem," able to be eradicated or minimized by means of *nursing* interventions.' If the answer was yes, the item was included.

The framework can be looked at from two perspectives, from above or below, in the following ways.

1   If the patient has a 'physical' illness, which will invariably have a non-physical component, it is looked at from above. The items in column 1 are potential primary (physical) problems, those in columns 2 and 3 are potential secondary (physical and non-physical) problems. For example, an elderly person with a fractured femur may be immobilized and will, at least, be experiencing an activity problem. In addition, he may experience an anxiety problem secondary to the primary *activity* problem.

2   If the patient has a 'non-physical' illness, which will invariably have a non-physical component, the framework is looked at from below. The items in column 3 are potential primary (non-physical) problems, those in columns 1 and 2 are potential secondary (physical and non-physical) problems. For example, an elderly person suffering from senile dementia will, at least, be experiencing a *reality (orientation)* problem. In addition, he may experience a *fluids (dehydration)* problem because of an inability to find and drink fluids.

3   If the old person is not known to be ill and is being assessed for the absence/presence of problems which require nursing intervention, then the entire framework will be used without reference to the labels which are printed above or below the main 'H' structure.

Using the Assessment Framework

When using any framework in order to compile a nursing history, the questions which need to be asked are:
(a)   Who will collect the information?
(b)   How will the information be recorded?
(c)   Who will record the information?
(d)   When will the information be collected?
(e)   From whom/where will the information be collected?

(a) WHO WILL COLLECT THE INFORMATION?

All members of the nursing staff group have a firm responsibility to collect information which is relevant to the provision and evaluation of nursing care. A firm recognition of the importance of this 'team effort' will minimize the risk of important data being lost.

Being familiar with patients' potential problems as outlined in Figure 11.1 will give direction to the information collection process. This requirement is particularly true for inexperienced or untrained staff who often ask, 'What am I supposed to be looking for?'

(b) HOW WILL THE INFORMATION BE RECORDED?

All *relevant* information which points to the existence of a problem must be recorded in writing as either a diary, nursing notes or on a form designed for the assessment phase of the nursing process. An example of such a form is shown in Figure 11.2 (see p. 123).

Additionally, enough relevant information which shows that a specific problem does *not* exist must be recorded in writing; for example:

Activity   Is able to perform a full range of physical tasks such as washing, shaving, walking unaided and using toilet.   *No problem.*

Alternatively, an assessment format for each potential problem (such as those shown in Chapters 12 to 29) might be completed and, if no problem is found, a comment such as '*Activity: No problem*' entered as a conclusion.

(c) WHO WILL RECORD THE INFORMATION?

Any trained nurse, or a learner under her *close personal supervision*, may enter a summary which is a composite view of the nursing team generally. Alternatively, arrangements might be made for all nursing staff to enter information on a less structured document, that information then being analysed by the nurse in charge who will then enter a conclusion/summary in a less detailed and more structured document.

(d) WHEN WILL THE INFORMATION BE COLLECTED?

Information on which an assessment is based begins to be collected before admission, or prior to the first nurse visit if the patient is in the community. Such data comes from a general practitioner's letter, details sent by a community or hospital nurse, as a result of a domiciliary visit by a doctor or via contact with relatives, friends or neighbours. Since the assessment process continues throughout the treatment period, information on which to base it must also be collected for the duration of the patients' nursing care. This data collection is a continuous activity which is undertaken at each opportunity that relevant information is available, certainly during *all* nurse–patient contact.

Although a formal and structured means of collecting information *may* be used during initial contact, in an office or treatment room in the form of taking a nursing history, for example, much of importance will be collected in more informal contact, when washing or chatting to a patient, for example, or when observing one or more patients from a distance.

(e) FROM WHOM/WHERE WILL THE INFORMATION BE COLLECTED?

Communication with, and observation of, the elderly patient is the richest source of information relevant to making a nursing assessment. Naturally, this data collection is made easier and is much more meaningful if you 'know what to look for', thus the advantage of using an assessment framework.

Relatives, neighbours, friends, other patients and nursing staff all contribute to our understanding of an individual's needs. Other professionals such as medical staff, physiotherapists, occupational therapists, social workers, psychologists, dentists and chiropodists, should all be regarded as potential providers of material.

When problems have been identified as a result of a detailed, comprehensive and systematic assessment you should, where possible, confirm these conclusions with the patient. In most, although not all, instances he is in the best position to confirm *or* deny that a specific problem is present. Examples of when he might be unable, or unwilling, to confirm that a problem exists when it in fact does, might be when a dependence problem has been identified or when a problem such as Reality (orientation) has resulted from a psychotic condition. Additionally, it is necessary to distinguish between the results of ageing and the effects of disease when making an assessment. In an excellent paper entitled 'Safeguard your elderly patient's health through accurate physical assessment', Hudson (1983) presents an excellent discussion of that facet of care. Much of the special skill which we as nurses have, concerns our ability to distinguish between significant and insignificant changes in our patients' behaviour. Time, knowledge, experience, awareness of each *individual* patient enables us to make professional judgements as to whether or not 'problems' such as anxiety, hostility and dependence fall within or outwith the normal range for him.

OTHER ASSESSMENT FRAMEWORKS

A number of assessment frameworks which relate exclusively, or partly, to the elderly have been developed with differing emphasis and various applications. The CADET assessment tool described by Rameizl (1983) deals with five basic functions: *C*ommunication, *A*mbulation, *D*aily living, *E*xcretion, *T*ransfer. Although limited to physical aspects of care, this system makes useful reading in terms of beginning to understand the need for, and use of, an assessment framework.

Using the CAPE system (Pattie & Gilleard 1979) nurses complete an observer rating scale for each patient and conduct a short interview with him. The patient is also required to undertake a number of tasks relating to the area being assessed. The CAPE system provides an excellent starting point, and a wealth of material, from which an assessment framework could be developed for local use in relation to nursing care.

The PGDRS system (Wilkinson & Graham-White 1980) was developed by nurses working in a psychogeriatric ward and, despite its brevity, is worth examining.

Prehn (1982) provided a behavioural analysis for disturbed elderly patients and focused on behavioural therapy as a treatment model. The central role of the nurse in identifying and influencing behavioural problems is highlighted.

In presenting a mental health charting instrument for use in nursing homes Pavkov and Walsh (1981) focus on non-physical problems to the exclusion of physical aspects. An excellent description of the meaning of descriptive labels such as 'Affect', 'Suspicion' and 'Delusions' is presented.

As the science of nursing assessment is still in a developmental stage, you are encouraged critically to examine a number of possible frameworks and begin to develop your notion of the ideal. Subsequently you must continue to develop and share your ideas with others through conferences/study days and publications in appropriate journals.

NURSING DIAGNOSIS

In general terms, the recording of a nursing history and making a nursing assessment are dependent on the use of fairly loose terms such as 'anxiety' and 'hydration', these and other such concepts having different meanings to different people. In using the assessment framework you will frequently find that, having collected information in relation to that particular topic, you will conclude that the patient has no problem in relation to it. For many patients, particularly those who are having their health care status monitored in the community, you may make no diagnosis other than that the individual has no health care problems which require nursing intervention. On other occasions, evidence of the existence of specific nursing problems such as anxiety or hydration, will emerge. It is always the case that these nursing diagnoses are made as a result of *evidence* of their existence being found, the word 'evidence' being very important here. From your knowledge of the concept of anxiety and hydration for example, you will be able to recognize evidence of problems in relation to these two concepts existing. The better your concept of the subjects as they relate to the elderly, the better will be your ability to identify problems in these areas. If you have a 'narrow' concept of these subjects, you will have a limited ability to recognize problems relating to them.

SOAPE MODEL OF THE NURSING PROCESS

In the model of the nursing process used in this text, the SOAPE model of the nursing process (Fig. 11.2), the identification and documentation of evidence which suggests a problem in relation to specific concepts is of extreme importance. Just as it is inadequate to simply record that the patient is 'anxious' or 'dehydrated' because these words having different meanings to individuals who have different concepts of them, it is also inappropriate to record only one piece of evidence upon which this diagnosis is based. Indeed, it is unusual to make a firm diagnosis based on only one piece of information (evidence), such a single piece of evidence may well be indicative of one of a number of problems; for example, imagine the following piece of evidence: 'Mr Jones urinated on the linen cupboard floor this morning'. This information could mean one of a number of things; that Mr Jones has an elimination problem; a reality (orientation) problem; a reality (perception) problem; a hostility problem; a communication problem, or that he has a dependence problem. Now imagine the following pieces of information, bearing in mind that they are parts of a concept, and constitute evidence of a particular problem relating to that concept. 'Mr Jones urinated on the floor of the linen cupboard this morning.' When asked why he had urinated in the linen cupboard, which is a small room with a brown door situated next to the toilet which also has a brown door, he replied, 'I did try to get to the toilet. Isn't this the toilet?' Thus, with a limited amount of further information (evidence), and with a well-developed concept of 'orientation', it is easier to identify the fact that Mr Jones is disoriented for place.

The collection and documentation of evidence relating to particular problems is an important part of all models of the nursing process, including the SOAPE model of the nursing process used in this text. In the example relating to Mr Jones, the *subjective evidence* (what Mr Jones said) is, 'I did try to get to the toilet. Isn't this the toilet?' The *objective evidence* (what the

Subjective evidence of problem: (What the patient says)
   For example: "I can't find the toilet."

Objective evidence of problem: (What the patient does)
   For example: Urinates in linen cupboard.

Assessment of problem: (Problem summary/label)
   For example: Disorientation for place, unable to find toilet.

Plan of nursing care: (Outline of nursing plan)
   For example: Teach patient to recognize distinctive colour of
   toilet door.

Expected outcome: (What you expect to occur as a result of plan)
   For example: Will manage to locate toilet at least once daily.

Fig 11.2   SOAPE model of the nursing process (Cormack 1980).

nurse saw or heard) was the fact that Mr Jones was seen to be urinating in the linen cupboard which had an identical door to the toilet which was situated nearby.

In some instances a very small quantity of subjective and objective evidence of the existence of a problem can be obtained, in which case it should all be recorded. In other instances large quantities of such evidence may be available, but only enough examples need to be recorded in order to illustrate it as clearly as possible. In all the examples used in this text three or more pieces of subjective evidence, and three or more pieces of objective evidence will be included. In reality, where quantities of evidence are available you must use your judgement in order to select those examples which are most typical and illustrative of the problem.

Some nurses who have a poorly developed concept of the subject being considered, as is understandably the case with beginners, ask the question, 'What do you have to ask the patient in order to establish whether or not a particular problem, anxiety for example, exists?' Implied in this question is the notion that, in order to establish whether or not a specific problem exists, a nurse must ask *the* question. Of course, there is no single question which can or should be asked in order to establish the existence of a particular problem. It is necessary to understand that the question which is asked is less important than the response, or the manner in which a patient responds to the question. A patient who is asked, 'How are you today Mr Jones?', may reply, 'Who is Mr Jones?'; or, 'Go to hell'; or, 'Why are you asking me all these questions?'; or, 'I have a terrible pain'; or, 'I think I am dying'; or any of a number of other responses. The ability to be less concerned with asking the 'right' question and being more concerned with the individual's response is a feature of a well-developed concept of the subject being assessed.

Assessment (or Nursing Diagnosis Label)

The initial phase of the nursing process, a nursing history or assessment, is a general examination of the patient in relation to a number of potential nursing problems. The information (evidence) which is collected will establish the existence or absence of specific problems. When a specific problem is found to exist subjective and objective evidence of it will be recorded (the S and O parts of this model of the nursing process). The A part of this model, *assessment*, is used to attach a label to that particular problem. A label such as 'disorientation' may be qualified by adding 'for place', and may be further qualified by recording the specific difficulties experienced by the patient. These difficulties may include 'is unable to find the toilet unaided, is unable to locate his own bed'. This label is no more than a summary of, and a conclusion based on, the materials contained in the S and O parts of the nursing process model.

Plan of Nursing Care

The ability to *plan* (P part of the model) appropriate nursing care is dependent on having developed a *nursing* concept of the topic, as opposed to having learned a layman's concept of it. Thus, you will have developed the ability to identify a range of strategies which can be used to eliminate or minimize specific problems, those relating to anxiety or dehydration for example.

The *Plan* section of the SOAPE model should contain a small number of specific nursing strategies which are designed to minimize or resolve specific problems. These should be short, sharp and specific and should be individualized for that particular problem, and for that particular patient. The number of examples used in this text will be three or more in number and will be used only to illustrate the fact that specific nursing interventions can be developed from a knowledge of nursing concepts.

Expected Outcome

The *expected outcome* (E part of the nursing process model used) requires you to identify what you expect to happen as a result of the previously prepared nursing care plan, *before* you actually implement it. In other words, the goals for that particular patient, goals which should be short, sharp and short term, will be set before the nursing care is actually implemented.

The number of expected outcomes (goals) used in each of the examples in this text will be three or more. The material for this part of the nursing process is taken directly from the S and O parts of the model. Figure 11.2 (see p. 123) illustrates the application of the SOAPE model of the nursing process in relation to a patient in whom a specific nursing problem relating to disorientation for place has been identified.

IMPLEMENTING THE GERIATRIC NURSING PROCESS

Trained professional nurses, with the support of supervised untrained staff, have the prime responsibility for implementing the nursing process. If other people are involved, nurse learners or other untrained staff for example, their contribution must be firmly monitored by trained nursing staff. The collection of information relating to a nursing history should be part of the responsibility of all nursing staff who come into contact with that patient; other staff such as doctors and occupational therapists, relatives and friends may make useful contributions. The contribution of the patient himself should be as great as he is capable of; some patients being far more able to participate than others. Where possible, patients should play a full and complete part in relation to all aspects of the nursing process including assessment, planning and implementation of nursing care, and in evaluating its outcome.

The nursing process, in common with nursing concepts, is a dynamic activity which is constantly changing, requires continuous evaluation and re-evaluation, and which requires the highest possible quality of professional nursing skill. As was stated earlier in this book, the provision of nursing care to the elderly also requires the highest possible level of professional nursing skill.

Many nurses view the nursing process as something which will interfere with their freedom of choice in relation to patient care. They fear that a prescribed 'recipe' of nursing care is part of the nursing process and that they will have a limited freedom of choice in relation to how they deal with patients. As will be seen in other parts of this text, this fear is unfounded and should not be regarded as a constraint imposed by the nursing process. The nursing process is about the organization and documentation of nursing care, requiring high-quality, specific nursing care to be delivered in relation to specific patient needs.

In relation to nursing care 'styles', particularly as they differ in relation to general and psychiatric nursing, it has become fashionable to talk about psychiatric 'ideologies'. These ideologies, or models of care, are reflected in very different approaches to nursing care which are taken by different nurses in one speciality, or by nurses in different specialities. Just as no distinction is made by the author between the delivery of nursing care to patients in the community, as compared with institutional care, absolutely no distinction is made between the delivery of care by psychiatric nurses, and the delivery of care by non-psychiatric nurses, and no distinction between 'psychiatric' and 'general' concepts of nursing care as they relate to the elderly person. It is extremely rare for an elderly person to require only 'physical' *or* 'emotional' nursing care. Nurses who care for elderly people must have a thorough understanding of both of these basic types of care and must be as at home dealing with, for example, concepts such as anxiety, orientation and trust, as they are with concepts such as pain, elimination and hydration.

Chapter 9 examined four major approaches to the delivery, as opposed to organization, of nursing care, these approaches being increasingly used by nurses in all disciplines who care for the elderly. Each has an important part to play in the delivery of comprehensive and holistic care which takes full account of the physical, psychological and social needs of the elderly population.

REFERENCES

Cormack D.F.S. (1980) The nursing process: An application of the S.O.A.P.E. model. *Nursing Times* (Occasional paper) **76** (9) 37–40.

Cormack D.F.S. (1981) Nursing care of the elderly in Scotland. *Journal of gerontological Nursing* **7**, 749–58.

Hudson M.F. (1983) Safeguard your elderly patient's health through accurate physical assessment. *Nursing* **13**, 58–64.

Pavkov J.R. & Walsh J. (1981) For nursing homes: A mental health charting instrument. *Journal of gerontological Nursing* **7**, 13–20.

Pattie A.H. & Gilleard C. (1979) *Manual of the Clifton Assessment Procedures for the Elderly.* Hodder and Stoughton, London.

Prehn R.A. (1982) Applied behavioral analysis for disturbed elderly patients. *Journal of gerontological Nursing* **8**, 286–8.

Rameizl P. (1983) CADET. A self–care assessment tool. *Geriatric Nursing* **4** 377-8.

Wilkinson I.M. & Graham–White J. (1980) Psychogeriatric dependency rating scales (PGDRS): A method of assessment for use by nurses. *British Journal of Psychiatry* **137**, 558–65.

FURTHER READING

Hampshire G. (1983) Defining goals. *Nursing Times* **79**, 45.

Rumbol G.C. (1982) The nursing process — a problem solving approach. *Journal of Community Nursing* **5**, 17–18.

Tapley K. (1982) Psychosocial needs and the geriatric patient. *Journal of practical Nursing* **32**, 22–3, & 48.

Wade B. & Snaith P. (1981) The assessment of patients need for nursing care on geriatric wards. *International Journal of Nursing Studies* **18**, 261–71.

Wilkinson I. & Zissler L.M. (1984) Standardised assessments for the elderly: Clinical applications. *Nursing Times* **80**, 1, 36−7.

Wilson-Barnett J. & Carrigy A. (1978) Factors influencing patients emotional reactions to hospitalization. *Journal of advanced Nursing* **3**, 221−9.

PART 2
GERIATRIC NURSING CONCEPTS

Eighteen concepts which are central to the delivery of nursing care to the elderly have been selected for inclusion in Part 2. The concepts, which appear in alphabetical order, are presented using a similar overall format which allows for some variation reflecting the nature of the topic, and the style of the writer. Each concept chapter includes: a brief introduction to, and discussion of, the concept; the presentation of selected factors relating to it; principles of care relating to that particular concept; a short profile of a patient who has a problem in relation to it; a nursing process outline applied to the problem; an example of nursing care delivery over a 24 hour period; and a means of assessing a patient in relation to that particular problem. Each of these sections is to be regarded as no more than *illustrative* of the way in which nursing care can be organized; for example, in relation to assessment, *selected* criteria which will indicate the presence or absence of a problem are presented. As with the notion of the 'concept', in terms of its uniqueness to each person and its capacity for growth, the contents of these chapters are offered as a starting point from which to develop *your* expertise.

The emphasis on particular parts of each chapter, and the order in which they appear, vary slightly in response to the nature of the concept, and as a result of the way in which authors perceive it.

Although each concept is dealt with in separate compartments (chapters), it is fully recognized that each item is affected by, and affects, all others. This separation of items has been done for the convenience of presentation and clarity. Similarly, the patient and nursing care examples used imply that one relatively well-defined problem may exist at any given time. In reality, as we all know, elderly patients invariably have a multiplicity of nursing needs (multiple pathology), you are asked to bear these two positions in mind when reading Part 2 and, more importantly, when undertaking the care of the elderly.

Patients used to illustrate nursing care in relation to each concept have been placed in an environmental context (home, hospital and so on) and have usually been given a medical diagnosis. This has also been done to aid presentation and clarity. In reality, *all* that is contained in Part 2 relates to *all* patients in *all* medical diagnostic groups, to *all* well elderly people, and to elderly persons in *all* environments.

Finally, the *nursing* emphasis in each of the chapters in Part 2 must be seen in the context of the full and collaborative multidisciplinary context within which we all work. Just as we expect to be consulted about, and informed of, decisions made by our medical and paramedical colleagues, they must form a full part of the process by which we organize nursing care. The focus of these chapters, in terms of the delivery of care, is the *geriatric* nursing process, reflecting the central position of the elderly person (rather than the nurse) in health care delivery. Medical and nursing staff work 'hand in glove', sometimes we, the nurses, are the hand, sometimes the glove; nowhere is this more true than in relation to the care of the elderly.

Chapter 12
Activity

Activity is the quality of being active and engaging in purposeful movements, which is one of the main ways in which human beings define and express themselves. In connection with nursing, one immediately thinks of the activities of daily living, such as, eating, washing and dressing. Many people when they become older have a restricted level of activity which seriously impairs the quality of their lives. The reasons for this are seldom simple and range from obvious causes such as arthritis, stroke or inadequate tissue oxygenation, to poor motivation and social isolation.

FACTORS RELATING TO ACTIVITY

Ageing

The newborn baby displays largely reflex activity but within a few weeks begins to assert itself by learning to control its movements. The child, in learning to walk freely without assistance from another person, achieves independent movement. This ability to move freely without assistance from other people or without aids is a highly prized capability. Loss of independent mobility is viewed by most adults as a regression back to childhood. Activity is basic to life and the enjoyment of living. Inactivity restricts the individual's ability to interact freely with his environment and so affects the quality of his life.

The structure of the human musculoskeletal system, controlled as it is by a highly developed central nervous system, enables human beings to perform an incredible range of movements. These are far more complex and varied than in almost any other form of life. Human beings can train their bodies to perform a huge variety of complex movements. From the infant learning to control its head movements, to the concert pianist playing a piano concerto is an enormous leap in terms of human development, but illustrates what humans are capable of.

Manual dexterity and muscle strength increase steadily throughout childhood and into adult life, reaching a peak in the twenties. After the age of about 30 years there is a slow but steady loss of muscle mass so that by 80 years of age some 30% is lost. There is also a corresponding change in overall muscle strength, though the degree of loss differs widely among different muscle groups, the loss being significantly less in muscles in which activity is maintained. The physical work capacity of the 70-year-old is only about half that of the 20-year-old. In addition to the decrease in muscular strength there is also a decrease in endurance and agility. The problem, of course, in assessing this phenomenon is to separate out the effects of ageing from the effects of disuse due to lack of motivation, joint stiffness, poor oxygenation and so on.

Disuse Phenomena

Who has not heard of a sportsman wanting to make a comeback? However, ask any sportsman how difficult it is to achieve fitness after some enforced lay-off and he will soon be telling you how hard it is to get back to form.

Experiments have shown that even in young, healthy adults, periods of enforced inactivity for as short a period as three weeks result in muscular weakness, decreased exercise tolerance, changes in the cardiovascular system, nitrogen and calcium imbalance. The longer the inactivity is prolonged, the greater the effects. The individual feels weak and out of shape! In addition to the physical changes, inactivity contributes to feelings of boredom and apathy. The person becomes anorexic resulting in a poor nutritional status which leads to further weakness. He becomes easily fatigued at even quite modest exercise and quickly loses the motivation to become more active. Even the anticipation of fatigue will discourage the individual from participating in activities. Inactivity and restriction of movements often lead to isolation from other people so that even the activities of daily living become neglected. This is a pattern, seen quite often in the elderly, in which a vicious cycle of inactivity leads to boredom, frustration, isolation and further inactivity.

Stereotype

The elderly person is often pictured as someone whose posture is stooped, with head and neck allowed to fall forward. His steps are short and shuffling with the feet barely leaving the ground. There is limited or absent arm swinging and a slowing down of movement. Whilst this is true of many elderly people, it is untrue of many others, or at least, is not the whole story. The reasons for change in posture are complex; sheer bad habit may be a contributing factor, combined with simple disuse phenomena. In other people, loss of the ability to maintain posture and to recover balance quickly may result in a particular style of gait. In addition, the aged person may have some loss of proprioceptive activity. In these circumstances joint and position sense from the limbs is lost or may not be as effective. As a substitute the elderly person may have to watch the ground for visual clues which he uses as a substitute. This is seen in an extreme form in some diseases, for example, tabes dorsalis in which the dorsal columns of the spinal cord are selectively destroyed.

Changes in the musculoskeletal system will also result in marked changes in posture and stature. There is a loss of body fluid so that the intravertebral spaces become narrower and the length of the spine is shortened. Also bone changes may lead to changes in bone shape; for example, the angle of the neck of the femur may become more acute, so altering the weight distribution in the pelvis. One common disorder of this kind seen in the elderly is osteoporosis; in this disorder there is a reduction in otherwise normal bone. There is, of course, with increasing age a gradual loss of bone density but in osteoporosis there is an additional increase in the amount of bone lost. Often there appears to be no underlying cause, but in some cases conditions such as Cushing's syndrome and rheumatoid arthritis may be present. Loss of bone density is a feature of immobilization but in this instance recovery takes place on remobilization. Osteoporosis rarely occurs in children or young adults and is most commonly seen in postmenopausal women. There is no satisfactory treatment. The sufferer should be encouraged to stay mobile.

Other chronic disorders of the musculoskeletal system, such as arthritis, may lead to marked changes in posture, either because the actual disease process causes deformity or due to pain. The majority of people as they grow older, however, maintain their posture and gait and only in extreme old age conform more closely to the common stereotype outlined earlier.

Prevention of Inactivity

If the stooping posture and shuffling gait are not inevitable, how can the ageing elderly person be helped to maintain his posture, mobility and independence? Being 'off the legs' is one of the most common reasons for the elderly person being detained in hospital or confined to his own home. From what has been said already, this is problematical for the individual's morale and self-esteem. The elderly person whenever possible should be out of bed and engaged in purposeful activity; by that we mean activity which provides for interaction with the environment in pursuit of goals which seem meaningful and worthwhile to the individual. For most elderly people, purposeful activity is preferable to contrived exercises. The problem lies in ensuring that the elderly person has enough exercise on a regular and preferably daily basis to maintain bodily functions at an optimal capacity.

Simply maintaining the activities of daily living, however well performed, may not, of course, be enough to provide adequate activity levels.

Individuals as they grow older typically withdraw from intense physical activity and take up a more passive lifestyle which is less demanding. Also, when the older person retires from active employment physical and social activity is reduced; this is especially true of men in our society. Women often continue to run the home and remain active, for example performing a wide range of domestic chores much as they have always done. All too often, men have been so engrossed in their work that they have never participated in other recreational activities or hobbies. When retirement comes they have little to keep them active and lack the motivation to learn new skills. Notice we have said, 'lack the motivation', not ability. There is now sufficient evidence available to show that being old is no bar to learning, given the right conditions and the will to try. However, we must not forget pressures from within society on the elderly person to withdraw, to conform, not to take risks and generally to 'act his age'.

Activity in Old Age

How active a person is when he becomes old is very much dependent on how active he was when young, and, on how well he looked after his body. There are of course a few factors which should be considered, such as the presence of some disease, diagnosed or not, which affects the oxygenation and perfusion of tissues, the genuine effects of ageing and the effects of disuse; sometimes called 'hypokinetic disease'. It is obviously dangerous for any elderly person suddenly to take up strenuous exercise if he has not been indulging in this for many years. However, it has been shown that the elderly can improve their physical activity by conditioning. What is important is that the elderly person has a thorough medical examination first, so that a programme of activity can be devised to meet his needs. By and large, elderly people do not readily take to the sort of vigorous physical exercise advocated for the young. Any attempts to increase an elderly person's activity must be carefully thought out if it is to be enduring. This is especially so when we consider the group who are most in need. It is not 'busy' elderly people who are at risk, they are used to exercise and have usually always been active. This is the group one finds walking, dancing, swimming, in yoga classes and running marathons! It is not this sort of *busy person* who has the problem though he may often be the key to involving his more indolent contemporaries. Very often it is the elderly person who no longer has a meaningful interaction with his environment who is in need of help; a person whose volition is low and whose goals in life have become lost or have been frustrated by physical, emotional and or social factors. For this group, more than any other, energy expenditure has to be channelled into what are, for them, productive and satisfying activites. They need to regain their self-esteem and motivation to improve their health and well-being. In any attempt to increase an elderly person's activity level, the professional must first of all obtain the approval and willing cooperation of the individual concerned. Furthermore, any activity programme must be considered within the context of the individual's environment; it is no use planning something like this without careful consideration of the whole person.

It follows from this, therefore, that it is not the prerogative of any one agency to harness the necessary and varied resources needed to cater for a wide range of human activities. This process demands cooperation between many agencies. The elderly person is every bit as much an individual as a young person *perhaps* even more so in terms of resistance to change.

As an example we will look briefly at a hospital setting. Invariably many professionals will be involved; doctors, nurses, physiotherapists, occupational therapists, and so on. In some circumstances one professional may have more to offer than another depending on individual needs. The team, therefore, needs to assess *the individual* so that his strengths and weaknesses can be ascertained. The team must never rush the individual; an unhurried approach which allows an atmosphere of acceptance and trust to develop should be aimed at. The person who is the object of the assessment should be involved in the decision making, using a mutual problem-solving approach, which leads to careful gradations of expectation. In other words, what does the old lady or gentleman want? There is no point in setting expectations too high. The elderly, like the young, need to be able to achieve any goals set, otherwise, frustration and distrust will surely follow.

Benefits of Exercise

Increasing physical activity has been shown to bring about significant improvements in bodily functions even in the elderly. Physical conditioning leads to an improvement in aerobic metabolism despite structural changes and functional decrement; for example, men in their sixties gain significant benefit from a 30 minute walk which raises the heart rate to 100–110 beats per minute. Physical activity has been shown to lower the blood pressure in many hypertensive individuals. It leads to loss of adipose tissue without the necessity of reducing calorie intake; for many older people, taking exercise is more acceptable than cutting down on food intake. Walking and other forms of physical activity also stimulate the gut and so help to reduce emotional tension, allowing the individual to relax more easily, which leads to a more natural sleep. Many elderly people do not sleep well and are prescribed sedatives which depress the central nervous system, so reducing the stimulus to take exercise.

Whether a person is young or old, activity plays an important role in tissue oxygenation and perfusion. By maintaining the tone of the heart muscle, and the muscles of the venous pump in the legs, circulation is greatly improved. This leads to better renal perfusion because of the improved cardiac output which, combined with the action of the venous pump, may go a long way towards alleviating dependent oedema, seen so frequently in the elderly. The activity has, of course, a direct effect on metabolism and influences oxygen uptake, heart rate and temperature; because of these effects the elderly in particular must embark on exercise programmes only after a proper medical appraisal. Obviously any sudden and extraordinary demands on the cardiovascular or respiratory systems which they were unable to meet would be disastrous. The consequences are seen, for example, following a fall of snow when the elderly person is tempted to clear it; the exertion plus the cold causing angina or even a myocardial infarction.

In terms of overall health and well-being the elderly person, indeed all of us, should be aiming to:
(a)   preserve normal posture;
(b)   preserve joint mobility;
(c)   prevent contractures;
(d)   preserve strength for ambulation;
(e)   preserve circulatory and respiratory function.

By keeping fit there is no reason why man as he ages should not lead a full healthy life, doing what he wants and needs to do. As long as the elderly person can function adequately and independently, even when he has multiple pathology, he may not regard himself as being in poor health.

PRINCIPLES OF CARE

Because activity levels vary so widely between individuals, prescribing appropriate levels is by no means easy. Whilst some will readily participate in any suggested activity, others may be reluctant. An important consideration is the dignity and self-esteem of the person. Nobody likes to be made a fool of or be forced to participate in activities in which one would prefer to take no part. For this reason any exercise regimen needs to be planned to suit the individual. Generally speaking, the older person prefers what for him are socially acceptable activities, such as walking, dancing, swimming, gardening, woodworking, weaving, housekeeping duties and so on.

Physical Disabilities and Limitations

These determine the nature of any activity permitted and its duration. If an aid is required, it must be one which the patient can learn to use readily and one which will complement and enhance whatever strengths he has. Footwear and clothing may have to be adapted, for example, support for a dropped foot may allow virtually normal walking. Any braces or physical support must be fitted by the appropriate professional; this ensures the fitting of an appliance selected to meet the individual's needs.

Environmental Considerations

It is important to create a safe environment for the elderly person to interact with. This includes such obvious factors as non-slip flooring, no loose carpets or other articles lying about. Good lighting is vital, especially on stairs and landings. Additional handrails should be added where appropriate, for example in toilets, by doors with steps, on ramps, stairs and landings. Nurses and other people must refrain from constantly rearranging or moving furniture around in the ward or home, as this leads to confusion and disorientation which may discourage the elderly person from moving around.

Daily Exercise

Times should be set aside each day for exercise, however limited the individual may be; there are few, if any, elderly people who will not be able to take any exercise. Opportunities to take exercise should be presented several times during the day and the patients encouraged to participate. The form of exercise is not important, the partaking of it is. Whenever possible, dayrooms, dining-rooms and bedrooms should be separate, so that patients, if able, can walk between the various parts of the ward.

It is important to foster independence in eating, washing, cleaning the teeth, hair care, dressing and undressing. In hospital the occupational therapist will assess the patient and suggest appropriate ways to assist him in becoming independent once more. It is essential that all responsible for the care of the patient are consistent in the amount of assistance given, so that steady progress can be made. It is best if the team agree on short-term goals, for example, the patient will be able to put on his socks by himself using an aid in three to four days. The occupational therapist can also arrange for activities such as weaving, pottery, polishing, etc., which are designed to encourage the use of and strengthen a particular part of the body. These activities are valuable in that something is produced for all the hard work, giving a sense of achievement. The physiotherapist will also teach the patient appropriate exercises to overcome specific disabilities or increase strength in general. It is essential that nurses, relatives and others encourage and assist the patient to keep up the exercises prescribed.

Exercise is often easier when people are enjoying themselves. For this, and other, reasons birthdays and other special occasions should be celebrated. This provides the opportunity for various 'party games' such as 'pass the parcel', dancing, singing and clapping the hands to music and so on. Also what about a bit of armchair football? All that is required is a largish beach-ball which can be kicked from person to person across the room or thrown. Other games which can easily be played and enjoyed from a chair or by patients whose mobility is restricted are quoits, skittles, darts, and so on.

PATIENT PROFILE

John Smith, aged 68 years, was born and brought up on the outskirts of a large town. He left school at the age of 14 and after 5 years working on various farms he joined the police. At the outbreak of the Second World War he joined the Navy and served on several ships until the end of the war. On leaving the Navy he rejoined the police and eventually completed 25 years as a village policeman. On retirement from the police force he did a variety of jobs until finally retiring completely when 63 years of age. Apart from an occasional attack of influenza and the common cold, he had kept very well and fit; indeed he was an active person who had used a bicycle in the course of his duties as a policeman. When aged 67 years, he became very ill with pneumonia and was unable to leave his bed for three weeks. The illness left him very weak and unable to take his weight on his legs. Being so weak, he required a lot of assistance in getting dressed and up into a wheelchair. He had become terrified of falling and refused to move on his own. The pattern of increasing dependence would undoubtedly have been broken in the weeks that followed but for one event; during the period in which he was starting to be mobilized his wife died suddenly. Mr Smith was grief stricken and unable to attend the funeral. In the weeks that followed his wife's death, Mr Smith was depressed and emotionally labile. He wept readily and became increasingly dependent on the nursing staff. He was, however, a big man, 1.94 m in height, and weighed 94 kg, so that lifting, moving, dressing, toiletting, etc., was not easy.

Mr Smith's refusal to help himself in any way and the general awkwardness of handling him, meant that he was far from popular with the nursing staff. Several nurses had complained of injuring their backs and shoulders when lifting and moving him. The doctors were also at a loss as to what to do next because they could find no medical reason as to why Mr

Smith should not be active and independent. What finally led to a very full re-appraisal was Mr Smith's refusal to use the toilet. He insisted he be allowed to move his bowels whilst in bed—not into a bedpan but on incontinence pads; this was, of course, unacceptable to everyone, so that obviously new tactics were required to help Mr Smith overcome his mobility problems.

ORGANIZATION OF NURSING CARE

Subjective Evidence (What the Patient Says)

- 'Hold on to me nurse; I am falling.'
- 'My legs are too weak; I cannot stand.'
- 'I am too tired to stay up all day.'

Objective Evidence (What the Nurse and Others Observe)

- Holds on tightly to the top of the bed, chair, etc., when being moved.
- Observed to move legs freely in bed.
- Looks frightened whenever he has to move from bed to chair.

Assessment (Nursing Diagnosis)

- Inactivity due to a morbid fear of falling.

Plan of Nursing Care

AIM

- To assist Mr Smith overcome his morbid fear of falling.

NURSING ACTIONS — 1st STAGE

Short-term objective

- The patient will dress himself and get up from bed to chair.
  Screen bed.
  Strip bed down to top sheet.
  Give Mr Smith his clothes.
  Leave for five minutes, give encouragement for any progress made in dressing.
  Give some assistance as required.

Leave for a further five minutes.
Repeat.

Note   Routine to be repeated daily until the patient regains confidence to dress and get up. Give praise and encouragement, however little the patient manages on his own.

Expected Outcome

● Able to dress himself and transfer from bed to chair unaided.

NURSING ACTION — 2nd STAGE

Short-term objective

● Will walk by himself (using a walking aid) from his bed to the dayroom, to the lavatory, etc.
  Supply walking aid (Zimmer frame) and explain its use.
  Assist Mr Smith to stand by his bed when he completes dressing.
  Encourage him to use walking aid.
  Reassure by providing good support (two nurses).
  Praise all positive attempts to use the walking aid—ignore any negative behaviour.

Expected Outcome

● Walks of his own volition using a walking aid.

NURSING ACTION — 3rd STAGE

Short-term objective

● Will walk using a walking stick or unassisted.
  Allow patient to walk along corridor using walking aid.
  Once walking confidently, suggest he tries with walking stick only.
  Provide reassurance and support.

Expected Outcome

● Will walk using walking stick as only aid and without other assistance and no longer be afraid of falling.

Long-term objective

● Will return to a reasonable level of activity so that he may once more lead an independent life.

Footnote

Mr Smith made, what can only be described as, a spectacular recovery. He responded to the new approach readily and his activity level increased very rapidly. Within four weeks of commencing the remobilization regimen he was ready for transfer to local authority accommodation. He had regained his self-esteem and independence. Whether he would ever have done so had his inactivity been allowed to continue much longer is something we will never know.

NURSING CARE OF A PATIENT WITH AN ACTIVITY PROBLEM (EXAMPLE)

07.30 hours	Awaken and encourage to lift himself up the bed using rope ladder on bed and 'monkey pole' overhead. Provide hot water, flannel, soap and towel for washing of hands and face.
08.00	Encourage patient to sit well up the bed (Fowlers position) for his breakfast. Allow to feed himself.
08.30	Provide with clothes after screening bed and removing top bed covers.
09.00	Walk full length of ward (using aid if necessary) before going to the dayroom. Nurse to supervise and aid if required.
09.30	Encourage patient to walk to the bathroom to wash and shave himself.
10.00	Return to dayroom in time for mid-morning tea or coffee.
10.15	Form appropriate and willing patients into large circle in dayroom and provide large beachball for game of handball or football or other activity of choice.
11.00	Keep group in circle initiate a discussion of current events—make sure all patients participate.
12.00	Lunch, encourage patient to walk from dayroom to dining room for lunch where he can feed himself seated at table.
13.00	If weather suitable, encourage patient to go for a walk outside along verandah—supervise.
14.00	Occupational therapy—designed to encourage meaningful activity (see Daily exercise pp. 137–8).
15.00	Tea break.

16.00	Encourage walk along corridors—up to fifteen or more minutes duration.
17.30	Evening meal in dining room. Encourage walk, but may be tired, assess to avoid overfatigue.
18.00–20.00	Watch television or participate in table games, e.g. cards, dominoes, or if not too tired skittles or bowling—ensure a competitive game.
20.00–21.00	Prepare for getting to bed, toilet, undressing, put away clothes, cleaning teeth. Late drink of hot chocolate or other preference.
21.00	Go to bed. Encourage patient to read or listen to the radio for an hour before retiring.
22.00	Settle patient down for night, encourage good posture, provide any aids which may be helpful. Ensure call bell is near, plus drink. Discourage smoking in bed. Unless unable to move or incontinent do not disturb during the night.

Assessment of Activity

The elderly person's activity status needs to be assessed so that problems are clearly identified. In relation to activity the musculoskeletal system must be assessed in detail.

GENERAL QUESTIONS

Would you consider yourself to be a physically active person?
If the answer is NO, allow the person to explain in his own words how he thinks he is not.
If the answer is YES, proceed with the next question.

What sort of exercise do you regularly take?
Again, allow the person to respond in his own words. Beware of exaggeration, many people think, for example, that they walk much farther than they actually do.

Do you have any limitations on the amount of exercise you take?
Let the person answer in his own words. Limitations may be real or imaginery and include breathlessness, pain, for example, intermittent claudication, joint pain or stiffness or other problems.

Do you normally use an aid when you are walking, for example, a cane or a tripod?
Let the person explain why he uses the aid. He may give important clues to non-physical problems such as a fear of falling.

Having assessed the individual in a general sense and established a good rapport with the person, the next stage is a systematic assessment of the following physical aspects.

POSTURE

Stands erect
Stoops
Stands unaided
Requires support (specify)

GAIT

Normal, swings arms
Slow, shuffling, arms hanging by side
Difficulty in initiating movements
Difficulty in stopping movements
High-stepping, broad-based gait
Excessive movements of trunk

BODY MOVEMENT

Normal
Slow
Incoordinated

JOINT MOBILITY

Full range, all joints
Limited range (specify joint and nature of limitation)

MUSCLE STRENGTH—UPPER LIMBS

	right	left
Normal power		
Mild weakness		
Severe weakness		
Spastic flexion		
Extension		

MUSCLE STRENGTH—LOWER LIMBS

	right	*left*
Normal power		
Mild weakness		
Severe weakness		
Spastic flexion		
Extension		

SENSORY STATUS

Vision
  normal
  impaired (specify)
Hearing
  normal
  impaired (specify)

FURTHER READING

Bozian M.W. & Clark H.M. (1980) Counteracting sensory changes in the elderly. *American Journal of Nursing* **80** (3), 473–6.

Callaghn W. (1981) Aids for the disabled. *Nursing Times* **77** (24), 1029–34.

Castledine G. (1979) Nursing assessment of the musculoskeletal system. *Nursing (Oxford)* **3**, 48–9.

Cooper S. (1981) Common concern: Accidents and old adults. *Geriatric Nursing* **2**, 287–90.

Gioiella E.C. (1980) Give the older person space. *American Journal of Nursing* **80** (5), 898–9.

Haleem M.A. (1978) Peripheral arthropathies in the elderly. *Nursing Times* **77** (44), 1799–801.

Hudson M.F. (1983) Safeguard your elderly patient's health through physical assessment. *Nursing 83* **13** (11), 58–64.

Imms F.J. & Edholm O.E. (1981) Studies of gait and mobility in the elderly. *Age and Ageing* **10**, 147–56.

Kenny R.A. (1982) *Physiology of Ageing*. Yearbook Medical Publishers, Chicago.

Kent S. (1982) Exercise and ageing. *Geriatrics* **37** (6), 132–5.

MacLennan W.J., Hall M.R.P., Timothy J.I. & Robinson M. (1980). Is weakness in old age due to muscle wasting? *Age and Ageing* **10**, 147–56.

Martin D. (1981) Enjoyable activity for everyone. *Geriatric Nursing* **2**, 210–13.

McCormack D. & Whitehead A. (1981) The effect of producing recreational activities on the engagement level of long-stay geriatric patients. *Age and Ageing*, **10**, 287–91.

Rienisch E. (1981) Quick assessment of hemiplegic functioning. *American Journal of Nursing* **81**, 102–4.

Chapter 13
Affect

The English essayist Joseph Addison remarked that 'the grand essentials to happiness in this life are, something to do, something to love and something to hope for.' The 'pursuit of happiness' has been a central concern of thinkers and writers down the ages, in all cultures. Their concern seems to be understandable, given the importance which most people attach to happiness as a key feature of their lives. Although most of us would like to live a long life, many of us would rather it were short but happy, than long and unhappy. When we talk about people's *moods* we often mean their relative state of happiness. Although mood or emotional state covers more than mere happiness, this is a central aspect of the concept. When, for example, we say that someone is 'moody' we usually mean given to sudden changes of mood, usually from a normal to a gloomy disposition. This gloominess, when experienced in a severe and continuous form, is often referred to as depression. However, in addition to mood changing in a downward direction, mood can also be lifted to an abnormal degree. People often experience a heightened state of happiness, when they feel that they can do anything, can solve any problem, and see no limits to their abilities or energies. When people are so unusually happy or exhilarated we often refer to them as being 'manic' or overexcited. Indeed 'happiness' is rather like a long line: at one end lies the state of gloom or despondency, *depression;* at the other end lies the excitable or exhilarated state we usually call *mania.* Somewhere in the middle lies the state of 'normal affect' which most people experience; some days we feel a bit down, on others we are extremely happy. However, in neither case do we ever drop to the depths or rise to the heights which are characterized by depression and mania.

The state of mania, or extreme excitement, is an unusual occurrence. Although many people often feel depressed, far fewer people experience the emotional 'high' of mania. This is as true of the elderly, as it is of younger people. Indeed, since the depressed state is found more often in older people, this chapter will concentrate on the lowering or flattening of affect, to the exclusion of the manic state.

Many people appear to experience 'depression' at some stage in their lives. This may be quite specific, as in feelings of sadness, or it may take a

145

more general form, involving difficulty in coping with life. Usually, they manage to cope with such temporary distress by using some simple 'coping strategy' to take their mind off their problems. When depression is evident in older people it may take a more complex form than the gloomy or despondent state experienced by younger people. Often this depression does not only involve disturbance of subjective experience, such as changes in the way they 'feel', it may also involve changes in behaviour and physiological functioning. It is important to note at this stage that although the elderly have a higher than average incidence of emotional disorder, they often receive less psychological help than other age groups (Eisdorfer & Stotsky 1977). This may be due partly to a traditional neglect of the needs of the elderly, often shown by the stereotyped roles which Western society projects for old people. It may also be related to the prejudices of old people themselves, who may be reluctant to accept psychological help because of the stigma attached to it.

It is important that we recognize that although many old people may be 'depressed' in the sense that they feel low, or unhappy, not all of them will be diagnosed formally as suffering from depression. In this chapter the author will consider the management of all elderly people whose mood is lowered or flattened, whether they are 'officially' depressed or not. Having said that, it is clear that depression, in its formal sense, is very common in the elderly (Post 1981). However, our understanding of the condition is very limited indeed. In common with other age groups some people recover spontaneously from their depressed state. Where the problem becomes 'chronic' in nature this may be a sign that a number of complex factors are involved; for instance, it may be that one or more psychological factors, such as grief reaction, are interacting with the peculiar processes of ageing. Depression in the elderly may, in effect, be quite different from depression in other age groups. Exactly how different is unclear.

Bereavement has often been proposed as a significant factor in the onset of depression. However, most old people lose family or friends late in life. Does this mean that all old people can be expected to become depressed? Since only a proportion of old people experience such problems, this should lead us to question our understanding of the way old people react to bereavement. Dimond (1981) suggests that old people react differently to the death of a loved one. They may be using coping skills acquired in earlier difficult situations to help them survive the loss. Although the depression of old age is similar to that found in other groups we should acknowledge that our understanding of this problem is sorely limited. Most of the care and 'treatment' strategies recommended in this chapter have not been built around the specific needs of the elderly, they are no more than generalizations from approaches used with other age groups. Although the use of such 'general principles' is not wrong in itself, it shows that more research is required to develop approaches which are specific to the needs of the elderly themselves.

Although the death of a loved one can serve as a 'trigger' for depression, other forms of *loss* may be equally important. Old people commonly lose their homes when taken into care. They may also lose various kinds of attachments: relationships with friends, pets, routines or even prized objects or situations. They can also lose control over their circumstances, especially when family, neighbours or caring agencies take over the running of their lives. Although this can be done with the best of intentions, it may lead to the sort of withdrawal and apathy which Seligman (1975) described as 'learned helplessness'. This is most often associated with the elderly in institutional care; especially where their lives are organized to meet the demands of the institution rather than their own personal needs. Finally, old people often experience a distressing loss of function when their senses begin to fail them or they lose the dexterity which they once took for granted. For many, this heralds the certainty of the 'final loss', of life itself. Although some may look forward to death, others may feel bitterness or resentment at the prospect of deterioration and death. The idea that the elderly might wish to protest, perhaps symbolically, against the inevitability of death is no more clearly illustrated than in Dylan Thomas' lines, written at his father's deathbed:

'And you, my father, there on the sad height,
Curse, bless, me now with your fierce tears, I pray.
Do not go gentle into that good night.
Rage, rage against the dying of the light.'

Although such forms of 'loss' may be unavoidable, it is clear that some people cope better than others with such inevitable happenings. The way a person interprets and reacts to loss may determine whether or not he becomes depressed. The person's attitude towards himself, his circumstances, and his future, play a large part in influencing how he feels. As Addison commented it has much to do with what the person does, who he loves and what he has to live for. If he believes that, 'I don't enjoy anything any more', or that, 'there's just no point . . . I'm going to die anyway', then it may be quite natural that he should feel apathetic and defeated, if not seriously depressed. However, depression in the elderly can be difficult to identify clearly. Although formal medical diagnosis is the responsibility of the physician, nurses are often expected to report on the patient's mood and behaviour. Furthermore nurses may be required to identify 'depressive' problems in patients who are not clinically depressed. They should, therefore, be aware of the significance of different signs and symptoms; for instance, old people often complain of difficulty in concentrating, poor attention or memory and may appear apathetic. These problems are frequently associated with confusion. They may also be indicative of depression. Identifying a depressive state may be further complicated if the patient is agitated, hostile or overtly aggressive. These problems are sometimes 'written off' as part and parcel of the process of dementia. However, they may also be signs of depression. Although the danger of failing to recognize a depressive state is ever present, some signs provide a more specific pointer to it. Especially important are expressions of hopelessness and worthlessness. These are often combined with feelings of inferiority and inadequacy and, in very severe cases, the patient may also express a willingness to end his own life.

Two distinct kinds of depression are evident in the elderly. The person may have suffered from a similar problem when younger; this might be a continuation or repetition of this earlier depressive state. In other cases the problem shows itself for the first time in old age. This latter example is most relevant to our discussion here, where depression appears to be linked to some aspect of the ageing process.

Depression in the elderly is often seen as involving an interaction between *life stresses* and certain kinds of physical activity in the brain. This may explain why they are so prone to this problem. Of those who become *clinically* depressed, a proportion will recover without relapse; some will have relapses but remain well in between; some will continue to suffer from a 'depressed invalidism'; whilst 10% or more will remain in a state of unremitting depression. Although electroconvulsive therapy and antidepressant drugs are the most common forms of treatment, in recent years more interest has been shown in developing various kinds of psychosocial therapy (Beck *et al.* 1979; Steuer & Hammen 1983). This chapter concentrates upon the use of such a psychosocial approach since this appears to be most relevant to the nurse's interpersonal role. It also appears to be the most appropriate approach for those elderly people who experience disturbance of affect, but who may not be diagnosed as clinically depressed.

FACTORS RELATED TO DEPRESSION

Ageism

The elderly, like the mentally or physically handicapped, are all too easily stereotyped. Staff often find it easy to sympathize with a young person's negative view of life. Similar views expressed by an older person may be taken as further evidence that old people tend to moan a lot. The reality is that old people, like young people, tend to become depressed because of the views they hold about themselves and their lives, not because they are old and getting older. Old people often express, or believe, the negative judgements which younger people make of them: 'I'm too old to start learning new things,' 'Us old folk are just a burden on everyone.' Again, the reality is that old people are not inferior to young people; they are just different by virtue of their age. You should take care not to reinforce such expressions of ageism, for example by being overly supportive, or patronizing, nor should you necessarily accept the patient's self-imposed ageist attitude.

Relationships

If the nurse is to avoid practising ageism, she must take care not to patronize the patient. He should be consulted about what he would like to do, or asked how he feels about decisions which affect him. He should be given the respect which his age demands. A good starting point to establishing a positive relationship is to ask the patient how he would like to be addressed. The common practice of calling all old people 'grandma' or 'grandpa' or even by their Christian name may be seen as overfamiliarity or even an insult. A close relationship is crucial if the elderly patient is to be encouraged to talk about the aspects of his situation which depress him. It is also important if he is to *avoid* becoming depressed, as in the case of an amputee or a patient with a terminal illness. In general it is best to *collaborate* with the patient at all times, rather than treat him as a dependent individual, even where this is manifestly the case. If you are overly supportive, this may be interpreted as further evidence of the patient's worthlessness, uselessness or hopelessness. Try to point out that although the staff are there to help the patient, this can best be done by helping him 'to help himself'. The relationship should be kept 'open', discuss briefly what you want to do in advance, asking for the patient's comments and, if he is agreeable, his assistance. Patients often feel that they are being manipulated by staff who plan every aspect of their lives from the security of the nursing station. In such cases the patient sees himself as having no part in the decision-making which influences his very existence. Where you decide that it might be beneficial for the patient to do something, like talk to someone from another ward, or write a letter to his family, you should suggest that he might consider trying one of two or three things; giving him the opportunity to pick one and carry it out independently. Then he can honestly say that *he* has done something to improve his own life. It is clear, however, that many nurses find such an 'indirect' approach to care less rewarding than providing a more supportive, 'mothering' type of care.

Perception

It has already been noted that the patient is likely to be depressed because he views himself, his circumstances and his future in a particularly negative way. He usually blames himself for things which have gone wrong; interpreting any failure as a sign of his inherent worthlessness or uselessness. A particular problem experienced by elderly people is the *selective life review.* Here the patient recalls all the unhappy or unsuccessful things which have happened to him in his life, excluding or ignoring all positive experiences. The patient tends to dwell on these bad memories, citing them as examples of his own failings or weakness. As a result of thinking in this negative way, the patient feels bad. These negative thought patterns can even influence the patient's physiological functioning; he thinks, 'What's the point in doing anything?' This leads to a reduction in activity level, which can lead to specific problems like constipation. Stated very simply, his problems are caused not so much by things which happen to him, as by the view he takes of them.

In helping the patient to overcome such problems, encourage him to challenge his distorted view of himself and his world. The simplest way to do this is to begin by identifying his problems; he may complain that he does not enjoy *anything* any more, or is unable to do *anything.* Then he should be encouraged to *test out* his belief in practice. This can be done by conducting a small 'experiment'; for example, if the patient says that he cannot concentrate sufficiently to read any more, then he might be asked to read a short passage aloud, taking care to select one which he *can* read. Some advice should be given as to how he should approach this 'experiment', with phrases like, 'Just take your time . . . say to yourself "I'm going to have a go at this . . . it's not the end of the world if I get stuck". Just relax, take your time, take a deep breath . . . off you go.'

Using simple tasks, such as reading, walking, recalling an incident from the past, you can challenge the patient's distorted belief that he is 'all bad' or 'a complete write-off'. The importance of testing out his beliefs cannot be stressed too strongly. It is not enough simply to reassure the patient that he should not be depressed, or that he is not 'all washed up'. Instead, he should be encouraged to find out for himself that there is little in the way of evidence to support his belief.

Education

As we have noted, many patients attribute their depressed feelings to the ageing process, you can play a central part in correcting such misconceptions. If there is some truth in what he says, as when he complains of failing eyesight, try to correct any exaggeration. Does this really mean that he is useless? Has he any other assets? Can he not simply get a new pair of glasses? Never subscribe to the patient's viewpoint simply for fear of upsetting him. Try to educate him as to the nature of his depressed mood; he feels depressed because of the negative way he looks at things which happen to him, or might happen to him, for example. Encourage him to see things as they really are, not as he *thinks* they are.

Resistance

Challenging the patient's viewpoint is rarely easy, many resist offers of help, even encouragement. Often this is because they feel unworthy of praise or help. Again, ask for 'evidence' that the patient is 'unworthy' or that he has not been successful at *something,* and is entitled therefore to some praise. Often patients feel that the nurse cannot help because she is too young. In either of these cases, avoid arguing or reasoning with the patient. Instead, acknowledge that he is unhappy about something; perhaps he feels that he is being manipulated by a 'mere youth.' You might say, 'OK, I think I understand how you feel. I know that this may seem a bit silly to you, or maybe you just don't want to do it, but perhaps we could just try it for a short while. We could try to work out these problems together and if you think that I don't understand how you feel . . . maybe because I'm too young or something . . . then just let me know. Who knows, we might be able to work it out there and then. What do you say?'

PRINCIPLES OF CARE

Depression in the elderly has much to do with the ageing process. However it may have much more to do with the old person's reaction to events common in old age. Nursing goals should always acknowledge the individual and his unique problems. However, there is likely to be some common ground between one depressed individual and another. Many will complain of similar somatic symptoms: lethargy, sleep disruption, loss of appetite. They may also share anxieties about the future. Most common of all will be expressions of 'negative self-concept': the patient may feel guilty about past actions, real or imaginary; believe that he is a burden on everyone; and feel ashamed about having some kind of 'psychiatric illness'. We should recognize the seriousness of depression in old age, taking care not to dismiss it as another aspect of ageing. Although helping such patients can be frustrating and unrewarding, there are a range of goals which can be set to suit most patients.

Symptomatic Relief

When the patient complains of distressing symptoms, such as anxiety, sadness, sleep disturbance, alleviation of this discomfort should be an immediate goal. At this stage you can offer advice about relaxation, teaching the patient how to monitor his feelings of tension, before and after using relaxation techniques. In the same vein he might be taught about the value of exercise, such as brisk walking or stretching, as an aid to relaxation, and of the negative effect of heavy tea and coffee consumption.

The patient may also be shown how to use 'distraction', especially when he experiences severe negative affect. He can be shown how to think about something distressing, rating how sad or tense he feels afterwards. Then he should be asked to transfer his attention to something in his immediate environment, studying perhaps a plant or a picture. He should try to give this his full concentration, collecting as much 'information' as he can. Then he should rate his feelings of sadness or tension again, with the likelihood that he will feel some reduction in distress. On the basis of this 'experiment' he should be encouraged to use this technique whenever he feels distressed.

Increasing Positive Activity

When depressed, the patient gradually withdraws from routine activities. Usually this is because he does not feel able to do things, or because he believes that he will not enjoy them. Once he has some control over his distressing symptoms he should be encouraged to increase his level of activity again. Here also, he should be encouraged to adopt an 'experimental' approach, testing out whether or not activities make him feel better or worse. A simple diary can be used to detail what the patient does throughout the day. This can also be used to record how he feels at different times in the day. This record may help him recognize that he feels slightly better when active, and more depressed when inactive.

If the patient reports feeling no pleasure when doing things, he should be encouraged to judge how much satisfaction or achievement he feels *after* doing something, especially something which he has recently been unable to do. Even simple activities, such as making his bed or making a pot of tea, can be used as the basis of *achievement* ratings. If the patient *can* complete simple tasks like these, his performance can be used as further 'evidence' that he is not quite as hopeless as he thought. As a final stage in these medium-term goals, the patient can be helped to plan his life, rather than waiting to decide what he will do on the basis of 'how he feels'. At first, he may make plans for later in the day, including activities which will give him a sense of pleasure or achievement. Then he might plan what he is going to do the next morning; progressing to planning the whole day ahead. Eventually he will be able to map out a flexible routine for most of his week. This plan can be used as an aid to overcoming feelings that 'things happen to him' rather than as a result of his actions.

Challenging Distorted Thinking

In the long term try to change the patient's views of himself, his world and his future. It is important that you do not simply reassure him. Ask the patient to give *evidence* of how he was a bad husband, or how he knows that he will not enjoy himself. In the long term the patient should be helped to recognize that he is *exaggerating* the importance of certain events and *ignoring* the positive experiences in his life. In some cases he may also be *predicting* that there will be some negative outcome, instead of waiting to see what the result of his action will be. This *challenging* process begins when the patient is encouraged to find out that he can do *something* to ease his distress. It is taken a stage further when he starts *experimenting* with his daily routine, instead of predicting how he will feel on any particular day. Finally he learns about the specific ways in which he distorts reality. Armed with this knowledge he stands a better chance of checking his negative thinking before it does too much damage.

PATIENT PROFILE

Mrs Jackson is 73 years old and has been in a psychogeriatric ward for about three months. She was admitted with a diagnosis of senile dementia following her return from a holiday at her son's home in France. She had gone to stay with him 'to avoid being alone at Christmas'. Her husband had died in December two years previously. Mrs Jackson had been in hospital the previous Christmas receiving treatment for her diabetic condition which became unstable. She returned home after a few weeks but reported feeling 'low in spirits'. This passed off quickly, and by her own report she coped well alone over the summer. However by Christmas she started to 'feel tired all the time; everything was an effort. I felt empty inside and just lost interest in everything.' Mrs. Jackson attributed these problems to her diabetes saying, 'I suppose its a touch of what I had before. I expect I'll get over it again.'

On the ward she spends a lot of time sitting alone, occasionally getting up to look out of the window. She says that at these times she is thinking about her husband, and how she misses him. She also worries about the future, and has discussed with the social worker the possibility of selling her house and going into a home or staying in hospital. She has commented on a couple of occasions that 'maybe I've just had it ... can't seem to cope ... being so helpless gets me down.' Her two sons both live abroad. They have asked her to come and live with them but she feels that she would be a burden. She presents no major management problem on the ward, where the team are heavily committed to caring for more dependent patients. She helps out a little in the ward if asked to, but rarely interacts with other patients. Over the last month she has become more withdrawn and complains of a painful tension in her neck and shoulders.

ORGANIZATION OF NURSING CARE

Subjective Evidence (What the Patient Says)

- 'I'm tired all the time.'
- 'I'm just a burden on everyone.'
- 'I just can't cope . . . maybe I've had it.'

Objective Evidence (What the Nurse and Others Observe)

- Spends a large proportion of her day aimlessly — appears preoccupied.
- Tearful when reading letters from sons; often tears them up after reading them.
- Does not mix with other patients. Avoids going out of ward.

Assessment (Nursing Diagnosis)

- Is experiencing specific emotional problems typical of a depressed state.

Plan (of Nursing Care)

- Encourage her to accept that she is 'depressed'. Explain that this is not related to her diabetic condition. Explain that she can help to overcome this by tackling these difficulties in a practical, problem-solving fashion.
- Encourage her to make simple decisions using a graded framework: beginning with simple ones, becoming more complex.
- Help her to reduce distressing symptoms, such as tension or sadness, by using relaxation or distraction.
- Encourage her to challenge her beliefs that, for example, she has lost all interest, by simple experiments.
- Help her to challenge her belief that she is a burden on everyone by inviting her to help with the social and recreational needs of the other patients.

Expected Outcome

- Will be able to tackle her problems in a more constructive manner.
- Will be able to plan her time more constructively.
- Will appear less tense and tearful.
- Will feel more useful.
- Will feel more able to cope with her life in general.
- Will mix more with the other patients.
- Will be more optimistic about the future.

NURSING CARE OF A DEPRESSED PATIENT (EXAMPLE)

07.30 hours	Prompt her to dress and prepare for breakfast. Remind her to monitor her mood throughout the day.
08.00	Ask her to take 'orders' for breakfast from her table, to help her to engage in simple conversation with other patients.
08.45	Ask her to help dry and stack dishes from the kitchen.
09.00	Spend 10 minutes discussing her 'plan' for the rest of the day. Invite her to pick one new target from a list of two or more 'possibles'. Review her problem-solving approach; discussing how she should break each task into small steps, talking herself through the action and praising herself at the end for completing it.
10.00	Remind her to record her anxiety level before and after the exercise session with the other patients.
10.45	Prompt her to serve coffee to the other patients, using this activity as a cue for conversation.
11.15	Encourage her to join in a reminiscing session with a small group of other patients.
12.00	Prompt her, as necessary, to 'chat' to the other patients at her table over lunch.
12.45	Discuss briefly how she is progressing with her diary record and pleasure and achievement ratings for the day.
13.00	Supervise her 'concentration' assignment; she reads aloud a short passage as a test of her concentration. Ask her how she feels about her performance; encourage her to evaluate it realistically.
13.15	She takes a walk with another patient in the grounds.
13.45	Ask her if she would like to help another patient paste family portraits in an album. Prompt her at intervals to disclose information about her own family.

14.30	Supervise a repetition of the concentration assignment; add about ten more lines of text. Discuss her performance briefly, asking her to give herself appropriate encouragement.
14.45	Invite her to *make* tea and serve this to a small group of more dependent patients.
15.15	Assist her in writing a letter to her son. Discuss briefly possible content, leaving her to begin writing. Return at intervals to give encouragement.
16.00	Relaxation session in armchair. Coach her in tension and relaxation of major muscle groups. Ask her to record anxiety level before and after session.
17.15	Tea, followed by helping another patient to set her hair.
19.00	Discuss briefly her 'social assignment' for the evenings: talking to three other patients about the 'Stars of the Music Hall'. Prompt her as necessary in self-instruction and anxiety control. Ask her for her comments on completion, encourage realistic evaluation.
19.45	Prompt her to prepare her 'activity schedule' for the following day.
20.15	Encourage her to watch television with other patients. Encourage her to 'ask' if she might watch a specific programme. Discuss her feelings about this afterwards. Encourage realistic evaluation.
22.30	Following her retiral routine, assist her to relax, prompting her only if necessary.
23.00	She retires to bed.
24.00–07.00	Observe her each hour, recording whether she is asleep, awake, or restless. If she complains of difficulty in getting to sleep, prompt her to rise and *repeat* her retiral routine, then return to bed. If she remains awake after 30 minutes prompt her to rise and sit and read for ten minutes in the dayroom before returning to bed. If she still remains awake, provide relaxation coaching *in bed* in a soft voice, with bedside light off.

ASSESSMENT OF AFFECT

As noted already, nurses need to be aware of the key signs of a lowering or flattening of affect.

Changes in mood.   The patient may report feeling sad or apathetic. In some cases the patient may say he feels fine but may look sad or distressed at times.

Negative self-concept.   The patient may reproach himself constantly for things which he has, or has not, done. Often there may be little evidence that he has anything to blame himself for.

Avoidance. The patient shys away from social contacts; spends a lot of time on his own. In particular he may avoid situations which once were highly pleasurable to him.

Physiological changes. The patient may complain of disruption to his sleep pattern: finding it difficult to fall asleep; sleeping fitfully; and especially wakening early in the morning. He may also complain of tiredness and loss of energy; loss of appetite and sexual desire; and may also find it difficult to remember things or concentrate upon what he is doing.

Activity level. In general, the patient's activity level becomes greatly reduced. He spends much of his time sitting inactive, or 'resting'. In some cases the patient may complain of *agitation* rather than lethargy.

Suicidal thoughts. In very severe cases the patient may talk a great deal about death or his desire for an 'early release'. In some cases the patient will actually express a willingness to end his own life.

It should be clear from these points above that depression is an 'umbrella concept'. It covers a variety of changes in the patient's functioning. Some of these involve changes in the patient's behaviour, his biochemistry or the way he perceives his life, his future and himself. Although it is often argued that depression, in general, is a psychological problem which *arises* from some biochemical imbalance, recent evidence suggests that psychological factors may be highly important in causing the person's flattening of mood. The nurse's assessment should attempt to give equal coverage to both the patient's physical and his psychological presentation. In addition to routine observation you may also need to assess the patient in finer detail; for example, by helping him to complete a depression inventory (Beck *et al.* 1979). This measures a core of symptoms which are associated with depressed mood, and which are relevant to most cultures throughout the world. Completion of such scales may be tiring for the patient, or tax his powers of concentration. Consequently, you should try to space out such assessments, thereby reducing the stress on the patient.

When interviewing the patient, be wary of accepting everthing the patient says as 'fact'. Many elderly people tend to be rather conservative and may give the kind of answers which they think the nurse wants to hear, for fear of upsetting anyone. Your line of questioning is also important. You should always try to use 'open-ended' questions, which cannot be answered by 'yes' or 'no' or even single words; for instance, 'How are you feeling this morning?', is preferable to, 'Are you still feeling a bit down today?' If the patient is very withdrawn, such questions may be inappropriate. Instead, you must try to gauge how he feels, from his appearance, asking him to confirm or discount your impressions. You might say, 'You took a long time getting up this morning, were you a bit apprehensive about going out today?' By following a line of 'hunches' it may be possible to establish, for example, that the patient is feeling a bit defeated as a result of his loss of motor skills, or due to difficulty in speaking. An effort should also be made to frame questions clearly and concisely. Avoid long rambling statements which contain questions within them. Remember that the patient may have difficulty in concentrating or in remembering facts.

In addition to completing a standardized depression inventory, or interviewing the patient, other simple means can be employed to build up a picture of the patient's mood state. His activity level can be 'sampled' by the nurse simply noting what he is doing at intervals throughout the day. This record might also include whether or not he engages in 'planned activities' which used to be enjoyable to him. These 'behavioural' notes, supplemented by a record of eating and sleeping patterns, will provide a fairly comprehensive picture when combined with the more subjective information on mood which is obtained through the interview or rating scale.

SUMMARY

The concept of depression in the elderly poses a dilemma for nurses and doctors alike. The problem does not merely involve unhappiness, but is a complex of difficulties which often may be confused with dementia or other aspects of the ageing process. Although treatment of depression is most often represented by antidepressant and electroconvulsive therapy (ECT) where the patient's problems appear to stem from psychosocial factors, a psychological approach may be more appropriate. This is relevant to the class of depressive disorder which may afflict elderly people, as a result of hospitalization; a state which may not be diagnosed specifically as depression.

The nurse's role in helping a patient overcome depressed affect involves helping to identify the patient's problems of living in specific detail. She then encourages him to use simple, practical procedures, for trying to overcome or come to terms with difficulties. You act as a guide, providing *occasional* support and encouragement. You provide feedback as a way of reflecting the patient's performance, so that he may evaluate it more realistically. The ultimate goal is to encourage the patient to change the beliefs he holds about himself, his life and the future. This can best be achieved by helping him to challenge his negative evaluations by progressing through a series of practical 'experiments'; these will test out his beliefs that he 'can't cope', or 'is a burden to everyone'.

Depressed people often hope that care staff will make them feel better. Staff often respond to such expectations by offering high levels of support and encouragement. Ultimately, this may maintain rather than lessen the depression. This chapter has suggested that you can best help the patient by helping him to learn to cope with his own depression. The patient gains an opportunity to learn how to deal with his own difficulties within an atmosphere of general support and encouragement.

REFERENCES

Beck A.T., Rush A.J., Shaw B.F. & Emery G. (1979) *Cognitive Therapy of Depression*. Guildford Press, New York.

Dimond M. (1981) Bereavement in the elderly: a critical review with implications for nursing practice and research. *Journal of Advanced Nursing* **6**, 461–76.

Eisdorfer C. & Stotsky B.A. (1977) Intervention, treatment and rehabilitation of psychiatric disorders. In Birren J.E. & Schaie K.W. (eds) *Handbook of the Psychology of Ageing*. Van Nostrand Reinhold, New York.

Post F. (1981) Affective illness. In Arie T. (ed.) *Health Care of the Elderly*. Croom Helm, London.

Seligman M.E.P. (1975) *Helplessness*. W.H. Freeman, San Francisco.

Steuer J.L. & Hammen C.L. (1983) Cognitive–behavioural therapy for the depressed elderly: issues and adaptions. *Cognitive Therapy and Research* **7** (4), 285–96.

Chapter 14
Anxiety

Anxiety, an experience with which we are all familiar, causes us to anticipate that harmful things are about to happen to us. Anxiety may be fixed and relate to a specific experience such as receiving injections, it may also be free floating in that it is not related to any specific experience.

Although anxiety is a primary symptom of some illnesses such as the neurotic disorders, it is sufficiently common as a component of all illness experiences for it to be included in this text. As with other concepts, anxiety is on a continuum which may range from a mild feeling of unease prior to admission to hospital, to a feeling of acute terror and panic which is experienced by a phobic person when confronted with the object of his phobia. The psychological symptoms include a general sense of anticipation of danger with or without a specific cause. The physiological symptoms are generally related to the autonomic nervous system and include tachycardia, muscle tension, increased sweating and a dry mouth. Other symptoms include a general restlessness, frequency of micturition, pacing and loose stools.

When people are anxious it is generally apparent from their behaviour that this is so. Additionally, in most instances, on being asked, 'How are you?', patients will reply with phrases such as, 'I'm very worried', 'I'm churning inside', 'I just can't stop thinking about the operation', and, 'Are you sure they won't make any mistakes?'

Because of their reduced ability to adapt quickly to change, the elderly are particularly susceptible to experiencing anxiety. Because they are less resilient and adaptable than younger persons, they often have considerable concerns about submitting to care of any kind, and to intimate forms of their particular. Although many are reluctant to admit to feeling anxious, which are invariably evident in their behaviour. The forms of behaviour excessive may prompt include hostility, distrust, disorientation, elderly person and a morbid fear of dying. Additionally, the anxious instructions ces difficulty in eating, communicating, remembering context of the ation, and in generally cooperating within the stem.

FACTORS RELATING TO ANXIETY

Personality Type

All of us are more or less anxious, dependent on our personality type. We have all met individuals who are relatively carefree and able to cope with even the most demanding situation. Conversely we meet individuals who are constantly 'on edge', fearful of change and having to adapt to new circumstances, and generally regarded as being 'anxious people'. This continuum ranges from the strong and stable personality on the one hand, to the neurotic type personality on the other.

Information. Involvement in Decision Making

It is generally accepted that the more information a person has about his future and circumstances, the less anxious he will be about them. Although it is accepted that, on occasions, the amount of information which may be available to a patient will be limited for a number of reasons, it is best to make available as much information as possible. Similarly, it is essential that patients generally, and anxious patients in particular, be fully involved in all decisions which affect them. Where informed consent is a necessary part of the delivery of health care we must make absolutely certain that our anxious patients are really fully *informed* of what they are consenting to, and of its consequences. Remember that people who are anxious have considerable difficulty in assimilating and remembering information which is given to them.

Demands Made by the Environment and People in it

Because of the energy that the anxious person must expend just to keep going, any additional demands which are made on him by the environment or people in it will seriously increase his anxiety level. For this reason our patients may become excessively dependent on us during the initial phases of their nursing care. By doing so they opt out of having to make decisions and dealing with demands on them which they see as being excessive. In the short term, at, least, it is probably as well to allow this excessive dependence with a view to decreasing it in the medium to longer term.

Stability of Environment and the People in it

The extent to which the evironment is unstable, ever changing and lacking in any predictable routine will increase levels of anxiety. Much movement, coming and going, stimulation and change of staff will do little to alleviate anxiety. This is particularly true in the elderly population who, by and large, are more at ease with a stable and *relatively* unchanging environment. This applies particularly to the need for stability in the staff group who are caring for the elderly person.

Availability of Support Systems

Anxious people tend to need the constant presence of support systems which may be used or may be of value simply because they are there. These support systems take the form of health care staff, other personnel and relatives who are willing to lend a sympathetic ear. The support is not so much in terms of what is actually said by the sympathetic listener, rather, it takes the form of the warmth and support which the anxious person identifies as being in, and coming from, a sympathetic listener.

Since we have all experienced anxiety in its many forms, and those things that reduce it, we are in a good position to *empathize* (experience *with* our patients) their anxiety. Similarly, from an experiential viewpoint, we are all aware of the general strategies which can be employed in reducing anxiety. The author is not suggesting that these strategies are the same for all patients, they will clearly have to be individualized to suit each patient's needs.

PRINCIPLES OF CARE

When caring for the patient who is anxious, it is essential to realize that much of what we can do to reduce anxiety takes place during our normal day-to-day contact with him. Additionally, we must appreciate that much of what we as individuals do, or do not do, can increase or decrease our patient's anxiety level. In general we are better able to reduce anxiety if we, ourselves, are confident, knowledgeable in our area of expertise, relatively non-anxious, and are generally seen to be in control of the situation in which we work. It has often been said that anxiety is contagious, meaning that if we are anxious this will cause our patients to feel likewise.

Recognition of Anxiety

Determining the presence or absence of unduly high levels of anxiety forms a central part of any meaningful nursing assessment framework. This continuous assessment process causes us to look for specific indicators of anxiety such as pacing, sweating, dry mouth, frequency of micturition and statement such as, 'Nurse, I'm very worried.' Once the general recognition of anxiety takes place, and has been recorded, more specific details such as the nature of the anxiety in terms of it being free floating or fixed must be sought.

On occasions you may be inclined to instruct anxious patients to, 'Pull your socks up!', or, 'Pull yourself together! it will be O.K.', or, 'I can't see what you are worried about, you will only be in hospital for five days.' This approach inevitably increases the problem and results in a feeling of guilt because the patient is being expected to control something which, in reality, is outwith his immediate control. It is, therefore necessary to recognize that anxiety is a real, serious and important problem to the patient, and one which you can do much to reduce.

Nurse – Patient Relationship

By using a supportive one-to-one relationship with the patient, it is usually possible to encourage him to talk about the anxiety and identify those experiences which make it better or worse. In the short term at least it is necessary to encourage him to talk about the anxiety as often and as freely as possible. Bear in mind that many older patients will feel reluctant to expose themselves in this kind of way, often feeling that they should keep their worries and concerns to themselves. This reticence to talk about their emotions means that you have to work very hard at encouraging older people to discuss what they feel to be their private affairs.

Sharing your perception of the patient's anxiety level with him will encourage him to verbalize more and will make him feel more inclined to share the experience with others. By making comments such as, 'You seem very worried today', or, 'I notice you've been very restless this morning', or, 'I see you haven't eaten your breakfast this morning', you will give the patient the opportunity to admit to feeling anxious.

Formalized One-to-One Therapy

In instances where the anxiety is of a prolonged and relatively serious nature, it could be necessary to organize a formal one-to-one psychotherapeutic process in which the patient meets with a nurse therapist on a regular and continuing basis (see Chapter 9 for a discussion of this type of intervention). Alternatively, a fairly informally structured one-to-one form of support may be necessary. Finally, the general availability of staff to the patient is beneficial providing that the patient *knows* that staff are available to him whenever he needs them.

Non-threatening Environment

An environment which is non-threatening in terms of being non-competitive, generally quiet, having low levels of activity and having staff who are experienced in and sympathetic to the care of the elderly will do much to reduce anxiety levels. Overcrowded, noisy and busy wards do little to relieve anxiety.

Specific activities such as walking, listening to favourite music, indulging in social chitchat, watching television or reading newspapers can help anxious patients to relax more.

Information

Because of the general hustle and bustle prevalent in hospitals, or because we sometimes feel that our elderly patients are not capable of handling it, there are occasions when we 'forget' to give our patients the information which they require to enable them to understand their care and treatment. Patients who are fully and appropriately informed of events and plans relating to them are much less likely to feel anxious. Whenever possible, patients should be included in all decision-making processes relating to them and, when they are unable to participate in this decision-making process, they should be fully *informed* of decisions which have been made on their behalf. This must be done bearing in mind that as levels of anxiety increase, the ability to understand and assimilate information decreases. We must, therefore, take additional time when giving information to the elderly anxious person.

Minor Tranquillizers

Although not specifically a nursing strategy, the use of minor tranquillizers is often initiated by nursing staff who report on the patient's anxiety to the medical staff. In recent years the unnecessary overuse of minor tranquillizers as a means of reducing anxiety in the elderly has come under close scrutiny. It is now generally felt that, in the past, we have not tried hard enough to use strategies which are alternative to the use of drug therapy in the form of minor tranquillizers. The lesson that we have learned is that, for the most part, these tranquillizers should only be requested when *absolutely necessary* and only after we have explored reasonable alternative means of reducing anxiety.

You should remember that anxiety is a problem commonly experienced by the elderly and is one which can be dramatically reduced by appropriate and sensitive nursing care. In terms of influencing anxiety on a day-to-day basis, nurses, and others who work under their general guidance, are ideally suited to minimizing this very serious problem.

PATIENT PROFILE

Mr Farington is a 72-year-old widower who was hospitalized three weeks ago following a mild myocardial infarction. His physical status is now described as stable, with the medical staff indicating that he is in no imminent danger from a further infarction. His prognosis is described as being good, with minimal permanent damage resulting from the infarction. On admission he was 8 kg overweight and smoked 10 cigarettes per day.

Prior to admission this man had no significant anxiety problem, being described by his nephew (his only close relative who lives locally) as being, 'a stable person with a strong and resilient personality'. Mr Farington describes himself as being, prior to admission, a fairly carefree person who was optimistic about the future. Since admission to the hospital Mr Farington has become increasingly concerned and introspective about his health, despite the fact that all the indicators are that his prognosis for a full recovery is a good one. During a recent conversation with the staff nurse he said, 'I'm finished. My health is in ruins', and, 'I'm so jumpy and nervous; I've never been like this before', and, 'I suppose you tell *all* "heart patients" that they will recover fully', and, 'The way I'm feeling now, I'll never get better'. He complained to the staff nurse about being 'kept in the dark' and not getting enough information about his medical condition.

Since his admission Mr Farington's daily cigarette consumption has gone up from 10 to 30 cigarettes per day and his weight has increased by a further 2 kg (he is now 10 kg overweight for his age, build and height). He complains of having to urinate frequently and says he uses the toilet about every half hour.

Mr Farington is described by nursing staff as 'fidgety', 'hyperactive', 'restless' and 'on edge'. His nephew reports that he often complains of a dry mouth and resultant difficulty in swallowing.

ORGANIZATION OF NURSING CARE

Subjective Evidence (What the Patient Says)

- 'I'm finished. My health is in ruins.'
- 'I'm so jumpy and nervous; I've never been like this before.'
- 'I suppose you tell *all* "heart patients" that they will recover fully.'
- 'The way I'm feeling now, I'll never get better.'

Objective Evidence (What the Nurse and Others Observe)

- Cigarette smoking has increased from 10 to 30 cigarettes per day.
- Urinates approximately every half hour during the daytime.

- Is unable to sit down for more than 5 minutes; paces the ward floor for the remainder of the time.
- Has difficulty in swallowing because of dry mouth.

Assessment (Nursing Diagnosis)

- Anxiety relating to current health status.

Plan of Nursing Care

- Give full and detailed information relating to all aspects of health status and treatment.
- Ensure that Mr Farington knows that staff are continuously available and will be willing to discuss his fears with him at any reasonable time.
- Encourage to discuss and verbalize his anxieties generally and those relating to his health status in particular.
- Engage in non-competitive activities, walking for example, which will allow him to engage in conversation which is not related to his health status concerns.
- Introduce him to a patient with a similar health background who is coping well and who is optimistic about his future health prospects.

Expected Outcome

- Will make more optimistic statements about his future health status, e.g. 'I'm looking forward to getting well and out of here'.
- Is less pessimistic and introspective about the future generally.
- Frequency of micturition decreases to hourly (in the first instance) during the daytime.
- Level of cigarette smoking decreases to (or becomes less than) the level at admission of 10 cigarettes per day.
- Frequency of pacing decreases and is able to remain seated for periods exceeding 5 minutes.

NURSING CARE OF PATIENT WITH AN ANXIETY PROBLEM (EXAMPLE)

07.00 hours Waken patient, if not already awake, and convey a general feeling of optimism, confidence and positiveness about the present health status. Convey to him that he is relatively well and is expected to function fairly independently.

07.30 Before breakfast spend a few minutes with him and talk about the general activities which will be undertaken during that particular day. Allow ample opportunity for questions and/or comments about health care generally.

07.45   During breakfast ensure that Mr Farington is able to proceed with minimal fuss or complication. The general hustle and bustle which invariably accompanies mealtimes in a hospital ward will undoubtedly cause his anxiety level to increase. In this patient's case the anxiety causes him to overeat, the resulting weight gain has done little to improve his future health prospects. This aspect of his anxiety problem has, of course, been previously discussed with him.

08.30   Allow and encourage him to help around the ward, ensuring that the tasks given to him are easily accomplished and present no particular challenge or difficulty. This approach will help channel his hyperactivity into a meaningful and productive outcome. Additionally, it will go some way towards keeping his mind off his health.

09.30   Prepare Mr Farington for the medical round which starts at 10.00, an event which causes him particular anxiety and which he has difficulty in coping with. Explain who will be on the medical round and what is likely to be discussed. If possible, ensure that the nurse who will be accompanying the medical staff is known to him and has had the opportunity to discuss his condition with him prior to the round. During the medical round ensure that his anxiety is made known to and discussed with the medical staff. Additionally, arrange that a special effort be made to reduce Mr Farington's inevitable anxiety at this time.

10.15   Allow him to help with the distribution of coffee and tea to other patients.

10.30   Spend some time with him on a one-to-one basis discussing his health status and introducing him to the health education literature which is available for patients recovering from a myocardial infarction. Remember, this is the first occasion on which this patient has experienced this particular problem and that his information about it will be rather limited. It is very likely that with suitable information about the effects and after-effects of myocardial infarction this person's anxiety level will decrease and, hopefully, return to its pre-admission level

11.00–12.30 This period is generally regarded as free time. Mr Farington should be made aware that if he requires the time and attention of staff, they will be happy to give this to him. It is not being suggested that he should be encouraged to become unduly dependent on the presence of nursing staff. Rather, it is being suggested that the knowledge that nursing staff are freely available to him will decrease the dependence which he has on them.

12.30   Encourage him to help with the distribution of meals and (as for breakfast) pay particular attention to calorie intake.

13.30   Mr Farington will be walking in hospital grounds with three other patients. The importance of exercise as a means of reducing weight, relieving tension and reducing the likelihood of a further myocardial infarction will have been part of the health education process in which he has been involved.

14.30   Free time.

15.30   Mr Farington's nephew visits, and, by prior arrangement with the nursing staff, encourages him to think positively and optimistically about the future. Following the visit the nephew is seen by nursing staff in the presence of his uncle and general progress discussed.

16.30   The next hour is spent in the hospital library where Mr Farington finds some respite from the general hustle and bustle of the ward environment. His need to 'get away from it all' is recognized by the staff who try, as far as is possible, to reduce the sensory input which results from general ward activity.

17.30   Teatime. He eats with two other patients who are also re-covering from myocardial infarction and who are relatively positive and optimistic about their future health status.

18.30   An individual nurse, with whom Mr Farington finds it easy to talk, meets with him and discusses his general progress. In particular they discuss his anxiety and the successes that he has had in controlling and reducing it. They also discuss the general nursing strategies which are being used to reduce his anxiety level and make him feel more comfortable and positive about the future. Part of this discussion relates to the agree-ment that he has reached with medical and nursing staff that the minor tranquillizers, which have been prescribed on an 'emergency only' basis, be given to him only if absolutely necessary. Since minor tranquillizers were prescribed one week ago he has taken them on two occasions only. Mr Farington is aware of the limited value of minor tranquillizers in his particular case and is very pleased with his ability to cope (with the help of nursing staff) without them.

19.00 Listens to his favourite classical music on a personalized tape recorder/radio with the use of earphones. This interest of Mr Farington's is important to him and serves a useful purpose in helping him to relax

20.00 Mr Farington is allowed to help generally around the ward with tasks such as cleaning locker tops and collecting used glasses and cups. He also reads the daily newspapers to a blind patient with whom he has formed a close relationship

21.00 He is allowed to help with the distribution of evening drinks

22.00 He prepares for bed and finds a hot bath an excellent way of relaxing prior to settling down for the night

23.00 Mr Farington tries to sleep without night sedation which was prescribed two weeks ago. He knows that he will receive his night sedation any time up until 01.00 if he has difficulty in sleeping. Additionally, he knows that the night nursing staff will be available throughout the night and be more than willing to talk with him if necessary.

ASSESSMENT OF ANXIETY

Activity

- Pacing, restless.
- Exhibits hand-ringing.

Features

- Looks anxious.
- Has furrowed brow, sweating palms.

Gastrointestinal

- Hyperacidity, anorexia, diarrhoea, dry mouth.

Urinary tract

- Frequency of micturition.

Communication

- Concentration poor, repeatedly seeks information.
- Dependent, poor short-term memory, difficulty in making decisions and in sustaining meaningful interaction with others.
- Disorientation.

Fearfulness

- Fear of specific or non-specific situations.
- Avoids potentially stressful circumstances.

Chemical Dependence

- Excessive or increased use of alcohol, tranquillizers or cigarettes.

Response to Others

- Irritable, on edge, tense, hostile.

Cardiovascular System

- Hypertension, tachycardia.

Complaints

Feeling anxious, tense, unhappy, nervous or churning inside.

FURTHER READING

DeYoung M. (1982) Planning for discharge. *Geriatric Nursing* **3**, 396–9.

Dickel H.A., Dixon H.H. & Shanklin J. G. (1955) Observations on the anxiety tension syndrome. *The Canadian Medical Association Journal* **72**, 1–6.

Hamner M.L. (1984) Insight, reminiscence, denial, projection: Coping mechanisms of the aged. *Journal of gerontological Nursing* **10**, 66–8, 81.

Hernan J.A. (1984) Exploding retirement myths through retirement counselling. *Journal of gerontological Nursing* **10**, 4, 31–3.

Lancaster J. (1981) Maximising psychological adaptation in an aging population. *Topics in clinical Nursing* **3**, 37.

Polletti R. (1984) Helping people to cope with stress. *Nursing Times* **80**, 47–9.

Pritchard P. (1981) Stress and anxiety in physical illness—the role of the general nurse. *Nursing Times* **77**, 162–4.

Rosswurm M.A. (1983) Relocation and the elderly. *Journal of gerontological Nursing* **9**, 632–7.

Thomas V.T. (1983) Hospice Nursing—Reaping the rewards, dealing with stress. *Geriatric Nursing* **4**, 22–7.

Vogel C.H. (1982) Anxiety and depression amomg the elderly. *Journal of gerontological Nursing* **8**, 213–16.

Wallace J. (1978) Living with stress. *Nursing Times* **74**, 457–8.

Watcher-Shikora N. & Perez S. (1982) Unmasking pain. *Geriatric Nursing* **3**, 392–3.

White P.H. (1983) Supportive Counseling in action. *Geriatric Nursing* **4**, 176–6a.

Chapter 15
Communication

Communication* is the process by which we transmit information to, and receive information from, other individuals or groups. The nature of the information is varied and may include facts, emotions, questions, requests or answers. Successful communication in dependent on successful sending of the message, and successful receipt of it. Invariably, the initiator of the communication is given some feedback from the recipient of it.

Communication, a dynamic social process, which involves an exchange of information between two or more people, is a highly complex concept. The means by which this information passes between individuals are many but include *overt* and *convert* forms. The overt form of communication is clear and easily understood by both parties, an example is when a teacher informs a group of students that a class has ended. Covert communication is less easily understood and often includes a hidden message or a hidden agenda. An example of covert communication is when you are asked by another partygoer, who is unknown to you, if you are enjoying the party. The overt component of this communication may be a genuine desire to know how you are enjoying the party. However, the covert component of that communication may relate to a desire on the part of the person asking the question to form some kind of relationship with you.

An important form of communication, particularly between nurses and patients, is the fairly direct type in which you physically present yourself to a patient and use words as a means of communication. This type of communication has two major components, the *verbal* and *non-verbal*. The verbal form of communication is expressed in words, such as, 'Good morning Mr Jones, how are you today?' The non-verbal part of this communication will relate to the way in which you, the nurse, say these words and the manner in which you physically present yourself during that communication; for example, if you rush past a patient's bed and direct that question to him without waiting for an answer, that type of communication is really a very different one from one in which you pull up a chair to the

*This chapter should be read and used in combination with Chapter 27 which contains a considerable amount of material relating to Communication.

patient's bedside, draw the screen for some privacy and ask the same question.

All our senses are used in our communication with others: we can communicate through touch, seeing, hearing, smelling and tasting. Although taste and smell are not often associated with interpersonal communication, it is important to remember that body odour can be a serious deterrent to meaningful communication, and that the use of food as a means of communicating with others is well recognized.

FACTORS RELATING TO COMMUNICATION

Personal Sensory Skill

Although communication is not entirely dependent on ones ability to speak and hear, the use of sign language being an obvious exception, these skills are of considerable importance in relation to the majority of old people. The changes which are associated with the ageing process (see Chapter 7) clearly demonstrate that the sensory abilities of the older person are significantly diminished. These deficits are demonstrated in circumstances where you have a small group of hard of hearing elderly people trying to communicate with each other. Invariably, they give up after a fairly short time because of the excess energy which is required to sustain such a communication.

Practice/Opportunities

As with all other skills, our ability to communicate with each other is dependent on practice and opportunity. Unless the elderly person is given ample opportunity to practice the communication skill which they possess, the ability to do so will decrease over time. Similarly, unless there is ample opportunity to practice these skills, the older person will not be able to perform well on the few occasions when the opportunity does arise.

Interpersonal Stimulation

The environment in which the older person lives must contain sufficient stimulation and experiences which can be the basis for interpersonal communication. If the environment is dull, routine, barren and lacking in experiences which will form the subject of the communication, it is unlikely to occur. Similarly, others in the environment have a responsibility to offer the older person every opportunity to communicate with staff, other patients and casual visitors to the ward.

Environmental Structure

The structure of the environment can do much to either increase or decrease patients' communication skills. The classic example of this is the seating arrangement in which we place many of our patients in day rooms and other places. If the seating arrangement is such that patients can sit in a circle or semi-circle and achieve some form of eye contact, see the lips of other people and are within reasonable distance of each other, then communication will be facilitated. Alternatively, if elderly people are sitting in a row with their backs to the wall they will find it exceedingly difficult to communicate with others, including the person who is sitting next to them.

Under most circumstances we communicate with other persons from a physical position which is similar to theirs, for example we might both be standing or both be sitting. Since many of our patients are either chairbound or, on occasions, bedridden we must be careful to place ourselves in a physical relationship to them that facilitates communication. This might be achieved by sitting or squatting near the patient who is seated or in bed. In either event we must make reasonably sure that we are within earshot of our patients and that they have a clear view of our faces generally and lips in particular.

Confidence and Self-esteem

Because communication is a two-way process, it is dependent on both parties having the ability and confidence to send *and* receive messages. Individuals who have a low level of self-esteem and confidence, whilst able to receive messages well, are seriously restricted in their ability to return the communication. How often have we heard an older person say, 'I wanted to ask him for an explanation, but I just didn't like to do it, or 'I didn't ask him to explain in case he thought I was being silly'. A special part of our, the nurses', role is to give our patients the confidence with which to ask questions, challenge the decisions made by ourselves and others, and seek clarification about decisions regarding them.

Anxiety

Anxiety is a serious barrier to communication both in terms of sending and receiving. Although it is widely recognized that a small increase in our level of anxiety will improve our ability to send and receive messages, any further increase in our anxiety level will seriously interfere with both these aspects of communication. Of all patient groups the elderly are particularly susceptible to the development of anxiety, and the subsequent interference with their ability to communicate.

Health Status

The general and specific health status of the elderly person will influence the extent to which he is able to communicate. If the older person is feeling weak, thirsty or hungry, if he worries about the future, is dizzy, in pain or unable to talk then his communmication ability in relation to subjects other than those problems will be seriously impaired.

A number of disease processes, such as cerebrovascular accidents (CVA), can seriously impair the ability to communicate. The three major types of communication problems experienced by the elderly as a result of disease processes are: dysphasia, dysarthria and dyspraxia.

Dysphasia refers to all areas of language use including understanding of the spoken word, speaking, writing, reading and possibly the use of non-verbal language such as the use of gestures. Dysphasia divides into two broad types which may or may not occur in isolation from each other: *expressive dysphasia* and *receptive dysphasia*. Expressive dysphasia causes the person to have difficulty in finding the 'right word', with expression being considerably reduced. The ability of the person to understand the 'messages' which he receives may be relatively unimpaired, his difficulty lies in expressing himself. Receptive dysphasia causes the person to have a poor understanding of communication input.

Dysarthria is a neuromuscular impairment of the organs (tongue and lips) which enable us to speak. The person is perfectly able to receive communication input, identify and prepare his reply, but has difficulty in making the sounds and saying the words.

Dyspraxia is a disorder of articulation in which the ability to make voluntary movements of tongue and lips is affected.

PRINCIPLES OF CARE

It should be clearly recognized that the elderly person may experience one or more communication impediments. A person's ability to communicate should be assessed during the admission process and be regarded as a crucial component of the overall delivery of health care. Any specific impediment to successful communication must be identified early and treated, where possible, by nursing and/or other means. Such impediments may include correctable hearing and visual deficits. Additionally, such things as ill-fitting dentures are a serious handicap to the ability of the older person to express himself verbally. During conversation you should stand where the old person can hear and see you, only give as much information at a time as can be assimilated, speak slowly and clearly, and allow time for your transmitted message to be assimilated by him.

All members of the health care team, including casual visitors to the ward, should be alerted to any known communication problem. Additionally, strategies which have been found useful in minimizing the problems as far as this particular patient is concerned should be made known to all who are involved with him. Thus, each individual will pay special attention to making their communication as clear and meaningful as possible.

The possibility of covert and/or non-verbal communication being misunderstood by an individual with a communication problem is very great. For this reason it may be necessary to make overt the covert, and pay particular attention to your non-verbal forms of communication. You need to constantly ask yourself, 'Is repetition and/or clarification of that last point necessary?'

In discussing this particular problem with the elderly person, it is essential that he be given the opportunity to identify strategies that he would like you to use and which minimize his difficulty in receiving information. Similarly, you should feel free to inform the patient of things which he/she does which enable you to understand him better.

The effects of touch as part of the communication process are not to be underestimated. A discussion of the effects of touch on communication with elderly confused patients can be found in a paper by Langland and Panicucci (1982). They concluded that: 'With an awareness and understanding of self in the relationship, the nurse can begin to consciously incorporate touch in developing the most effective means of communication with individual clients who may be confused and/or elderly.'

Our success in communicating with our patients is of fundamental importance if we are to optimize the quality of their health care. The importance of forming a close one-to-one interpersonal relationship with the person who has a communication problem is considerable. The range of communication problems which our elderly patients have includes the mild embarrassment which may be experienced by an elderly patient when asked if their bowels have moved recently, the person who has loose dentures and is also hard of hearing, and the profoundly demented patient who has an extremely limited quantity and quality of communication skill.

PATIENT PROFILE

Mrs Jenkins is a 72-year-old married lady who was recently admitted to the local general hospital (medical ward) for stabilization of her diabetes mellitus. Although otherwise physically and mentally well, Mrs Jenkins is hard of hearing and experiences considerable problems with her loose fitting dentures which she has had for the past 35 years. Her hearing problem is irreversible and progressive. This lady lives in town with her husband and twin sister, neither of whom work. Her sister and husband both lead a fairly active social life but Mrs Jenkins rarely leaves the house for any social purpose. In the four-week period prior to admission she had only been out of the house on one occasion, a visit to her general practitioner.

Since admission she has been rather solitary and has rarely left her single room unless it was unavoidable, for meals and to use the bathroom for example. If a nurse or other patient enters her room and tries to initiate conversation, Mrs Jenkins becomes rather anxious and embarrassed and makes clear attempts to terminate the conversation as quickly as possible by saying things such as, 'I'm deaf; I can't talk to you', and, 'Tell my husband what you want me to do; he'll let me know', and, 'I never wear the hearing aid; it makes funny noises'.

Although able to communicate verbally with her husband and twin sister, Mrs Jenkins is, apparently, unable and/or unwilling to communicate with other people.

ORGANIZATION OF NURSING CARE

Subjective Evidence (What the Patient Says)

- 'I'm deaf; I can't talk to you.'
- 'Tell my husband what you want me to do; he'll let me know.'
- 'I never wear the hearing aid; it makes funny noises.'

Objective Evidence (What the Nurse and Others Observe)

- Never wears her hearing aid.
- Never initiates conversation.
- Terminates conversations as quickly as possible.
- Only leaves her single room when it is absolutely necessary.
- Makes considerable use of written communications when interacting with nursing staff.

Assessment (Nursing Diagnosis)

- Communications problem (hearing deficit and ill-fitting dentures).

Plan of Nursing Care

- Refer to dentist.
- Refer for hearing tests and, if necessary, new or adjusted hearing aid.

- Refer to speech therapist for communication (speaking and hearing) exercises.
- Encourage to wear hearing aid.
- Plan specific conversation practice with nursing staff.

Expected Outcome

- Will wear hearing aid at least one hour a day.
- Will initiate one or more conversations daily.
- Will leave room on one or more occasions each day for purposes other than those which are absolutely necessary.
- A reduction in the written communications to nursing staff.
- Will spend at least half an hour each day in communications practice with nursing staff.

NURSING CARE OF PATIENT WITH COMMUNICATION PROBLEM (EXAMPLE)

07.30 hours   Waken and engage in short conversation such as, 'Good morning', or, 'It's time to get up', or, 'How are you today', or, 'Breakfast will be ready in half an hour'.

08.00   Encourage Mrs Jenkins to eat breakfast with other patients in the dining room and sit her near to the patient with whom she is most able to communicate. This arrangement has been made with the permission of Mrs Jenkins and the patient concerned.

09.00   Conversation practice with a member of the nursing staff.

09.30   Visit to speech therapy department.

10.15   Coffee time and further interaction is encouraged with other patients.

11.00   Hearing aid practice. Mrs Jenkins has agreed to work hard at wearing her hearing aid constantly between 11.00 and 12.00. She makes notes of any problems associated with this and these are discussed with a member of nursing staff at a later stage.

12.00   Free time.

12.30   Lunch. During this time Mrs Jenkins is encouraged to eat with other patients in the ward dining area. As at breakfast time she sits near a patient with whom she can communicate fairly easily.

13.30   Visit by her husband who stays for most of the afternoon. Mr Jenkins is fully informed of, and involved in, the process which has been designed to minimize his wife's communication problem.

16.00	Mr and Mrs Jenkins meet with a member of staff and discuss her progress generally and her communication difficulty specifically.
16.15	Free time.
17.00	Evening meal. Arrangements and objectives as for breakfast and lunch.
18.00	Mrs Jenkins reads in her own room for part of the evening and watches the television with other patients for the remainder.
22.00	Before preparing for bed, Mrs Jenkins meets with the night nurse and reports on her progress for the day.
23.00	Bed time. No further specific intervention is necessary in relation to the communications problem during the night-time.

Deafness, which is a rather invisible disability, is a relatively common problem associated with the ageing process. The extent to which it interferes with communication is considerable and can, in many instances, be reduced considerably by the intervention of nursing and other staff. The social isolation which invariably results from deafness is both considerable and painful.

Communication difficulties, from whatever cause, are as important to us and our patients as all of the other problems associated with the concepts discussed in these chapters. *All* patients in *all* areas of health care are at risk in relation to this problem and the nurse must always have an open mind and be alert to the existence of communication problems in every patient with whom she comes into contact.

ASSESSMENT OF COMMUNICATION

Interpersonal Skills

(See assessment of interpersonal skills in Chapter 27.)

Vision

- Normal/abnormal visual ability.
  ? need to be seen by optician.
- Suitability of spectacles, willingness to wear them.

Hearing

- ? need for testing.
- Indicates difficulty in hearing.

- Use/suitability of hearing aid.
- Wax in ears.

Mouth Condition

- Mouth dry/dirty.
- Dentures fitting well/poorly.
- ? Difficulty in formulating words.

Voice

- Pitch, tone, clarity.

Comprehension

- Ability to understand communication input.
- Intellectual deficits.
- Anxiety level.
- Memory defects.

Pathology

- ? suffering from diseases which place him at high risk; for example, dementia, cerebrovascular accidents, respiratory infections and acute confusional states.
- Any experience of pain.

Drug Therapy

- ? being prescribed drugs which sedate or interfere with ability to communicate; for example, insulin, tranquillizers, analgesics.

Activity

- Able/unable to move freely among, and communicate with others. High risk if bedfast or chairfast.
- Movement of head, neck and shoulders will facilitate communication.
- Hyperactivity and agitation will reduce communication skill.
- Pacing, frequency of micturition.

Facial Appearance

- Tense, worried expression.
- Difficulty in smiling.

Expressions of Anxiety

● For example, 'I'm worried', 'I just can't stop thinking about it', 'I've got butterflies in my tummy,' and so on.

REFERENCE

Langland R. & Panicucci C. (1982) Effects of touch on communication with elderly confused patients. *Journal of gerontological Nursing* **8**, 152–5.

FURTHER READING

Blodi F.C. (1981) Eye problems of the elderly. *Ophthalmologica* **181**, 121–8.

Burton D. (1984) Social and communication needs of the deaf. *Midwife, Health Visitor and Community Nurse* **20**, 54–8.

Dreher B. (1981) Overcoming speech and language disorders. *Geriatric Nursing* **2**, 345–9.

Ernst P. & Shaw J. (1980) Touching is not taboo. *Geriatric Nursing* **1**, 193–5.

Frank S. (1984) The touch of Love. *Journal of gerontological Nursing* **10**, 28–35.

Gardiner P.A. (1979) Visual difficulty in old age. *British Medical Journal* **1**, (6156) 105–6.

Hanebuth L. (1981) The dying of the Light: Nursing strategies for the patient who is going blind. *Journal of practical Nursing* **31**, 25–8.

Hart G. (1983) Strokes causing left VS. right hemiplegia: Different effects and nursing implications. *Geriatric Nursing* **4**, 39–43.

Heron C. (1983) Communication problems. *Nursing Mirror* **157**, ix–xi.

Koch K.H. (1981) The deaf and hard of hearing. Some hints. *Nursing Times Supplement* (5th August, 1981).

Koshy K.T. (1983) The art of listening. *Nursing Times* **79**, 38.

Levene B. (1983) Hearing Loss — the invisible disability. *Nursing* **2**, 525–9.

Meikle M. (1981) Listen, I want to tell you something. *Nursing Times Supplement. Hidden Handicaps* 5th August 1981).

Miller M. & Dobson M. (1984) Stop, Look and Listen. *Nursing Mirror* **158**, 40–1.

Richardson K. (1983) Assessing communication. *Geriatric Nursing* **4**, 237–8.

Rouchneen M. J. (1983) Ear syringing. *Nursing* **2**, 530–2.

Sofaer B. (1983) Pain relief — the importance of communication. *Nursing Times* **79**, 32–5.

Sullivan N. (1983) Vision in the elderly. *Journal of gerontological Nursing* **9**, 228–35.

Synder L.H., Pyrek J. & Smith K. C. (1976) Vision and mental function of the elderly. *Gerontologist* **16**, 491–5.

Veeramah E. (1981) Communication with psychogeriatric patients. *Nursing Times* **77**, 1220–1.

Chapter 16
Death and Dying

For the first time in the history of mankind people born today have very good prospects of living a full human lifespan of approximately eighty-five years. The major causes of death in the past, infectious diseases, nutritional deficiencies and hormonal disorders, have virtually been eradicated. Of the major diseases, as opposed to trauma, which kill people today, arteriosclerosis and cancer are both disorders which affect the elderly more than the young. Both are increasingly amenable to treatment and, perhaps even more important, largely preventable. Given that this is the case the individual's expectation of a long life is heightened. Death, and least of all one's own death, is not something to be contemplated too seriously and certainly not something to be discussed openly! People's attitudes towards death are more tangled and evasive than almost any other topic. So much so that one of the major problems in dealing with the dying person and his relatives is that of communication.

FACTORS RELATING TO DEATH AND DYING: PRINCIPLES OF CARE

Communication

The reason why communications are so difficult between the dying person and those near to him, including nurses and doctors, are very complex. Part of the problem relates to changes in the cultural and societal attitudes towards death. We are all hooked on living so that death has become a taboo subject, something to be hidden away. The trend throughout this century has been to remove people to hospitals for terminal care, that is, to die. This means that the majority of people have never lingered with the dying person or witnessed death. Most people have no experience in caring for the dying person. A slight reversal of this trend has become evident in Westernized societies over the past two decades with the provision of hospices which provide comprehensive and sensitive care of the dying person and his grieving family. It is particularly appropriate for the person whose illness is beyond the furthest boundaries of the curative process. The emphasis being on symptomatic relief and caring. The provision so far is only available for small numbers so that for the majority of people death in a hospital of one sort or another is most likely.

Very often in hospitals there is a problem of inadequate communication between members of the caring team. Doctors and nurses need to discuss frankly how a particular patient is to be managed. The doctor on diagnosing a terminal illness must decide whether the patient is to be told of the diagnosis or not. One must remember, however, that prognosis in the elderly is never easy. The elderly by definition are survivors; people who have overcome or escaped many illnesses to which their contemporaries have succumbed. They often have a remarkable capacity to adjust to chronic illness such as extensive cardiac and pulmonary diseases. Even some cancerous tumours are relatively slow growing in the elderly. At what stage, therefore, one talks of 'terminal care' is a difficult clinical decision to take.

Should the doctor decide not to inform the patient he should give his reasons to the nursing staff. This should include what he told the patient and his relatives especially if his decision was influenced by them. By doing so, nursing staff faced with questions from the patient can give appropriate replies. Each patient must be assessed on an individual basis. This is what makes decisions about what to tell him so difficult. There is no way of telling how the person will react to the knowledge that he is dying if told. The caring team must avoid blanket rules and decisions, but try instead to establish a good relationship with the patient and his relatives. If we believe in the dignity and worth of an individual, we must surely accept the need to allow him some discretion if extreme life support measures are to be used. It should be the basic right of any ill person (or his spouse) to make 'informed decisions' on care and treatment. But what are informed decisions in a technological age? What might have seemed extraordinary and outrageous treatment a few years ago are now commonplace. This makes it difficult to tell the patient what is for the best.

Part of our communication problem, of course, is that patients are strangers to us. This may work to the nurses advantage in some cases in that people will often confide in strangers, but be reluctant to confide in those nearest and dearest to them. Basically caring for the dying requires commitment and, at times, intense involvement without loss of objectivity. This is not without risk to the carer who may feel vulnerable and exposed so that mutual support from other members of the team is essential. Nurses unable to face the reality of the situation may use a variety of blocking tactics; for example, they may appear to be very busy so that the patient refrains from asking questions. One must always remember that being ill and in hospital brings with it a loss of individuality and a feeling of helplessness. Patients often feel isolated and alone amidst the turmoil of activity around them. The patient needs to be given every opportunity to express his feelings. This is only possible if people are receptive to his attempts to communicate. Remember one cannot 'not communicate' so that both verbal and non-verbal cues should be acted upon. This of course is a two-way process and the individual patient must sense that the nurse is receptive and willing to listen. A busy, hurried attitude effectively blocks communication and enhances the patient's feeling of loneliness and isolation. Be patient; give the dying person time to translate his fears, etc., into words. Some people find it difficult to express themselves at the best of times. Much depends on the individual's personality and what he knows of his illness and prognosis. Some patients may be quiet and withdrawn, others abusive or aggressive or even excessively cheerful. Responses such as this represent an incongruity of affect. They are very often out of keeping with the person's normal self and cause him great hurt and anguish because he will very often immediately regret the harshly spoken words. The nurse who fails to recognize this may even feel personally insulted, and so create yet more barriers to effective communication. It is not only the literal meaning of the words that is important, but also the way they are spoken and even more importantly the 'latent content' or hidden meaning which may be equally important. This is sometimes referred to as 'metacommunication' and is an important aspect of many human inter-actions, especially when dealing with the dying patient.

Physical and Psychological Factors

When all reasonable methods of care have been exhausted and death is inevitable the nurse is the principal care giver. The relationship between the nurse and the patient is, therefore, of great importance in the overall management.

Opportunities to establish rapport with the patient can easily be created whilst providing basic nursing care. Few nurses really appreciate the unique opportunities they have for communication when assisting the patient with the activities of daily living. Assisting the patient to bathe, brush their hair, clean their teeth, shave, put on make-up, and so on, can all be used as a means of establishing rapport and gaining access to the patient. The opportunity for such physical contact is denied to most other professionals or, at least, severely circumscribed. Generally they have no reason for such 'intimate contact'. Physical contact of this nature, that is when providing basic nursing care, combined with a genuine interest in the patient as an individual, leads to a relationship of trust and understanding. The patient should be given the chance to talk about whatever he wants. Hence discussion need not all be gloomy but may be about events in the person's life: a review of life's achievements; his successes and failures; events he can look back on with pride and pleasure; marriage, family, success at work, in helping others, wartime contributions. It may become apparent that the patient has some unfulfilled dream or ambition which even after many years is still causing conflict so that he needs to be helped to resolve this by exploring his successes in life. There are also few families that have not at some time experienced internal strife. Often the exact details are long forgotten and only the bitterness remains. Such unresolved conflicts can cause great anguish so that attempts should be made, if the patient and family wish it, for the dying person and the loved one to resolve their differences and say their farewells. It is too late at the funeral! Many a bereaved person is haunted for many years by unresolved quarrels which may even on occasion taint the whole family's relationship. Helping people to resolve problems of this nature or to make meaning and sense of their lives is of course far from easy, requiring, as it does, the sort of profound involvement few of us are really capable of.

In answer to direct questions nurses should reply as honestly and simply as possible. If you do not know the answer you should say so. If the patient has cancer, for example, facts relating to where the tumour is, why they have particular symptoms, the effects of treatment and so on are what he wants to hear. He needs to make sense of his situation within a meaningful frame of reference. On many occasions the patient will ask the same questions of several members of staff, either because of disbelief, anxiety or fears of the unknown. Various coping mechanisms may be produced in an attempt to control fear and anxiety. These may be direct, where an attempt is being made to alter the patient's relationship to his environment, or palliative, where attempts are made to reduce or eliminate body, motor and effective stress (Porritt 1984). Various unconscious defence mechanisms may also be apparent such as denial distortion, projection and even regression (Tatro & Marshall 1982). Pertinent here also are the five stages of psychological preparation proposed by Kubler-Ross (1970) whose pioneering work is well known. In her research she interviewed 200 patients who were dying and identified five stages which the majority experienced. The first is *denial and isolation* ('No, not me, it cannot be true'). The second stage is *anger*. This is displaced in all directions and often projected into the environment and the people in it. This is a particularly difficult stage for the family and others who are caring for the dying person. The third stage is *bargaining,* in which the individual negotiates with those around him and possibly with God. It is during this stage that the individual tries to make sense of it all. The fourth stage is that of *depression*. He can no longer deny his illness and is overwhelmed with grief. The final stage is that of *acceptance*. This occurs if the patient has the time and opportunity to work through the previously described stages. Not all dying persons will go through each stage, this depends on many factors including individual personality, time available, support systems and so on. Additionally, not all persons will experience these stages of dying in the order in which they are presented. Dying, like all aspects of living, is a highly individual process.

Death is potentially the loneliest experience any of us will ever have to face. From an individual standpoint we are ill prepared to cope with the reality of it and usually have little in our past experience to call upon. This leaves the individual and his family in a vulnerable position. There is often a great tendency for medical and nursing staff to take over completely the life of the patient, especially the elderly patient. Perhaps this stems from the deep-seated guilt feelings that a cure has not been effected. There is often a failure to consider his wishes as if he had no wishes or desires left. Very often also there is a lamentable lack of involvement of relatives. Opportunities should be provided to enable the patient and significant others such as relatives, friends and care givers to spend time together. In an open-bedded area screens should be provided to give privacy and freedom from interruption. Without privacy it is difficult for the patient and his loved ones to share the last few precious days and hours together in a meaningful way. At times like this people find it difficult to find the right words to say, so that physical contact becomes important. If nurses and others are constantly jostling around the patient, the relatives may be inhibited about touching; however, this should be encouraged. When words are hard to find, great comfort can be gained from simply holding the person's hand. Try to involve the relatives in some aspects of care, such as giving a drink, washing the hands and face, etc. Physical action of this nature should be seen as mediating factors in facilitating meaningful interaction.

Providing comfort measures is of course very much part of the nurse's function. In the last few days and hours these are geared towards supporting deteriorating body systems and in providing symptomatic relief. Limbs become weary and stiff and may often become very cold and swollen. Changing the patient's position, passive limb movements, support of a limb on a soft pillow and a soothing back rub are all very comforting.

Thirst is often a problem and needs to be alleviated. Fluids of choice are given. If possible sit the patient up, well supported by pillows, to enable him to drink naturally. Oral hygiene is vital to basic comfort. As the muscles become weaker the patient may experience difficulty in keeping false teeth in position. The problem is not readily solved and is usually worse where weight loss has been considerable. Whenever possible the teeth should be worn and perhaps the use of some fixative will help to keep them in position.

Elimination can be a nightmarish problem in the latter stages. Patients fear loss of control above all else. Especially those very elderly, ardently independent old folks, who have always held a firm rein. Care given at this time should never appear demeaning or as if the individual is a child. It is the maintenance of self-esteem that the nurse must enhance. This is only possible if one has a deep respect for the dignity of others.

Pain

Some dying patients will undoubtedly experience pain as part of the dying process. It is perhaps pain that people fear more than anything else about dying. However, dying can be painless if approached in the right manner. The hospice movement has been very successful in developing techniques and methods for the relief of pain. These methods are equally applicable in the hospital or home.

The general principles are, first, to identify the cause of the pain. This is essential if rational measures of pain relief are to be adopted. Second, analgesia on a regular round-the-clock basis prevents pain breakthrough. This reduces anxiety and raises the patient's pain threshold, so that lower optimal doses of analgesia are required. Third, oral analgesia is preferable whenever possible and especially in the thin cachectic patient, where injections would be difficult and painful. Fourth, do not give too frequent doses of analgesics as this is demoralizing and may interfere with sleep, etc. It is best to increase the dose rather than the frequency. Finally, the aim is to provide a balance between a painfree state without undue drowsiness or euphoria. Always start off with the simple analgesics such as paracetamol and if the pain worsens work up to drugs such as Brompton's Cocktail. This is an old, well-established pain relieving concoction which is given orally and is very effective. Addiction is not a problem; the problem is giving enough analgesia to relieve pain whilst still enabling the patient to remain alert and able to participate in life and perform as many of the activities of daily living unaided, that is, within the limits of his physical capability. In providing analgesia the nurse must not forget the emotional, social and spiritual aspects of stress, any one of which can increase the patient's pain through lowering the pain threshold (Waterhouse 1982). The patient's relatives are always grateful if the patient's pain can be controlled, as it enables them to communicate more readily. To watch someone die in pain merely compounds their grief.

Patients on analgesics, especially narcotic-type drugs and their derivatives, will almost certainly become extremely constipated if appropriate measures are not taken. Additional fibre in the form of bran or some other bulking agent must be given. If not, the patient will experience great difficulty in emptying the bowel, which will lead to unnecessary discomfort, and possibly distressing loss of control. Whenever an analgesic is prescribed for regular use, other agents to prevent constipation should be prescribed simultaneously.

Once the patient has died, care and support of the relatives is very necessary. Relatives should be given access to the body if they request it, and all documentation necessary should be completed with a minimum of fuss. Personal items should be given back to the relatives after careful checking that all is in order. It reflects badly on the nursing staff if items are lost or mislaid at this time.

Spiritual needs

An important aspect of the nurse's role is to ensure that the patient's spiritual needs are met. Assessment of spiritual needs is, to say the least, difficult and something many nurses feel uncomfortable about. Stoll (1979) offers constructive advice on how to assess a patient's spiritual needs; not only when he is dying but as an integral part of a holistic approach to patient care. No attempt should be made to influence the patient; the assessment is purely to ascertain his wishes so that appropriate arrangements can be made. Henderson (1960) in her booklet, *'Basic Principles of Nursing Care,'* lists helping the patient worship according to his faith as a basic right of all patients. Many patients confronted by death or serious illness may turn to religion even though it has not been a dominant aspect of their lives previously. In the case of those for whom religion has been an important aspect of their way of life, the prospect of dying may be easier.

As in all other matters the patient's wishes and those of his relatives should, as far as possible, be granted. It is not the nurse's prerogative to offer judgement but to care for the individual regardless of his religion or other beliefs.

PATIENT PROFILE

Mr Harry Watt, an 81-year-old retired instrument maker, started to have recurrent digestive problems some six to eight months before seeking medical aid. Investigations carried out, when he eventually sought aid, revealed an extensive cancer of the stomach. The surgeon was only able to perform palliative surgery to relieve an obstruction and to make Mr Watt feel more comfortable. He was simply told that he had had an operation to relieve an obstruction. His wife was told he had a tumour and that life expectancy was from four to six months. Mr Watt had been initially reluctant to have surgery, fearing he might not survive, and worrying about how his wife would manage if he did not recover from the operation. Mr and Mrs Watt never openly discussed the nature of the illness; somehow or other it did not seem essential that they did so. After over 50 years of marriage they had few secrets and a very good understanding of each other. On return home from hospital, Mr Watt was reasonably well and continued more or less as he had done since retiring at 65. He managed some gardening and enjoyed his other hobby of building and repairing model engines. He was aware that he was not as fit or as well as he had been but at 81 years old accepted the situation philosophically.

It was not until about a month before he died that the services of a district nurse were required. Mr Watt began to experience difficulty in the activities of daily living, especially in getting up, dressing and using the lavatory. Mr and Mrs Watt refused a home help and between the help of neighbours and the district nurse, Mr Watt was able to spend all his remaining days at home except for the last two days of his life when home nursing became too much for his wife and neighbours. Pain had also became a problem. Two days before he died he was admitted to a local hospice-type facility where he died peacefully.

ORGANIZATION OF NURSING CARE

Subjective Evidence (What the Patient Says)

- 'I am getting so stiff and weak.'
- 'I am becoming a burden to everyone.'
- 'Old age doesn't come itself.'

Objective Evidence (What the Nurse and Others Observe)

- Obvious weight loss.
- Unable to get up from lavatory seat on his own.
- Difficulty with basic activities of daily living.

Assessment (Nursing Diagnosis)

- Patient's physical condition deteriorating rapidly.
- Extreme wasting and loss of mobility.

Plan of Nursing Care

- Patient should try to live each day to the fullest of his physical and mental capacities. (See also Chapters 12, 20 and 22.)
- Spend *time* with Mr Watt and his wife individually and together.
- Encourage them to talk about Mr Watt's position and future (be prepared for a willingness by Mr Watt to be given an honest answer to the question, 'Am I dying nurse?').

- Meet any reasonable request for things other than those provided as part of normal provision of routine care.
- Give maximum amount of care and support required in relation to physical/non-physical activities of daily living.

Expected Outcome

- An open awareness of the prognosis will emerge.
- Fewer negative comments about such things as 'being a burden' will be made.
- Maximum flexibility in the provision of care will be achieved.
- Mrs Watt will feel involved in care and, following her husband's death, will feel positive about her contribution towards his care.
- The physical and emotional problems associated with the dying process will be minimized.

NURSING CARE OF DYING PERSON (EXAMPLE)

07.30 hours Early morning cup of tea. Although every reasonable encouragement will be given to drink, refusal will *not* be met with vigorous nursing interventions. Flexibility of routine to meet individual requirements is essential.

08.00 Mr Watt gets up, washes and dresses. Assist as necessary. As far as is possible, a nurse (who may well be assisted by a visiting relative) who has formed a close relationship with Mr Watt will spend as much time with him as possible. Nursing the dying person is one of the more time-consuming of nursing activities; he must be given all the time he needs.

08.30 Breakfast—whatever the patient fancies. Because eating and drinking will become increasingly difficult, the provision of food must be very flexible. A stock of favourite items could be kept in the refrigerator.

09.00 Reads newspapers, etc. Inclusion in decisions and normal activities is essential, so often the dying person is excluded and rejected by the mistaken notion that he is unable to participate.

10.00 He is assisted to walk around the garden or simply on to back porch, as able. Remember, he will want to do something, and feel exhausted by it a few minutes later. Ample assistance should be available to cater for these 'changes of mind' and to ensure that he is never alone when he prefers company.

10.30 Mid-morning tea or coffee, followed by exercises (see Chapter

12). Although vigorous/curative exercises are clearly not required, continued efforts should be made to sustain the quality (although not necessarily the quantity) of his life.

11.00–12.00 Attention to hygiene needs by district nurse, time to talk. 'Talking time,' which is part of every nurse – patient contact, requires you to be available, relax and give him the opportunity to talk about whatever he wants to talk about. Look for clues that indicate he wants to talk about his health/terminal status; for example, he might say, 'I wish I was away,' or, 'I hope my wife will be OK', or 'What do you really think about all this nurse?'

12.00 Lunch.

13.00–1500 Lie down for two hours rest.

15.00 Afternoon tea — visit by minister or neighbour for a chat. Free and open visiting including (if necessary) during the night-time seems reasonable *providing* it meets the requirements of the patient; for example, if he has slept most of that day, it might be best for his wife to visit him at night.

16.00 Participates in hobby if able.

1700 Evening meal.

18.00–20.00 Watch television, participates in games, etc.

21.00 Prepares for bed. Quiet period for chat with wife or other visiting family members or friends. You have a role to play in balancing the needs of Mr Watt, who will tire easily, with those of family and friends, who will wish to spend much time with him. Close nurse – relative/friend contact is necessary; you will have to guide and advise them.

During all of the activities mentioned above, Mr Watt will be given the opportunity, indeed encouraged, to discuss his circumstances and future prospects. If he indicates a wish to know if he is dying, or if he hints at this, he needs to be given a full opportunity to arrive at an understanding and acceptance of his terminal state.

ASSESSMENT OF DYING PATIENT

Awareness of Prognosis

- Patient has/has not been informed.
- Patient's relatives informed.
- Patient's relatives have requested patient is not told.
- Brief statement relating what patient has been told.

Orientation

- Alert and orientated.
- Alert but disorientated.

Consciousness

- Altered level of consciousness.
- Unconscious.

Affect (Mood)

- Responds normally to human interaction.
- Excessively cheerful (incongruence).
- Depressed.
- Withdrawn.
- Hostile.
- Emotionally labile.

Pain

- No complaints of pain.
- Complains of mild pain.
- Complains of moderate pain.
- Complains of severe pain.

Independence

- Able to perform all basic activities of daily living.
- Requires assistance with activities of daily living.
  Specify which: . . . .
  . . . .
  . . . .
- State problem/s for each activity of daily living.

Elimination

- Continent of urine and faeces.
- Incontinent of urine only.
- Doubly incontinent.
- Incontinent at night-time only.
- Catheter in situ.

- Constipated.
- Faecal impaction (spurious diarrhoea).

Hydration Status

- Taking adequate fluids orally.
- Unable to take adequate fluids orally.
- Requires tube feeding.
- Requires i.v. fluids.
- Nausea.
- Vomiting.
- Oral hygiene.

Integument

- Skin intact.
- Pressure sores—specify site, degree.
- Fistula, drains.
- Oedema.
- Other skin lesions, e.g. bruising.

Spiritual Needs

- Does/does not want clergy to visit.
- Committed to specific religion/faith – specify.
- Arrangements made.

Relatives

- Supportive and attentive.
- Not generally supportive.
- Coping/not well.
- No known relatives.
- Friends only.
- No visitors.

Where specific problem/s have been identified the reader should refer to the appropriate chapter for a more detailed assessment.

REFERENCES

Henderson V. (1960) *Basic Principles of Nursing.* International Council of Nursing, Geneva.

Kubler-Ross E. (1970) *On Death and Dying,* 1st edn. Tavistock, London.

Porritt L. (1984) *Communication: Choices for Nurses.* Churchill Livingstone, Melbourne.

Stoll R.I. (1979) Guidelines to spiritual assessment. *American Journal of Nursing* **79** (9), 1574–7.

Tatro S.E. & Marshall J.M. (1982) Regression: A defense mechanism for the dying older adult. *Journal of Gerontological Nursing* **8** (1), 20–2.

Waterhouse M. (1982) Don't despair—dying can be painless. *The Australian Nurses Journal* **11** (6), 40–2, 53.

FURTHER READING

Kay J.M. (1983) To cure sometimes; to comfort always. *Nursing Times* **79 (40),** 61–3.

Knight M. & Field D. (1981) A silent conspiracy: coping with dying cancer patients on an acute surgical ward. *Journal of advanced Nursing* **6** (3), 221–9.

Lunt B. & Hillier R. (1981) Terminal care: present services and future priorities. *British Medical Journal* **283,** 595–8.

Pett D. (1979) Grief in hospital. *Nursing Times* **75** (17), 709–12.

Pike C. (1983) The broken heart syndrome and the elderly patient. *Nursing Times* **79,** (7), 50–3.

Scott R.S. (1983) Our patients' the teachers. *Journal of gerontological Nursing* **9** (9), 493–7;.

Summers D. (1984) Living with dying. *Nursing Mirror* **158** (2), 14–21.

The International Work Group in Death, Dying and Bereavement (1979) Assumptions and principles underlying standards of terminal care. Occasional Paper *Nursing Times* **75** (17), 69–70.

Turnbull R. (1982) Caring for the ageing: the nurse's relationship with the dying person. *The Australian Nurses Journal* **11** (10), 51–3.

Wagg B. & Yurick A.G. (1983) Care enough to hear. *Journal of gerontological Nursing* **9** (9), 498–503.

Chapter 17
Dependence

Henderson (1966, p.15) suggested that the unique role of the nurse was to:

'... assist the individual, sick or well, in the performance of those activities contributing to health or its recovery ... that he would perform unaided if he had the necessary strength, will or knowledge. And to do this in such a way as to help him gain independence as rapidly as possible'.

This statement indicates the central importance of 'dependence' as a problem requiring nursing intervention. Henderson quite clearly states that nursing interventions, of any kind, should only be performed if the patient is unable to perform the task himself. Despite the importance of dependence and independence to nursing, as evidenced by the writing of Henderson, the topic is given scant attention in many contemporary texts. The following anecdote illustrates the reluctance which many staff have in helping patients achieve an optimal level of independence.

An 83-year-old ex-patient of the author had been hospitalized for some months for the treatment of depression. It was clear that she would eventually be discharged to live a fully independent life. When asked if she would be willing to make her bed in the mornings, she replied, 'Yes'. When this proposition was subsequently put to the rest of the staff on the ward an enrolled nurse protested that: a hospitalized patient should not be expected to make her own bed; that an *old* patient could not be expected to make her own bed; that an *ill* patient could not be expected to make her own bed; and that the ward would look untidy if she were allowed to do so. In the event the lady made her own bed, with minimal encouragement and assistance from staff, and was discharged a few weeks later in a state of virtual independence.

From a developmental viewpoint independence begins early in life and results in increasing autonomy. Although no-one is ever completely dependent or independent, the very dependent infant becomes more independent as he matures. In due course the adult is *relatively* independent.

In this chapter the word 'dependence' relates only to those circumstances in which an individual is unwilling, or unable, to reach the level of independence of which he or she is capable. It is recognized that some individuals are able to achieve a greater level of independence than others, and that there is considerable variation between individuals. It is also recognized that dependence/independence run on a continuum and that there are different levels of dependence/independence. As will be seen later in this chapter all persons who require nursing care assistance experience a degree of 'normal' dependence. It is important that we all recognize the existence of that dependence, the potential anxiety and distress which it may cause, and the need to make patients as independent as possible as quickly as possible.

FACTORS RELATING TO DEPENDENCE: PRINCIPLES OF CARE

A wide range of factors relate to the concept 'dependence', and a few will be presented here. Those discussed are not treated exhaustively and are only intended to illustrate the complexity of the concept 'dependence' and to show how these related factors might be considered in treating it.

Innate Abilities

There must be clear awareness, on the part of the patient and on the part of his care givers, of the level of functioning of which the patient is capable. This awareness will result from knowledge of the patient and his personality, knowledge of his illness and the extent to which it affects dependence, a knowledge of the current physical and non-physical health status of the patient, and a knowledge of him in terms of his day-to-day functioning. Unless there is a very realistic awareness and expectation of the patient in terms of the skills of which he is capable, it is very easy to underestimate those abilities, allowing him to become increasingly dependent, or to over-estimate his abilities and label him as being 'dependent' when in fact he *is* functioning at his highest possible level.

Diagnosing and monitoring a patient's level of dependence/independence requries a high level of skill and knowledge of the subject. In many instances you will have to be the final judge of whether or not a person has a dependence problem; for example, when he is unwilling or unable to admit to having such a problem, or in circumstances where his relatives are also unable or unwilling to admit to the existence of it. Remember, this is not the type of problem which patients will readily admit to experiencing, it may be that they may have a subconscious motive or reason for being pathologically dependent at this particular time. It is a problem area which needs to be dealt with in a particularly sensitive and understanding manner.

Iatrogenesis

Iatrogenesis is the term used to describe those illnesses or problems which are produced by the very staff and/or environment which *should* minimise these problems. Although much of the literature on the subject focuses on the role of medical staff in causing iatrogenic problems, undesirable effects of drugs for example, there can be no doubt that nursing staff play a major part in causing the iatrogenic problem 'dependence'. Another feature of much of the literature is that it takes full account of a range of physical iatrogenic problems, deep venous thrombosis resulting from prolonged bedrest for example, but takes limited account of non-physical problems such as dependence. The range of iatrogenic problems caused by nursing staff is large, and includes many disabling conditions such as dependence or dehydration following prolonged confinement to geriatric chairs.

It is not suggested that nurses are intentionally causing iatrogenic problems, but that these may be the result of a lack of awareness of their potential to cause them. The need for a high-quality and well-educated nursing staff group to care for the elderly, and to avoid causing iatrogenic problems was implied by Wells (1980, p.129) when she wrote:

Nurses in geriatric wards . . . are well meaning about the wrong things . . . The central problem in geriatric nursing is the central problem in all nursing: nurses do not know why they do what they do.'

Thus, *nurses* must carry much of the responsibility for causing iatrogenic problems relating to both physical *and* non-physical areas of health. The reasons for this situation result from educational deficits, the fact that a large nursing input is made by relatively untrained staff, the covert nature of many potential problems, dependence for example, and the high status given to nurses who are seen as being busy and 'doing everything' for their patients. If one accepts the definition of the unique function of the nurse made by Henderson (1966), then it is of the utmost importance that we always do as little as is safely possible for our patients in all circumstances. In short, you must only provide nursing care for your patients when they are unable to do things because they lack the necessary strength, will or knowledge.

Institutionalization

The concept of 'institutionalization' was made popular by Barton (1959) in his book *Institutional Neurosis*. Although other writers had recognized the problem earlier (Myerson 1939), Barton was the first to produce a comprehensive discussion of its cause, treatment and prevention. In describing the term institutionalization, which he in fact labelled institutional neurosis, Barton (1959, p.2) was at pains to point out that the syndrome could occur inside *and* outside institutions. He wrote:

'... the adjective "institutional" does not imply that institutions are the only cause of the disorder, but signifies only that institutions are the places where it was first generally recognised ... probably hermits, some house-wives and old age pensioners are afflicted with similar symptoms'.

The syndrome, which might just as easily have been labelled 'institutional dependence', is characterized by lack of initiative, apathy, lack of interest and submissiveness. The person is often described by nurses or other care givers as being 'dull', or 'institutionalized', or 'lacking in initiative', or 'gives no trouble', or 'cooperative', or 'solitary'. Institutionalization can be pre-vented and successfully treated; the following eight strategies can be used as preventive measures, treatment measures, they also clearly reflect the cause of institutionalization.

1 Stimulate the patient's interest in things outwith his immediate environ-ment.

2 Provide a friendly, permissive and relaxed atmosphere.

3 Use a minimum of sedative and tranquillizing drugs.

4 Make it possible for the person to have friends and enjoy personal events such as birthdays.

5 Ensure that nursing staff and other care givers have an appropriate level of education and experience.

6 Ensure that the patients are never teased, mistreated or made the subject of amusement.

7 Provide a daily routine which includes useful occupation and activities. *Encourage independence.*

8 Ensure contact with the 'outside world' and the people in it.

All elderly people, particularly those who are receiving institutional care, are at high risk in relation to institutionalization. Every effort must be made to ensure that the individual's environment is 'therapeutic'. This relates to the atmosphere within the ward which is created by the caregivers; for example, staff-patient contact and interaction must be frequent, positive and goal directed in order to ensure that the related problems of dependence and institutionalization do not occur.

Patient Role

For many people entry into the 'patient role' or 'sick role' is perceived as a situation in which they must, of necessity, become extremely dependent on nursing staff and other health givers. Indeed, many nurses also see this as a situation in which the individual moves from the 'non-sick role' (in which he is extremely independent) to the 'sick role' (in which he becomes extremely dependent). If one accepts the notion of dependence existing on a continuum, then it is easy to see that extreme dependence (even for a patient) is highly undesirable.

An important feature of the way in which nurses place patients in a sick role relates to the use of dependence as one means of controlling the patient. Nursing staff control is increased as the patient is more dependent; it is decreased as the patient becomes more independent. Some nurses may find this control, and enforced dependence, being used as a means of reducing their anxiety levels when dealing with patients. However, it is important that we extend our notion of 'patient' and 'sick role' to encompass the notion of dependence/independence existing on a continuum, and encompass the belief that we must foster and encourage the highest possible level of independence in all of our patients in all circumstances.

Rehabilitation

The author's definition of the word rehabilitation is: *The process of maximizing a person's independence either by prevention or active intervention as a means of treatment. The process should begin and coexist with the health care delivery being provided by staff or other care takers in all environments. The contribution of staff includes diagnosis, planned intervention, evaluation and documentation of the rehabilitation process.*

If you accept that 'maximizing a person's independence' is the central feature of rehabilitation, then you must also accept that rehabilitation is the business of all nurses, in all circumstances, at all times. In recent years it has become fashionable to develop specialist rehabilitation nurses, rehabilitation wards, and rehabilitation units. It is the author's view that, with very few exceptions, the creation of specialist rehabilitation nurses, wards and units has had a negative effect. The effect has been to lessen the awareness of nurses generally of their crucial role in the rehabilitation process. If one is not a 'rehabilitation nurse' or does not work in a 'rehabilitation ward' then one might be forgiven for thinking that rehabilitation is the business of some other person or of some other ward. The reality is that rehabilitation, maximizing independence, is the business of all nurses.

It is, of course, recognized that different patients will require differing rehabilitation goals. As with dependence, the experience and education of the nurse will enable her to set realistic and attainable rehabilitation goals for each patient.

Quantity and Quality of Staff

Although it may seem improbable, it is likely that the extent to which nurses encourage patients to be dependent on them increases as the quantity and quality of staff decreases. The series of events resulting in this outcome is as follows. If staff are well trained and available in appropriate numbers, they can afford to spend time encouraging a patient to do things for himself, and waiting for him to do so rather than doing them for him. If staff are relatively untrained and in short supply, it is much easier and quicker to do things for the patient rather than spend time encouraging him to do them for himself. Thus, the quality and quantity of nursing staff who care for the potentially dependent patient are crucial in either causing him to be more dependent, or encouraging his independence.

The innovation and determined efforts which can be made by appropriately trained staff to encourage independence are considerable. Such innovations frequently develop from a recognition that many health care systems are over protective of the patient, and seriously restrict his independence. Isaacs (1979a) in a paper entitled 'Don't trust him — he can't cope!' discussed the successful operation of a self-medication scheme for elderly people in hospital. In a later paper (Isaacs 1979b) entitled 'Don't get up — you'll fall' discussed the often questionable reasons which nurses give for immobilizing patients, for example to reduce their own anxiety levels.

Minimizing Dependence: General Strategies

Although there is no recipe for minimizing dependence that can be applied to all patients, the following general strategies may be used as guidelines.

Evidence of dependence must be fully documented, as must the nursing care to be used, nursing goals, and expected outcomes.

Patients should be allowed to function as independently of their immediate enviromments as possible. They should be encouraged, indeed expected, to accept as much personal responsibility as possible and to be as assertive as possible.

Dependence never exists in isolation from other underlying causes; for example a person might find the notion of independence very frightening and something which raises anxiety levels. Dependent patients should be encouraged to identify, acknowledge and verbalize this problem and explore alternative ways of behaving.

It should be recognized that behaving in a dependent manner is something that the patient may need to do at that particular time. The dependence only becomes problematical if it is either excessive or continues beyond a reasonable time period. Moving from relative dependence to relative independence may well be a painful and long process for some individuals, a process which may be facilitated by the use of a formal and structured one to-one psychotherapeutic interaction between patient and nurse.

Finally, it must be recognized that all patients are at risk in regard to becoming pathologically dependent. This applies equally to institutionalized and non-institutionalized persons. The importance of identifying dependence problems and fully discussing them with the person concerned cannot be overemphasized.

PATIENT PROFILE

Miss Gonsella is aged 81 years and has been resident in a nursing home for four years. She is normally vitually totally independent within the context of living in an institution (nursing home). However, in recent weeks she has become increasingly dependent on the nursing home staff and other residents. Evidence of this increasing dependence can be illustrated by describing a recent conversation which she had with one of the nurses.

Nurse: 'I think I hear the dinner bell Miss Gonsella.'

Miss Gonsella: 'Will you take me along in a wheelchair nurse; I don't feel like walking today?'

Nurse: 'I'll help you to get to the dining room; I'll help you to *walk* there.'

They walk to the dining room together.

Miss Gonsella: 'I see there is fish and pork chops on the menu. What do you think I should have nurse?'

Nurse: 'I'm not sure, just have whichever you prefer.'

Nurse leaves Miss Gonsella and returns to the ward. Miss Gonsella does not collect her own meal as is her normal practice, instead she makes her way to a table and asks another patient to collect her meal for her.

From the above description it is clear that evidence of a dependence problem exists. The evidence is both subjective (relating to what Miss Gonsella *says)* and objective (relating to what she does).

ORGANIZATION OF NURSING CARE

Subjective Evidence (What the Patient Says)

- 'Will you take me along in a wheelchair nurse; I don't feel like walking today?'
- 'I see there is fish and pork chops on the menu. What do you think I should have nurse?'

Objective Evidence (What the Nurse and Others Observe)

- Does not collect her own meal as is normal practice.
- Encourages other patients to collect her meal for her.

Assessment (Nursing Diagnosis)

- Dependence.

Plan of Nursing Care

- Do as little as possible for patient.
- Positively reinforce *any* independent act.
- Discuss dependence problem.
- Encourage discussion of dependence in group therapy meetings.

Expected Outcome

- Will become more independent generally and will walk and make choices.
- Will continue to move around ward without help.
- Will collect own meals.

NURSING CARE OF PATIENT WITH DEPENDENCE PROBLEM (EXAMPLE)

07.30 hours Miss Gonsella, who sleeps in a single room in the nursing home, is wakened by her own alarm clock which she has set the previous night. It is expected that she will get up, use the toilet, dress and prepare for breakfast without any assistance. If she does not appear for breakfast at 8 a.m., visit her room and encourage her to get ready. If she cannot, or will not, prepare herself for breakfast, give a considerable amount of encouragement, and minimal assistance.

08.00 At breakfast she will be expected, as is normal practice, to collect her own breakfast and cutlery. After breakfast she will be expected, as is normal practice, to clear away her cutlery and dishes.

09.00 Miss Gonsella will be encouraged to make her own bed and tidy her own room. If necessary, given minimal assistance from nursing staff.

09.30 She will participate in the group therapeutic activity which occurs each day to the week. Miss Gonsella will be encouraged to discuss her dependence on staff and other patients. The nurse leading the group will, as far as is possible, encourage open discussion of this problem as it affects Miss Gonsella and other patients, and will move the discussion towards exploring possible solutions.

10.30   She will assist two other patients in the preparation and distribution of mid-morning tea. As with other activities, a nurse will supervise the tea preparation, and will give minimal assistance.

11.00   Meeting with personal nurse therapist, a daily event, to discuss problems generally and dependence in particular. Miss Gonsella, in common with all residents, has been allocated a personal nurse with whom she meets daily in order to discuss any current problems.

11.45   Free time, hobbies, newspapers, radio.

13.00   Lunch. (As for breakfast.)

14.00   Rest period.

15.00   Prepares for, and helps with, distribution of afternoon tea as in the morning.

15.30   Out walking with visitors for a short period. Visitors, who come three times weekly, have been included in discussions regarding Miss Gonsella's dependence and care (with her permission). They will give general and firm encouragement to her in terms of independence.

16.00   Visiting continues.

16.30   Bath or shower. Miss Gonsella has indicated that she wished to have a bath or shower by saying to a nurse, 'Do you think I should have a bath *or* shower, will you help me?' The nurse helps her to decide and offers to provide supervision and minimal assistance.

17.30   Evening meal. (As for breakfast.)

18.30   Free time, hobbies, newspapers, radio.

19.30   Brief discussion with nurse about progress to date, problems/ successes, plans for next day.

20.00   Washes, irons personal clothing (with supervision and minimal help from another resident).

21.00   Free time before preparing for evening drink distribution as in the morning.

21.45 – 23.00 Free time, preparing for bed.

23.00   Retires, with access to an emergency call button for calling for help from staff. During the past few weeks has called for help

4 – 5 times per night (for example to obtain a drink). This frequency has now been reduced to 2 – 3 times per night and, with the present nursing strategies, is expected to reduce to 'real emergency' calls only.

ASSESSMENT OF DEPENDENCE

Each item should be considered in terms of what the person is *able* to do; for example, if he is physically incapable of walking, then his chairfast state is his optimal level of functioning. However, if he is capable of walking, but will not or cannot, due to causes other than physical inability, he might be regarded as being dependent.

Activity

- Bedfast.
- Chairfast.
- Walks up to five yards.
- Walks to toilet.
- Walks outwith ward.
- Fully mobile.

Self-help/Helping

- Seeks help from others (relatives, staff, other patients).
- Proficient in self-help skills.
- Helps others.

Toilet/Personal Hygiene

- Requires no help/prompting.
- Requires prompting.
- Requires help.
- Needs to be washed, shaved, bathed, taken to toilet.

Eating/Drinking

- Selects own food.
- Cooks/carries own food.
- Eats without/with help.
- Requires feeding.

Domestic Tasks

- Cleans, tidies, washes, makes bed.
- Washes/cares for own clothing.

Medications

- Full personal control of medications.
- Requires assistance/supervision.
- Expects others (relatives, staff) to take full control.

Assertiveness

- Takes initiative/makes decisions.
- Seeks help/approval in decision making.
- Relies on others to make decisions.

Interpersonal Relationships

- Assertive: initiates interactions, plays dominant role in one-to-one and group interaction.
- Passive: waits for others to initiate interaction, avoids communicating with others.

Patient/Person Role

- Maintains individuality and independence, plays active part in decisions relating to health care, questions professional judgements and decisions.
- Plays passive role, accepts all decisions without question, insists that others 'know best' and should decide.

REFERENCES

Barton R. (1959) *Institutional Neurosis.* John Wright and Sons Ltd, Bristol.

Henderson V. (1966) *The Nature of Nursing.* Macmillan, New York.

Isaacs B. (1979a) Don't trust him—he can't cope! *Nursing Mirror* **149,** 24–5.

Isaacs B. (1979b) Don't get up—you'll fall. *Nursing Mirror* **149,** 40–1.

Myerson A. (1939) Theory and principles of the "total push" method in the treatment of chronic schizophrenia. *American Journal of Psychiatry* **95,** 1197–1204.

Wells T. (1980) *Problems in Geriatric Care.* Churchill Livingstone, London.

FURTHER READING

Barton E.M., Baltes M.M. & Orzech M.J. (1980) Etiology of dependence in older nursing home residents during morning care. *Journal of Personality and Social Psychology* **38**, 423–31.

Bassett C., McClamrock E. & Schmelzer M. (1982) A 10–week exercise program for senior citizens. *Geriatric Nursing* **3** (2), 103–5.

Davies A., Goldberg B. & Wilkinson I. (1984) A methodology for manpower planning. Occasional Paper. *Nursing Times.* **80** (2), 44–6.

Cheadle A.J. (1978) Long–stay rehabilitation. *Nursing Times* **74**, 1382–4.

De Young M. (1982) Planning for discharge. *Geriatric Nursing* **3** (6), 396–9.

Dreher B. (1981) Deciding with the elderly. *Geriatric Nursing* **2** (2), 122–6.

Gajus M.J. (1980) A programme for long–stay patients. *Nursing Times* **76**, 203–7.

Harnkes D.D. (1984) Self care. Assessing the aged client's need for independence. *Journal of gerontological Nursing* **10** (5), 26–31.

Hicks C. (1984) An aid to better community care? *Nursing Times* **80** (2), 8–10.

Murray E.W. (1979) Why not night hospitals? *Nursing Mirror* **149**, 10.

Manley R. (1983) Dependence with dignity. *Nursing Times* **79** (50), 14.

Riffle K.L. (1982) Promoting activity: An approach to facilitating adaptation to ageing changes. *Journal of gerontological Nursing* **8** (8), 455–9.

Stevenson J. & Gray P. (1981) Rehabilitation for long-term residents. *Geriatric Nursing* **2** (2), 127–31.

Torrance M. (1983) To do or not to do? *Nursing Times* **79** (43), 24–5.

Williams L.V. (1979) Occupational therapy for the elderly. *Nursing Times* **75**, 167–9.

Chapter 18
Elimination

Elimination of bodily wastes is one of the basic requirements of all living organisms, this chapter relates to two forms of waste, urine and faeces. When something goes wrong with the processes of defaecation and micturition there is a marked effect on all other activities of life. For the elderly, one of the most distressing and incapacitating disorders of elimination is incontinence. It should always be remembered that incontinence is a symptom of something else that is wrong, and *not* an inevitable process of ageing. This chapter will concentrate on urinary incontinence and on constipation, and on the many things nurses can do to prevent their occurrence in the elderly.

Incontinence can be defined as, 'passage of urine or faeces at an inappropriate time and in an inappropriate place'. Often in elderly people, one small change in circumstance or physical condition can tip the balance between the socially acceptable and acquired behaviour of maintaining continence, and unsociable and demeaning episodes of incontinence. A careful nursing assessment should unearth the cause(s) of incontinence and action can very often be taken which enables the patient to regain continence.

Acquiring the habit of normal micturition in our society is a complicated process and requires many basic skills (ask any parents trying to potty-train their children!). In order to be continent one must be able to:

1 perceive that one's bladder is full;
2 decide whether it is an appropriate time to empty the bladder;
3 'hold on' if necessary;
4 find a toilet and physically move to it;
5 manipulate clothing and correctly position oneself;
6 start flow of urine;
7 use toilet paper and readjust clothing;
8 wash hands.

To be continent and socially acceptable we must be able to perform each step in the correct order, and in the correct place.

Urinary incontinence is a problem which increases with age. A recent survey (Thomas *et al.* 1980) found that 11.6% of women and 6.9% of men

207

over the age of 65 years suffered from urinary incontinence.

The major problem with faecal elimination in the elderly is constipation. A liquid discharge and faecal soiling may be associated with constipation, this is an overflow from a large impacted mass of faeces in the rectum and should not be treated as diarrhoea. True diarrhoea is a symptom of a pathological complaint and should be referred to a doctor. The presence of an impacted mass of faeces can be found by making a rectal examination.

Two important factors are necessary in disease-free adults to achieve normal defaecation: a balanced diet and regular exercise. Any changes in diet or patterns of exercise are likely to lead to bowel problems, this is why constipation is so common in the elderly patients in long-term care.

FACTORS RELATING TO ELIMINATION

Physical Disorders

URINARY

Obviously any physical disorder of the urinary system is going to make incontinence more likely. This can be because of obstruction somewhere in the urinary tract caused by, for example, bladder stones, carcinoma, or an enlarged prostate in males; or by obstruction from outside the urinary tract, for example a constipated impacted rectum, or uterine fibroids in females.

In women a weakened pelvic floor (often related to a poor obstetric history) can lead to stress incontinence where urine escapes from the bladder when extra stress is placed on the pelvic floor muscles by coughing, laughing or even moving. Elderly females may also have oestrogen deficiency which can lead to urethritis, frequency of micturition and incontinence. Urinary tract infections cause frequency by irritating the bladder and can cause urge incontinence. The patient may be unable to 'hold on' long enough to reach the toilet.

Other physical disorders can make the whole process of passing urine 'correctly' very difficult or impossible. Impaired mobility might prevent someone from reaching the toilet in time and lead to incontinence. It may be that walking has become slow and painful because of corns or ingrowing toenails, in which case a chiropodist is the best person to cure the incontinence. Arthritis and rheumatism often limit mobility and dexterity so the patient is unable even to adjust clothing before sitting on the toilet. Deteriorating eyesight, perhaps due to cataracts, can stop the patient from walking to the toilet for fear of tripping and falling.

FAECAL

Any physical disorder to the large intestine is going to cause problems with defaecation. If a person has haemorrhoids, he may well become constipated because opening his bowels has become too painful.

Impaired mobility leads to lack of exercise, which means peristalsis in the bowel is not stimulated, resulting in constipation.

Neurological

URINARY

In the elderly a cerebrovascular accident (stroke) is one of the most common neurological traumas which can occur, this may damage the part of the brain which controls the bladder. Continent adults are able to pass urine only when it is convenient to do so by consciously inhibiting contraction of the bladder. When a person has had a stroke he is aware of the need to pass urine but, because of damage to the brain, is unable to control and inhibit the bladder. He has only a few minutes (or less) to 'hang on' before the bladder contracts and urine is voided.

When dementia and brain damage occur, patients are often not aware that they need to pass urine, or if they are aware do not know the correct place to go and urinate in a basin or waste paper bin.

Any disease or trauma to the spinal cord or bladder nerve endings can lead to incontinence, for example, following spinal injury, multiple sclerosis and diabetic neuropathy.

One of the effects of ageing is a gradual loss in the ability to inhibit bladder contractions. In severe cases this can lead to a condition of an uninhibited neurogenic bladder, where small amounts of urine are passed frequently.

FAECAL

Damage to the bowel's nerve supply can lead to severe problems of constipation where a patient is unable to voluntarily initiate a bowel movement. Again, in dementia, there may be a lack of awareness of a full rectum, or the patient is unable to find the toilet.

Psychological Disorders

URINARY

In the elderly, psychological upheavals, such as the stress caused by admission to hospital, often lead to episodes of incontinence. The patient may be too frightened to ask to be taken to the toilet, or even too embarrassed to ask a busy young nurse for help. If the shame and trauma of one incident of incontinence is compounded by an unsympathetic remark by a nurse such as, 'Oh, you have been a naughty girl, Mrs Smith', the problem may come to be expected by both patient and staff.

Bereavement is a major trauma for the elderly and may leave someone so low and depressed that even the effort of going to the toilet is too much. Loneliness can have the effect of making someone so miserable that they become incontinent, as can low self-esteem, causing the person to feel that somehow they must be wet and smelly.

Boredom often leads to incontinence in a long-term institution. Places where efforts have been made to stimulate the interest and involvement of patients in various activities have found that episodes of incontinence dramatically drop.

FAECAL

People do become obsessed with their bowels and in order to achieve regular bowel movements, some take daily purgatives and laxatives. These are often unnecessary and patients frequently become overdependent on them.

Privacy is essential to most people when visiting the toilet. In a busy ward it may be difficult for a patient to achieve enough privacy, which can lead to constipation because of embarrassment and inhibition. Anxiety and depression can also lead to constipation.

Environment

URINARY

Hospital wards are confusing places for the elderly, and toilets may be few and far between. All too often the path to the toilets is littered with ward equipment, and some patients give up the attempt to find and forge a path to the ward toilets. Hospital toilets can often be inhospitable places: cold, draughty and lacking in privacy. It is not really surprising that many patients would prefer to wet themselves than suffer in a cold and dingy toilet.

Official Department of Health and Social Security (DHSS) statistics say there should be one toilet to every four patients. This frequency has been rarely achieved in hospital wards, especially in long-stay geriatric wards (Chamberlain & Stowe 1982). Many elderly people are still living in houses with outside toilets; icy weather or any problems with walking make visits outside very difficult and incontinence more likely.

FAECAL

In problems of constipation the environmental factors outlined for urinary incontinence also apply. Private, comfortable and easily accessible toilets are needed.

Diet

URINARY

Fluid consumption is one of the most important dietary components to consider when looking at problems of urinary elimination. Frequently, when elderly people have an episode of incontinence they feel they ought to decrease their fluid intake. This exacerbates the problem because the urine becomes concentrated and is more likely to irritate the bladder and make it more prone to infection, thus increasing the problems of urgency and the likelihood of incontinence.

Very few people drink too much, although late night drinks increase the possibility of night-time incontinence. Providing enough fluid is taken during the day, drinks after about 20.00 hours can be safely cut out if nocturnal incontinence is anticipated.

FAECAL

Constipation in the elderly is often due to an ill-considered diet. A good fluid intake is also vital to ensure smooth movement of faecal matter through the large intestine.

The fibre content of our diet makes up the faecal bulk and a diet high in fibre will lessen the likelihood of constipation (Leaves 1982). The elderly often find it difficult to maintain a high-fibre diet. Bran is unpalatable and really needs to be mixed or cooked with something else, whilst fresh fruit is often tricky to manage when wearing false teeth, and wholemeal bread can be hard to chew. Some old people living at home cannot shop for themselves and find it difficult to keep a stock of fresh vegetables. Hospital food is often low in fibre, white bread being more common than brown bread and, unless they are given fresh fruit by visitors, patients are unlikely to receive any with their hospital meals.

People who have a diet lacking in fibre form small, hard faeces which are painful and difficult to pass. Their bowel movements can be infrequent and irregular and they will tend to be constipated.

Drug-induced Disorders

URINARY

Several drugs commonly taken by the elderly have an effect on the urinary tract and result in episodes of incontinence. Diuretics are often an important form of therapy, but fast-acting diuretics can be too much for some less mobile patients. Drugs may take longer to act in the elderly because of a decreased metabolic rate. If a diuretic is given in the morning, it may not have any effect until the night resulting in night-time incontinence, giving the diuretic at night may allow diuresis to occur the next morning.

Sedatives given at night could put the patient so heavily to sleep that they sleep through any desire to void and are incontinent.

FAECAL

Many drugs are known to cause constipation; those commonly taken by the elderly include some pain killers, hypotensives, iron tablets and aluminium antacids.

Iatrogenic Problems

URINARY

In a hospital, one 'accident' can lead to a patient being labelled as incontinent. As has been mentioned previously, many things can trigger off an incident of incontinence.

When a patient is admitted, he is frequently worried or confused and instructions as to where to find the toilets are not taken in. Insecure patients need frequent reminders on where to find the toilets. Patients are concerned that they will have to 'fit in' to a hospital routine and will only be allowed to pass urine during a bedpan round, such patients should be reassured that we, the nurses, are willing to provide toilet facilities whenever they are asked for.

An elderly patient has very little time to hold on once he feels the urge to micturate, so unless we quickly offer toilet facilities that patient is liable to be incontinent. Offering a commode is sometimes not seen as a major priority of nursing care. What happens all too often is that a patient is labelled as 'incontinent' and is then fitted with incontinence pads. This leads the patient to the not unsurprising conclusion that, since the pads are provided, they must be the correct place in which to pass urine (Ramsbottom 1982).

FAECAL

It is all too easy for constipation to develop in elderly patients. Using a commode behind bed-curtains is not a very private affair and some patients find it acutely embarrassing. This can lead to constipation. Nurses working under pressure do not give the patient enough time or peace and quiet if they are always hurrying on to the next task.

PRINCIPLES OF CARE

Urinary

Once a person has been found to be suffering from incontinence all efforts should be made towards finding the cause. It is likely, in the majority of causes, that incontinence can be reduced if not completely stopped. A thorough nursing assessment should be made and, if necessary, medical advice sought.

First of all, an estimation of the degree of incontinence needs to be made. This can be done by charting a patient's micturition patterns over several 24-hour periods. Many charts have been designed for this purpose, any adopted for use should be simple and flexible. A typical charting procedure would be for the patient to visit the toilet at regular intervals, say every two or three hours, when a record would be made of whether the patient is wet or dry and whether or not urine is passed. Frequent toiletting may not be necessary at night, but regular checks do need to be made. After a few days of charting, any patterns of incontinence will become clear. Regular toiletting may indeed cure the incontinence; the frequency can be altered to meet the patients' needs.

Once it has been established that the patient does have a problem with incontinence, attempts can be made to find the cause. From a nursing point of view, regular two-hourly toiletting is a heavy commitment, and common sense indicates that for a successful and accurate record to be made, only one or two patients on a ward should be charted and assessed simultaneously. Any attempt to keep track of a whole ward of patients is doomed to failure.

Much can be found out about the possible causes of a patient's incontinence by considering the factors mentioned in the previous section.

PHYSICAL DISORDERS

Most physical disorders will require further medical investigation, but nurses should be able to initiate some assessments. A mid-stream specimen of urine can be taken to check for urinary tract infections which can be treated with antibiotics. A rectal examination should ascertain whether the patient has severe constipation which requires treatment. A general assessment of the patient's ability should show whether he is physically capable of going to the toilet independently, or outline the degree of assistance required.

Simple actions can be taken, such as moving the patient to a bed nearer the toilets if walking is a problem, or providing a commode by the bed if night-time trips to the toilet prove difficult. If the patient is at home, provision of an accessible toilet or commode should be made.

For someone with a dexterity problem, advice can be given about suitable clothing. For women, loose skirts are easier to manage than tight ones; corsets and layers of underwear should be discouraged; loose-legged knickers where the crotch can be pulled to one side are a possibility when a patient has urgency or impaired dexterity. For men, increasing the length of the fly opening may allow easier positioning of a urine bottle.

For women with weak pelvic floor muscles, pelvic floor exercises can be easily taught by a nurse or physiotherapist. All women should learn how to exercise their pelvic floor muscles and should be taught to routinely stop and start their flow of urine whenever they micturate.

NEUROLOGICAL DISORDERS

One of the effects of ageing is a decrease in the bladder's ability to 'hold on'. When caring for elderly people, requests for bedpans or commodes should be met as quickly as possible to avoid incontinence. For demented patients, the best way of achieving continence is to establish a regular pattern of toilet use. This should be planned to meet an individual's needs. Some patients only need to visit the toilet before or after meals, whilst others may need to go regularly every two hours.

It has been suggested that toiletting regimens will only work for patients who are able to hold more than 150 ml in their bladders without unstable contractions occurring (Castleden & Duffin 1981). The bladder capacity and diagnosis of the medical cause of incontinence can be made using various cystometric techniques.

Patients who have had a stroke may eventually regain bladder control and will need a great deal of support and encouragement during their re-habilitation.

PSYCHOLOGICAL DISORDERS

Time and patience are needed. Many elderly people feel that incontinence is 'bad' and 'dirty' and it is important that nurses do not make comments which reinforce that view. Positive encouragement should be given on a regular basis. For patients living at home, it is often the relatives who need most support and encouragement.

The elderly need time to talk through their problems and the support of a sympathetic and knowledgeable listener can make a great deal of difference.

Allowing patients to wear bright clothes and sit in comfortable armchairs gives them confidence. Encouraging participation in various activities is stimulating and may reduce incontinence due to boredom or depression.

ENVIRONMENT

Continence is much easier to achieve in a brightly lit and cheerfully coloured atmosphere than in a dark and dingy room. It helps to have toilet facilities clearly marked, perhaps the doors could be painted in a different colour? Some hospital and residential units have painted yellow lines on the floor so patients can follow them to the toilet areas.

For patients living at home where there is still an outside toilet it may be worth making enquiries about whether a grant is available to provide an inside lavatory. Otherwise a commode can be provided, as long as there is someone available to empty it.

DIET

You need to check that a patient is taking enough fluid. It is all too easy in a hospital ward for tea cups to be whisked away before a patient has had a chance to drink the contents. At least nine cups of something fluid are needed every day. A good, balanced diet should be taken to reduce the effects of constipation.

DRUG INDUCED

An awareness is needed of the effect various drugs have on the body. If, for example, it is thought a patient no longer in severe heart failure has inadvertently been left on a strong diuretic, it is worth suggesting that a less potent diuretic be prescribed. Obviously, a patient who is on diuretic treatment will need frequent provision of toilet facilities.

If an analgesic is thought to lead to constipation, perhaps the prescription can be changed to a less constipating variety.

NURSING FACTORS

Many medical and nursing staff are too willing just to supply patients with pads and pants and leave it at that. Pants, pads and aids do have an important role in the management of incontinence but they should be used to help a patient regain both continence and confidence. Part of caring for an incontinent patient is being able to give advice on the correct use of suitable aids. There is a vast range of products to choose from and it is difficult to keep up to date with the changing array. There are few guides available, the best is probably the *Association of Continence Advisers Directory of Aids*. Most health districts have a continence adviser in post and she is the best person to approach for advice (Blannin 1980).

Equipment can be provided which makes visiting the toilet much easier, such as raised toilet seats and grab rails on either side of the toilet. Commodes or chemical toilets can be provided for patients at home. Portable urinals can be provided for patients, but bedpans are very awkward to manage and should be avoided. Men often manage with a urinal bottle fitted with a non-spill adaptor.

There are many body-worn pads available. When used correctly, pads do not replace regular visits to the toilet but should give confidence to someone trying to regain continence. The type of pad chosen should be suited to the degree of incontinence suffered by the patient. Patients also like to be offered a choice of garment (Shepherd & Blannin 1980). Less bulky pads are suitable for stress or dribbling incontinence. Pads which slip into a pouch or pocket in specially designed marsupial pants are popular with many elderly women. These will cope with moderate urinary incontinence but not with faecal incontinence. They are easy to pull up and down and make toiletting simple. Large plastic-backed pads held in place with special stretch pants can cope with larger amounts of urinary and faecal incontinence. They may be harder to manipulate when toiletting patients.

Men are able to wear appliances or sheaths which divert urine into a drainage bag; no similar satisfactory devices have been manufactured for women. Sheaths held in place with an inner flexible lining are possibly the most comfortable. Men with a retracted penis will not be able to use sheaths.

For those still incontinent after all other forms of treatment have been tried, an indwelling catheter may be the answer. With careful management these can free patients from the indignity of being continuously wet (Kennedy 1983). Long-term catheters made from silicone or silicone elastomers are best if the patients are able to tolerate them. These can last for up to three months *in situ* without needing to be changed. Small-sized catheters with small balloons should be used, preferably 12–16 Charriere with 5–10 ml balloons. For females, the shorter-length female catheters allow drainage bags to be discreetly hidden on the thigh.

Body-worn drainage bags are preferable, these can be hidden under clothing and should not restrict movement. Leg bags strapped to the calf are suitable for men. Women need bags which can be attached to the thigh. These can be supported in a number of ways: in knickers with a special pocket; in special holsters; or supported on a holder suspended from a waist belt.

Catheterized elderly patients need a high fluid intake, a minumum of 2000 ml daily. For patients with gritty urine, regular bladder washouts may be needed. Patients on long-term catheterization may develop chronic urinary tract infections which are best left untreated if the patient shows no symptoms, otherwise the bacteria will soon become resistant to antibiotics.

Faecal Elimination

As mentioned earlier, constipation is the major problem of faecal elimination in the elderly. Nursing care must be directed towards prevention of constipation.

Principles of care are to improve mobility and/or promote exercise and to ensure patients are taking a diet including plenty of fibre. Ensuring peace and privacy in toilet areas also helps.

Evaluation of the patients' drug regimen may show that some drugs are having a constipating effect. If possible, these prescriptions can be altered.

If a patient is found to have severe constipation, efforts must be made to clear the bowel before regimens of care can have any effect. Often these patients have very impacted faeces which will not be cleared by laxatives or administration of an enema. A course of enemata will be required, this can be very exhausting for the patient. Some patients even need to have a general anaesthetic in order to remove a mass of faeces.

Patients who have had severe constipation sometimes need a regular routine of a daily enema or glycerine suppository to stimulate bowel evacuation.

PATIENT PROFILE

Mrs Owen is an 81-year-old widow who has recently been admitted to a geriatric assessment ward following a fall during which no bones were broken. She has been living on her own since her husband died seven years ago, and has three children.

This lady was slightly confused on admission and seemed unsure of her surroundings. She has no history of confusion and her only previous admission to hospital was for a cholecystectomy 20 years ago.

Mrs Owen is able to walk unassisted but is very reluctant to do so. As she walks she tends to grab hold of beds and chairs to steady herself. She has a healthy appetite but nurses have reported that she is unwilling to drink. She reports having regular bowel movements at home because she takes daily aperients. At home, Mrs Owen also takes occasional painkillers to cope with her arthritis as she says her hands are sometimes painful and she has problems with dressing.

Since admission, both day and night staff have reported incidents of urinary incontinence which Mrs Owen had not experienced before admission. On further questioning, Mrs Owen became upset and tearful. Incontinence is obviously a problem which has been bothering her for some time. 'It's my age, isn't it dear? I'm afraid people won't come near me because of the smell.'

ORGANIZATION OF NURSING CARE

Subjective Evidence (What the Patient Says)

- 'By the time I get to the toilet, it's sometimes too late and I'm wet.'
- 'I don't drink much, but I'm still wet.'
- 'I don't like to bother the nurses to ask for a commode; they seem so busy.'

Objective Evidence (What the Nurse and Others Observe)

- Tearful when questioned about incontinence.
- Incontinent twice during each day on average.
- Sheets are wet every morning.
- Walking is slow and unsteady, has difficulty in reaching the toilet in time.

Assessment (Nursing Diagnosis)

- Incontinence due to decreased bladder control and an inability to 'hold on' for long.

Plan of Nursing Care

- Reassure patient and give her time to talk and discuss the problem.
- Explain urge incontinence is due to anxiety and decreased bladder capacity.
- Start on two-hourly toiletting and charting regimen.

- Enlist help from physiotherapist to improve patient's mobility.
- Encourage patient to drink more: a minimum of 2000 ml daily.
- Institute regular, planned visits to the toilet to reduce episodes of incontinence.

Expected Outcome

- Patient more relaxed and prepared to seek help if further problems develop.
- Episodes of urinary incontinence cease or reduce.
- Patient is willing to increase fluid intake to 2000 ml daily.
- Can reach the toilet without being incontinent.
- Can walk from sitting-room to toilet unaided.

NURSING CARE OF PATIENT WITH INCONTINENCE PROBLEM (EXAMPLE)

07.30 hours	Remind to visit toilet, chart results, i.e. whether patient wet or dry and whether urine passed. Throughout day, offer praise if patient dry and if wet give reassurance that problem will be cured.
08.00	Encourage Mrs Owen to wear loose-fitting clothes and check on her ability to dress herself. (Dressing practice.)
08.30	Give 500 ml jug of water/fruit juice and instruct her to drink it all in addition to any drinks such as tea.
09.30	Remind to visit toilet, chart results. Obtain mid-stream specimen of urine.
10.30	Observe patient with physiotherapist. Give her encouragement with walking.
11.30	Remind to visit toilet, chart results. (Undressing/dressing practice.)
13.00	Check on amount of water drunk from jug, give fresh water if required. Give 500 ml jug of water/fruit juice and instruct her to drink it all in addition to any other drinks such as tea.
13.30	Remind to visit toilet, chart results. (Undressing/dressing practice.)
14.30	Talk to Mrs Owen about her problems, give reassurance that her incontinence can be cured. If patient remains anxious, suggest use of pads until she is more confident. Help to select type of pad. Show her how to put them on and give advice on how often to change them.
15.30	Remind patient to visit toilet. Chart results.

16.30	Discuss incontinence, and the nursing care strategies being used, with Mrs Owen and her daughter who is visiting.
17.30	Remind patient to visit toilet. Chart results.
19.00	Last hot drink of the day. Check that patient has drunk all 1000 ml.
19.30	Remind patient to visit toilet. Chart results.
21.30	Remind patient to visit toilet. Chart results.
22.00	Settle patient for the night.
23.30	Check bed for incontinence. Chart results.
01.30	Check for incontinence. If awake, offer toilet facilities.
03.30	Check for incontinence. If awake, offer toilet facilities.
05.30	Check patient for incontinence. If awake, offer toilet facilities.

ASSESSMENT OF ELIMINATION

- Unable to maintain continence.
- Partially able to maintain continence, state type and frequency of incontinence.

Bowel

- Establish patient's normal frequency of bowel opening.
- History of previous problems.
- Query use of laxatives.
- History of any physical or neurological disorders.
- Find out if defaecation associated with pain.
- Extent of mobility and dexterity.
- Determine the fibre content of the diet, is it too low?
- Find out whether the patient is taking any constipating drugs.
- Make a rectal examination to determine whether the patient is impacted. If true diarrhoea present, refer to doctor.

Bladder

- Establish patient's normal daily pattern of micturition.
- History of previous problems.
- History of any physical or neurological problems.
- Establish when incontinence occurs.
- Is incontinence:
  (a) Stress related — urine leaks when patient coughs;
  (b) urge related — a sudden onset of the desire to pass urine and an inability to hold on.

- Find out current frequency of visits to the toilet.
- Assess extent of mobility and dexterity.
- Note awareness of bladder fullness.
- Assess daily fluid intake; is it less than 2000 ml?
- Has the patient suffered any recent psychological trauma?
- Toilet facilities — determine ease of access and distance from patient.
- If urinary tract infection suspected, obtain mid-stream specimen.
- Routine examination of urine.
- Refer to doctor for further medical investigations as necessary.

REFERENCES

Blannin J.P. (1980) Incontinence towards a better life. *Nursing Mirror* **150**, 31–3.

Castleden C.M. & Duffin H.M. (1981) Guidelines for controlling incontinence without drugs or catheters. *Age and Ageing* **10**, 186–90.

Chamberlain M.A. & Stowe J. (1982) Bathing in hospital. *British medical Journal* **284**, 1693–4.

Kennedy A.P. (1983) Care of the elderly catheterised. *British Journal of geriatric Nursing* **2**, 10–15.

Leaves A. (1982) A question of fibre. *Nursing Mirror* **154**, 43–5.

Ramsbottom F.J. (1982) The use of incontinence underpads in hopsital. *Nursing Times* **78**, 1868–9.

Shepherd A.M. & Blannin J.P. (1980). A clinical trial of pants and pads used for urinary incontinence. *Nursing Times* **76**, 1015–16.

Thomas T.M., Plymat K.R., Blannin J. & Meade T.W. (1980). Prevalence of urinary incontinence. *British medical Journal* **281**, 1243–5.

FURTHER READING

Brocklehurst J.C. (ed.) (1984) *Urology in the Elderly*. Churchill Livingstone, London.

Disabled Living Foundation (1984) *Association of Continence Adviser's Directory of Aids*. Disabled Living Foundation, London.

International Rehabilitation Medicine (1982) **4**, 1. (Whole issue on incontinence.)

King M. (1984) Aids for incontinence. *Nursing Mirror* **158** (7), 30–6.

Mandelstam D. (ed.) (1980) *Incontinence and its management*. Croom Helm, London.

Watson A. (1983) Kanga pads on trial. *Nursing Mirror* **157**, 48–50.

Chapter 19
Hostility

Nursing is an activity that depends heavily upon the interaction of nurses and patients. The idea of 'good nursing' suggests that a 'good' or positive relationship exists between nurse and patient. In a very few cases it could be argued that the demand for such a relationship is not very high: for instance, where the patient is comatose, or so ill that he is unable to communicate. Nursing, in such situations is all 'one-way traffic'. In all other situations the patient responds to the actions of the nurse; she, in turn, responding to the patient's responses. The verbal, non-verbal and physical behaviour of nurse and patient forming the basis of this reciprocal relationship. This chapter discusses situations where positive relationships are not in evidence and considers possible reasons for this disharmony and suggests ways of resolving this problem.

In its most extreme form *hostility,* especially in a political sense, is seen as a state of war between two peoples. At the very least it is a situation which is characterized by unfriendliness. Any person who 'begs to differ' runs the risk of being branded as hostile, especially by the person with whom he has disagreed. The situation is not uncommon in nurse–patient interactions. Any patient who argues, tries to make his opinions heard, if not respected, or otherwise 'challenges' the authority of the nursing team, may be viewed as hostile. In some situations this 'challenge' may be punctuated by strong language or invective, depending on the patient's background or upbringing. Where such hostility becomes extreme it may be described as *aggression,* where one party is openly waging war on the other. Before proceeding further it may be appropriate to distinguish aggression more clearly from other kinds of hostility.

Hostility can be expressed in a number of ways. Common to all of them is an underlying air of disharmony. The two people concerned may refuse to speak to one another. If they do converse they may neglect to express common courtesies, quibble over trivia, or generally express non-cooperation by subtler means; an example might be 'elective deafness', pretending not to hear what has been said, or suggesting that one had assumed the comment was addressed to someone else. Such tactics are intended to intensify the hostility, scoring points in the battle without actually displaying aggression. Such strategies are to be found in a number of interpersonal situations, especially where cooperation is a necessity, for example between union officials and employers, or between nurse and patient. Hostility, in its broadest sense, involves interpersonal warfare where the blows are struck most often by symbolic means. The person most often causes offence by *not doing* something, rather than by any direct form of action.

Aggression, on the other hand, usually involves a direct attack. This might be verbal, where someone shouts, swears or otherwise abuses the other person. This might involve making derogatory comments, of a sexist or racist nature, or some kind of personal attack, which would commonly be construed as insulting or offensive. Aggression can also involve physical assault. This might involve minor attacks such as nipping, scratching or spitting, or more fully fledged acts of violence using some kind of weapon. Some forms of physical assault often also have psychological effects, which may be more potent than the actual assault. A slap in the face, especially in a public place, may be more damaging on a psychological level than is commonly assumed.

Hostility and aggression, therefore, belong to the same family of interpersonal behaviour; they belong to the practice of political disharmony. They also appear to exist on a continuum. If you imagine a line measuring 'extremity', at one end stands the simpler forms of non-cooperation already mentioned. The line extends through more and more severe forms of non-cooperation, where a range of 'frustrating' tactics are used, until it passes into the area of actual abuse, or aggression, where verbal and then physical abuse is evident. At the furthest extreme of this continuum stands the violent attack with a dangerous weapon.

This chapter concentrates upon the hostility end of this spectrum for two reasons; first of all, if hostility can be avoided or resolved, the risk of aggression is reduced. Of course, a small number of patients will make wholly unpredictable attacks on staff, however the number of such patients is relatively small when compared with the 'communication breakdown' syndrome found in many care settings. Second, the incidence of hostility, in its broadest sense, appears to be quite high. At one extreme are the situations where nurse and patient are not collaborating as much as they could. This may result in the patient failing to benefit, as much as he could, from the care relationship. At the other extreme, non-cooperation may be more obvious: the patient refusing to take medication or dress himself. Such an individual is often declared 'troublesome' and a specially designed care plan, often restrictive in nature, is implemented as a result.

Hostility, although clearly a problem in itself, may also be seen as a sign of other problems. Often the 'awkwardness' of old people is seen as another indicator or symptom of senility. If an 'organic' explanation of this kind is ruled out, such difficult behaviour may be attributed to some kind of 'death wish'; the patient has grown old, is losing his faculties, friends and independence, and is impatiently awaiting his demise. Undoubtedly, for some people in some situations these explanations may be appropriate. However, we might do well to avoid using them as general principles to explain the hostility of all old people. One major problem is that both these 'explanations' *blame* the patient. Blame may be a strong word but although the problem exists *between* two people, the explanation is rooted firmly in only one of them. This is either the patient's physical make-up, which is crumbling, or his psychological state, which has become negative. Gasek (1980) suggests that nurses, and indeed doctors, tend to employ these explanations because of the medical model under which they trained. This model commonly depicts the elderly person as a helpless, innocent victim of one disorder or another. It tends to see the patient as existing in an interpersonal vacuum; the patient's behaviour is always seen as arising from *within* the person. It is either his physical state or his mental state which is the cause of his behaviour. In general, this model rarely sees the patient's behaviour as a function of his interaction with those around him. The consequences of this narrow viewpoint are very important. Nurses might do well to consider the weaknesses of this view, and seek alternative explanations if we are to ever change the nature of our interaction with the patient.

First of all, the medical model assumes that the patient is not, in any way, responsible for his problems. Hostility is seen as a function of some condition, like dementia or 'mental illness'. As a result we tend to treat the patient as a very dependent individual; making allowances for him as we would a child. We might well 'explain away' his behaviour saying, 'He can't help it; it's all part of his condition. He is dementing very rapidly.'

Since the patient is not responsible for his actions he is assigned to a strictly 'passive role'; he is a helpless, hopeless patient and treated as such. If the patient is treated in this manner, he will ultimately get the message that he is hopeless. He will soon think, 'I can't do anything for myself.' Such an attitude will, of course, breed more irresponsible behaviour.

A third consequence of this model is the tendency to separate the patient from his condition. Staff who discuss the 'Alzheimer' are using a kind of medical shorthand, but one which presupposes that the condition operates independently of the person who *has* the condition. Such an attitude further reinforces the notion that the condition, not the person, controls his behaviour. Gasek (1980) points out that the ultimate consequence of this viewpoint is that the patient, or should we say 'his condition', is confined to an institutional web, where he is maintained and manipulated 'for his own good'.

The final consequence is perhaps most important. Since the patient cannot control the condition, which lies at the root of the problem, we see no reason to involve him in the planning or execution of his care. He is unlikely to be consulted about even the most basic aspects of his existence. If he tries to make his wishes heard, he may be seen as intruding upon a professional preserve. He will receive a clear message that the carers are not concerned with what he thinks about his care (Gasek 1980).

The outcome of this chain of consequences is that the narrow 'medical model' tends to alienate the patient, not only from staff but also from the condition which is assumed to be the root of the problem. The kind of care which strict adherence to such a narrow viewpoint breeds, first categorizes and then patronizes the patient. As a result, nurse and patient never work *together;* the outcome being either docile passivity or indignant hostility.

It is clear that in some cases the 'medical explanation' of the patient's behaviour is appropriate. However, for the majority of patients who fail to coexist harmoniously with their carers, other factors may influence or cause the problem. In general, it could be argued that the patient's hostile behaviour arises out of a series of complex interactions between the patient, his carers and other aspects of his 'environment'.

FACTORS RELATED TO HOSTILITY

Staff Attitudes

In some situations hostility may begin as an expression of dissatisfaction on the staff side. Over a period of time this is reciprocated by the patient, who is then labelled as hostile: this problem often being attributed to his condition (for example dementia). Hemsi (1982) has commented that 'aspects of the patient's behaviour may cause intense irritation — such as the constant repetition of the same question or following others around. This may lead to outright rejection. Sometimes there is unalloyed hostility . . . the deteriorating behaviour merely making the feeling acceptable and respectable.' Two major attitudes appear in situations where hostility is present.

Hostile and belittling: staff express the attitude that the patient is deteriorated, hopeless and perhaps even that aspects of his behaviour are repulsive.

Compassionate and loving: here staff show caring concern almost despite the reactions they get. Often the more difficult the patient is, the more caring they become.

It is often thought that both attitudes stem from anxiety. In the first case staff may feel that the patient is making demands which they cannot fulfil.

This results in frustration, even anger. However, such feelings are suppressed, emerging as hostility. In the second example the staff may fear that they may end up that way themselves, or that their parents may be similarly institutionalized. Their caring concern is a kind of symbolic sacrifice, offered in the hope that they, or their loved ones, will be spared a similar plight.

From these two attitudes spring four ways of dealing with hostility (Gasek 1980).

Authoritarianism: here staff exercise the 'rule of law' to control the patient, and may appear domineering, arrogant, disrespectful if not downright rude.

Confrontation: here staff try to resolve the problem 'once and for all.'

Both these actions display an underlying anxiety; staff may fear that their authority is being questioned and try to strengthen their status or use their position to resolve the problem, by 'intellectual force.'

Stoicism: here staff try to remain neutral and emotionally uninvolved. They do not, however, show compassion for the patient.

Martyrdom: here staff 'give in' to the patient; doing whatever he wants. This total submission rarely lasts.

A more appropriate alternative is to adopt a problem-solving approach. The patient's behaviour should not be seen as a threat or personal attack, but as a challenge. Can you uncover the reasons for his hostility and assist him to resolve the problem? In some cases the problem may lie in the patient's environment, such as sensory deprivation; in other instances it may be a function of prejudiced attitudes on the part of the staff. In trying to resolve the problem you should:

(a)   listen to the patient's point of view;
(b)   look for meaning in his hostility;
(c)   agree to compromise — within limits;
(d)   always explain what you are doing and why;
(e)   try to include the patient in any decision-making.

Stereotypes

As has been noted, stereotyped attitudes can be a major source of frustration for the elderly. One specific bias is the belief that 'disturbed emotional behaviour' is an example of the natural and inevitable outcome of old age, and nothing can be done about it. Such beliefs produce a vicious circle. If we assume that an old person cannot be helped, we will *neglect* to help him, which will lead to an exacerbation of the problem, making him appear all the more 'unhelpable'.

The elderly share many of the characteristics of disadvantaged minorities: negative stereotyping; restricted opportunities; and segregation. The most important stereotyping is in the view that emotional instability is normal in old age. As a result, a problem, like hostility, only receives attention when it is very severe or disabling; by that stage the problem may be beyond help, thus confirming the negative stereotype that 'there is nothing we can do to halt this kind of deterioration' (Pfeiffer 1976). In spite of the fact that most old people do not deteriorate greatly in old age, society still embraces the distorted view that anyone over 60 years old is somehow 'over the hill.' Although people should not have to apologize for their age, all too often we act as though they should.

The Patient's View

The process of ageing, even for the most fortunate, involves loss. There are few compensations for growing old. The elderly often have to group themselves in clubs, holiday parties and in sheltered housing to avoid a society which is becoming increasingly 'gerontophobic'. The old person is not likely to share the negative view of his younger counterpart. He knows that although he has lost some of his abilities, many are still intact. He will also be acutely aware that many artists, writers, musicians and politicians do not seem to fail with age the way people expect him to do. The personality of the old person also *does not* change with age; we simply change in our attitude towards him. He knows that his mind has not 'gone' but he suspects that we think that it has. He knows that we tend to view him as a 'doddery old fool', of no use to anyone, dependent on others for his every need. We do not say explicitly but our actions may well communicate this. The patient may feel that he has awoken from a bad dream, only to find his youth gone, his abilities and faculties wasting and a host of strangers reinforcing his failing independence. The loss of dignity and self-respect, not to mention lost friendships, and the feeling that he is becoming a burden on his family or the State can produce feelings of depression, but it can also produce anger and resentment. He may resign himself to his fate, trying to deny these deeply felt emotions, or he may become irritable, picking fault with trivia rather than discuss the things which really bother him.

Environment

Finally, the patient's environment can also function as a factor in stimulating or maintaining the problem of hostility. The immediate physical environment may be a problem to him, he may: miss the newspapers he used to read; be unable to hear the television or radio; or be unable to have it turned off; he may find his chair or clothes uncomfortable; or find his diet unapppetizing or inadequate. Such 'everyday' problems can serve to frustrate the patient. As indicated above, he may fail to complain specifically about these problems, expressing his dissatisfaction in a more prolonged, and unsuccessful, fashion through the medium of hostility.

The staff routine is part of the social environment of the patient. For many patients the 'routine' may be the very core of their life, especially in an institutional setting. It is worth asking, 'For whose benefit does the routine operate?' Many routines satisfy the needs of the staff, in terms of the fulfilment of their duty, but may meet very few of the patients' needs. Although, inevitably, some compromise must be reached, you should be seen by the patient as working 'for him', rather than dealing with him almost as a by-product of the running of the ward. Only in this way can resentment be avoided.

PRINCIPLES OF CARE

The best approach to hostility is preventive; you should try to avoid the kind of problems already mentioned, or, at the very least, try to reduce their effects. The simplest way to ensure that the patient sees you as 'genuinely caring' is to discuss *all* aspects of his care with him, asking for his opinion and negotiating with him over any disagreements. On a longer term basis, try to help the patient come to terms with his frustrations or feelings of resentment and help to strengthen his self-esteem.

Discussion

If you suspect that the patient 'resents' being manipulated, or processed or generally treated like an object, then your goal is clear: *propose* certain ways of organizing his care and ask the patient for his comments, advice or criticisms. The nature of the response to this invitation will depend largely on the personality of the patient and his present level of ability to make such a contribution to his own care. However, through such an approach you are giving the patient some say in his own affairs, making him aware of everything which *might* happen to him, and capitalizing on his assets. The patient is not only being given an opportunity to comment on his care, he is also being treated with respect. If the patient is a former bank manager or a retired nurse, he may not take kindly to a very junior nurse planning every aspect of his daily life, especially the more personal aspects of it. You must gauge your 'approach' to this discussion on the basis of your assessment of the patient, judging how much responsibility you can give, or how much you can afford to relinquish.

Negotiation

The nurse cannot, however, hand over responsibility for his care to the patient. In many situations you can allow him to comment, and make suggestions, in others you may have to try to coax him into accepting something which is generally thought to be in his best interests. In such situations, if the patient is unhappy about 'being told what to do', then some compromise may be necessary, or nurse and patient may need to come to some 'contractual arrangement'.

If you suggest, for example, that the patient might take a walk, perhaps to help rehabilitate a leg following a fracture, you should *propose* this and await the patient's comment. 'Well John, how is the leg this morning? Do you think you could manage a walk out on to the terrace with me? The sun's not too hot yet.' If his response is negative, you should give him a *rationale* as to why you would like him to do this, whilst *acknowledging* his feelings. 'Yes, I can imagine that it is pretty stiff, but that's exactly why I would like you to exercise it a bit. I'm a bit worried that always sitting around will delay the recovery ... walking on it will help improve the circulation, and may actually help ease the pain a bit. What do you say?' If the patient is still resistant, you should try to *compromise,* beginning by reducing the target slightly. 'Well OK, maybe you feel that it's too early for walking outside, but how about just walking with me to the door of the ward and back? *(Smiles)* See I'm trying to meet you halfway'. If the patient still resists, you may need to 'do a deal with him'; arranging a kind of contract. 'OK John, you don't seem keen at all do you? But I must make it clear to you, the reason I want you to walk with me is for *your* health not mine. *(Smiles)* Do you remember the other day that I said I would help you paste some of those old photographs in your album? well what do you say we do that *after* we have been for a bit of a walk. *(Laughs)* OK, you can say I'm holding you to ransom, but I think that's a fair exchange. What do you say?'

It is important that the nurse remains firm, without sacrificing her sense of humour. In the example above the nurse compromised and then negotiated a 'fair exchange'; she did not take offence at the fact that John was being difficult, seeing this instead as a challenge to be resolved. She also acknowledged John's feelings throughout, making no attempt to deprive him of his reasons for refusing.

Expression of Anger

This chapter has taken the view that hostility may arise from unhappiness or dissatisfaction: this can lead to an undercurrent of anger which the patient may feel unable to express, 'bottling it up' and releasing only small amounts in the form of niggling, or uncooperativeness. Where this is the case you should try to encourage him to acknowledge his anger and to deal with it in more direct terms. Essentially, you are giving the patient the freedom to 'be angry', a liberty he may not allow himself at present. You should try to 'sell' him the idea that by *identifying* what angers him, you can help him to cope better with such frustrations. You will have to sell this concept, since the patient may believe that expressing anger is taboo.

Encouraging the patient to say 'what is on his mind' is rarely easy. He may claim that 'nothing is bothering me'. If you simply pursue the question, this may provoke further hostility. Instead you should take an example of a 'hostile incident' which has occurred recently, attempt to interpret the patient's feelings at the time and present this for discussion, with a view to changing the nature of the interaction.

You might say: 'John, you know when we were doing your exercises on your leg this morning, I got the impression that you weren't too happy. It's not like you to be so quiet. Would you like to tell me what was bothering you?' The patient may well resent this intrusion into 'his thinking' and react negatively. Or, he may simply say that nothing was bothering him. You may reply: 'I understand how you feel: you resent me reading your mind like that, but maybe there is something bugging you, and you think that you shouldn't talk about it. What I'm saying is, let's get it out into the open so that we can work together to solve it.' If the patient still does not show willingness to cooperate in this discussion, you can make some 'suggestions' about what might be troubling him, taking care not to threaten him further, or to make him feel that he is a bigger problem than he already thinks he is. 'You know, some of the men in here get pretty fed up with us nurses "bossing them around" as they say. I guess it's only natural. Many of them — like you — have been pretty independent all their lives. I suppose it's a bit frustrating to have things done for you, when you're so used to doing for yourself?' By trying to relate the patient's 'assumed problem' (resentment) to other patients, you are reducing the feeling in the patient that it is only he who is frustrated: you are giving his problem some kind of respectability. You can continue this 'modelling' approach by suggesting that the other men on the ward have found it useful to talk about their grumbles and grievances with staff, being able to sort out solutions. In some cases it may be appropriate to discuss such a problem with another patient, preferably one who has resolved a similar disagreement with staff himself.

Building Self-esteem

In a few cases the hostile attitudes of the patient may be typical of his fundamental personality: relatives may tell you on admission that, 'Dad has always been a difficult man', or that, 'you'd better watch Mum; she'll run you off your feet if you're not careful.' In such cases, beware of over-interpreting the patient's behaviour. However, in most cases the hostility expressed by the patient will be a form of coping strategy: he is unhappy or frustrated and needs to be helped to overcome such deep-seated emotional difficulties. (See Chapter 26 for a discussion of self-esteem.)

As we have discussed, the patient who is losing his faculties and who is 'in care' may not always share the same view of himself as his carers do. However, he will begin to reflect on his 'state of decay': especially in the care setting where he has a lot of time on his hands. If he begins to think that he is a burden on everyone, or that he is a nuisance, his self-esteem will be dealt a very serious blow; the stoical or authoritarian attitudes of staff will merely deepen his despair. In addition to helping the patient work out ways to get on better with his carers, staff should also be trying to help him to take a more positive view of himself. The patient is not a 'write-off'; there is still life in the old dog yet. Instead of concentrating all our attentions on solving his problems, giving him the message that he is 'all problems', we should try to capitalize on his assets. If the patient is encouraged to use what skills or aptitudes he has, he will receive some positive feedback, which will serve to raise his self-esteem. The staff should try to organize the patient's day so that it revolves around the experience of 'positive' experiences, rather than around the staff treatment of negative aspects of the patient.

PATIENT PROFILE

John is a 68-year-old man who has been in a home for the elderly for two months. He was admitted from a hostel for the mentally handicapped where he lived for ten years. Prior to this he spent all his life at home with his parents, and latterly his unmarried sister. John is probably only mildly mentally handicapped: he can read a little but his writing is poor and child-like. He worked for over 20 years as a gardener in a large mansion house near his home. He was transferred to the home for the elderly as a result of a deterioration in his physical condition, following a mild cerebrovascular accident. He has a very slight right-sided hemiplegia, which has handicapped his walking, and a moderate receptive and expressive dysphasia.

John has tried to maintain his independence since his admission, but has had numerous rows with the staff over being 'in the wrong place at the wrong time'. He has been reported as abusive although never physically aggressive. He also tends to 'sulk': refusing to get up in the morning and ignoring staff when they talk to him. He spends a lot of time just sitting looking out of the window into the gardens. Over the last two weeks he has refused to go to the physiotherapist for his exercises: on one occasion locking himself in a toilet cubicle.

ORGANIZATION OF NURSING CARE

Subjective Evidence (What the Patient Says)

- 'No, get away' (when approached by staff).
- 'Stupid, stupid' (when asked to participate in physiotherapy programme).
- 'I've not done nothing' (when he locked himself in toilet).

Objective Evidence (What the Nurse and Others Observe)

- Turns his head away when staff talk to him; is often silent for long periods; rarely initiates conversation except to express needs.
- Refuses to take medication (aperient); also refuses meals on occasions.
- Isolates himself from other patients.

Assessment (Nursing Diagnosis)

- John is hostile towards staff: this is probably related to his frustrations over loss of independence and occupational activity.

Plan of Nursing Care

- Encourage John to 'talk' about how he feels.
- Help him to communicate better through using a sign/symbol board.
- Provide him with some occupational activity, e.g. indoor gardening.
- Give him more information about what is going to happen to him, *well in advance,* along with a simple rationale.
- Where he is uncooperative, allow John time to 'come out of it': never reprimand him or take 'punitive' action.

Expected Outcome

- Will communicate more with staff about needs and feelings.
- Will spend more time in positive activity.
- Will be less resistant to engagement in routines.
- Will exhibit less incidence of hostility than previously.

NURSING CARE OF THE HOSTILE PATIENT
(EXAMPLE)

07.30 hours	Check that John is up, wish him a 'Good morning' and *invite* him to help you set the table for breakfast, after he has dressed.
08.15	During breakfast discuss briefly what you would like him to do that day: e.g. go to physiotherapy, see the psychologist.
09.00	Using the signing board as an aid, discuss in detail *why* you want him to do the physiotherapy: ask for his thoughts and feelings.
10.00	Encourage him to show another resident how to transfer potted plants.
11.00	Ask John to take *you* down to the physiotherapy room so that you can sit in on his session.
11.15	Ask him to explain to you how to do the exercises which the physiotherapist has shown him.
12.00	Invite him to tell the other men about his physiotherapy session using the sign board as an aid — nurse and other men translating.
12.45	At lunch ask what his plans are for the afternoon. Negotiate with him over going to see the psychologist to do 'more tests'.
13.30	Ask if he would like any help with writing a letter to his sister: use the session to discuss his feelings about being in a home. Encourage him to view this as another 'home' where he can settle down.
15.00	Prompt John to go to the office to meet the psychologist: ask him to give you a 'brief report' when he comes back.
16.30	Discuss with John his experiences at the psychology session. Encourage him to see such 'tests' as all part of a plan to make him more comfortable in the home.
17.30	Over tea ask what he would like to do at evening: give him a choice of games with the other men or some purposeful independent activity.
18.30	Spend 15 minutes reviewing his 'progress' since he entered the home. Emphasize all his 'gains' and invite his comments on his feelings at present.
19.30	Assist in game of Monopoly, acting as interpreter at John's invitation only. Use session as opportunity to let John show other men what the symbols on the sign board mean.
21.00	Ask John to help you prepare supper for other men — setting out cups and saucers on trays, etc.

21.30   Negotiate which programmes to watch on television before retiring. Attempt to 'strike a bargain' with him.

23.00   Check that John is ready for bed and that he does not feel hostile about retiring at this hour.

23.00–07.30 Monitor John's sleep at hourly intervals — recording same. If he is restless and awake, invite him to get up for a few minutes to discuss anything which is troubling him. Encourage him thereafter to plan to work through his problems, practically, the following day.

ASSESSMENT OF HOSTILITY

The first priority in assessment is to beware of surface behaviour, or superficial explanations. It is not enough merely to describe the patient's behaviour: we need to establish its meaning. What might be the purpose or *function* of his hostility: is it intended to gain more staff attention, less staff attention, is it intended to maintain his independence? The assessment should aim to project such 'explanations' or hypotheses, so that some change in these factors can be arranged, which might reduce the problem.

An appropriate starting point for the assessment might be the specific details of the patient's interaction with staff. What sort of things does he say and do in response to the behaviour of the nurse? Below is a very short transcript of an interaction between nurse and patient.

Nurse: 'Come on John, are you not up yet?'
Patient: 'You never get a minute's peace in this place.'
Nurse: 'What do you mean 'peace', everyone else is up. You're not the only patient here you know.'
Patient: 'Well if you're so damned busy then b..... off and leave me in peace.'
Nurse: 'Don't worry, I'm going but I'll be back in five minutes and I want to see you up.'
Patient: 'Get away you silly young fool.'

This exchange of 'unpleasanteries' can tell us a lot about the relationship between John and the nurse. He appears to resent the nurse telling him what to do. She appears to resent him wanting peace and quiet. John appears to become abusive in order to get rid of the nurse, and although she 'threatens' him she actually fulfils his wishes. It seems fairly certain that when they meet again, hostility will resume, if not increase.

The nurse needs also to look at the way John might be *interpreting* her behaviour. She should try to gauge what kind of message her 'caring behaviour' actually communicates. Perhaps John is thinking: 'I'm just upsetting that girl's routine . . . I'm just an old fool who can't look after himself . . . She thinks I should be grateful for what she does for me . . . She must think I'm awkward on purpose . . . she should be in my shoes.'

In addition to trying to clarify the 'meaning' of the hostility the assessment should clarify *where, when* and *with whom* it is a problem. Does John only 'cause trouble' in the morning, at night, at mealtimes or at bathtime? Might his hostility at these times have something to do with specific 'needs', for example for peace and quiet, which are not being fulfilled at these times? Are there any *situations* when he is more hostile than in others? Does he appear more irritable in the dining area, at the television, when he is alone or when he is with other patients? Perhaps he finds the noise of the dayroom unsettling, or perhaps he cannot hear the television, or is dissatisfied with his diet? If the patient can answer such a question, the simplest strategy is simply to ask him 'what do you not like about . . .' Finally, it is worth considering that the hostility may be specific to one member of staff, or, alternatively, that only one member of staff gets on well with him. In either case it is important to establish what that nurse does and says which produces this effect. Once this is established the other members can learn from her mistakes or from her 'example' of good practice.

It is also important to obtain some kind of record of 'hostility' so that an evaluation of any specific nursing plans can be made. The easiest way to do this is to record the frequency of 'hostile incidents' each day. The content of the measure depends upon what sort of things the patient does or says, which are viewed as hostile. They might include: swearing at staff; refusing to take medication or meals; refusing to talk, go to the bath, or go to bed or get up. A simple checklist, covering all the kinds of things which he usually does, can be used to provide a general measure of 'hostility', represented by a rough frequency record of how many times he did each of these things in one day. This kind of record, if maintained each day, will provide a measure *across time* of the patient's progress or regression.

Two other points are worth mentioning on the subject of assessment. First, hostility can be a sign of another problem. Before you spend much valuable time studying the problem in the manner indicated, you should consider this seriously. Williamson (1978) suggests that the 'unlikeable patient', who may exhaust and exasperate staff and make himself very unpopular, may be suffering from a depressive disorder. Secondly, the assessment, if it is to come up with any kind of *positive plan,* should look beyond the patient's problematic side. As Davies and Crisp (1980) suggest, the assessment should emphasize his assets as well. Perhaps the best way to help the patient overcome such a problem might be by encouraging him to maintain his present level of capability and help him to continue to develop. This has often been referred to as a 'constructional approach' (Fleming *et al.* 1983).

SUMMARY

In this chapter we have discussed 'hostility' as arising out of interpersonal difficulties, especially in situations where the elderly person feels restricted in opportunity or denied status which they held prior to coming into care. Staff should attempt to encourage an atmosphere of cooperation: one which reduces the 'us and them' character of much nurse-patient interaction. The patient should be given an opportunity to participate in his own care, and also to realize that, on occasions, compromise is necessary. In general, the team should encourage the patient to maintain his independence through use of a positive 'constructional' approach.

REFERENCES

Davies A.D.M. & Crisp A.G. (1980) Setting performance goals in geriatric nursing. *Journal of advanced Nursing* **5**, 581–8.

Fleming I., Barrowclough C. & Whitmore B. (1983). The constructional approach. *Nursing Mirror* **156**, 21–3.

Gasek G. (1980) How to handle the crotchety elderly patient. *Nursing* **80**, 46–8.

Hemsi L. (1982) Psychogeriatric care in the community. In Levy R. & Post F. (eds) *The Psychiatry of Late Life*. Blackwell Scientific Publications, Oxford.

Pfeiffer E. (1976) Psychotherapy with elderly patients. In Bellak L. & Karasov T.B. (eds) *Geriatric Pyschiatry*. Grune and Stratton, New York.

Williamson J. (1978) Depression in the elderly. *Age & Ageing* **7**, 35–40.

FURTHER READING

MIND (1979) *Mental Health of Elderly People*. Mind, London.

Schow R.L., Christensen J.M., Hutchinson J.M. & Nerbonne M.A. (1978) *Communication Disorders of the Aged: A Guide for Health Professionals*. University Park Press, Baltimore.

Wisocki P.A. & Mosher P.M. (1980) Peer-facilitated sign language training for a geriatric stroke victim with chronic brain damage. *Journal of Geriatric Psychiatry* **13**, 89–102.

Chapter 20
Hydration

Hydration is a word that is used rather loosely by nurses. Literally it means the union of a substance with water; as used by nurses and others it is used to mean that there is a normal volume of water in the body. It follows, therefore, that dehydration refers to a decrease in water volume. The term is often used synonymously with hypovolaemia. Hypovolaemia refers to a deficiency mainly in the extracellular fluid volume (ECFV), the intracellular fluid volume (ICFV) often being near normal. It is quite possible for someone to have an ECFV (water) deficit that is hypovolaemia. This can occur because of inadequate water intake, or excessive sweating. More often, however, the problem is more complex as other solute levels are also disturbed. This is especially so with conditions such as vomiting and diarrhoea. Under normal circumstances fluid and electrolyte problems are very rare. Indeed most of us never give the problem a thought, no more than we think of breathing. The body has indeed a very remarkable ability to maintain fluid and electrolyte homeostasis. However, normality falls within a relatively small range in many instances, and in some pathological conditions can lead to serious disturbances of homeostasis in a very short time. This is especially so in the older person whose adaptive capacity is reduced and less responsive than that of younger persons. This will be discussed in greater detail later (see pp. 240–1). First we will look briefly at the normal control of fluid and electrolyte balance in the body.

FACTORS RELATING TO HYDRATION

This section looks briefly at normal fluid balance, how it is maintained and the problems the elderly person has in maintaining homeostasis.

Maintenance of Fluid Balance

The problem of maintaining fluid balance within the body is a formidable one. Just think what the body has to cope with. Each day we ingest a wide variety of materials in various quantities. These materials will seldom, if ever, exactly match the body's needs; for example, if someone drinks 3 l of beer he will have an excess of fluid in his body, on the other hand, if someone is working in a very hot environment, for example, an iron foundry, he may lose 3 l of fluid during the course of a shift and have a fluid deficit. In the first case the body fluids will be diluted and the osmotic pressure of the body fluids will be decreased. In the other example the volume of body fluids will be concentrated and the osmotic pressure increased. How does the body overcome these two quite different problems? The body has osmoreceptors which detect changes in the osmolality of the body fluids. These osmoreceptors are located in the hypothalamus in the brain and, when stimulated, indirectly stimulate the posterior lobe of the pituitary gland to produce or cease production of a hormone called vasopressin or antidiuretic hormone (ADH). ADH acts on the kidney tubules by altering their permeability. In the first case mentioned above, there is an excess of fluid and the body wants to get rid of it, therefore, the supply of ADH is cut off and the kidney then passes a very dilute urine. In the other case mentioned, the body needs to conserve body fluids and in this circumstance large amounts of ADH are required to prevent fluid loss and the kidneys pass a very concentrated urine. The kidney has indeed a remarkable ability to alter the concentration of urine in its effort to maintain fluid and electrolyte homeostasis. In the healthy adult under 45 years of age the kidney can concentrate urine up to four times that of the plasma whilst, if the need is to dispose of water, it can produce urine which is only one-tenth the concentration of plasma.

The second important mechanism is the regulation of salts, in particular sodium, potassium and chloride. This is achieved by the actions of yet another hormone on the kidney, namely aldosterone. Aldosterone is produced by the cortex of the adrenal gland and increases the reabsorption of sodium by the kidney tubule. Receptors in the kidney detect changes in salt concentrations and, if low, respond by producing renin, which is converted to angiotensin. This substance acts on the adrenal cortex stimulating it to produce aldosterone. If sodium levels are low, the kidney conserves it, and if high, more is passed in the urine. The kidneys, therefore play a key role in maintaining fluid balance.

FLUID BALANCE

In the normal, healthy individual, whether young or old, fluid intake and output are approximately equal as shown in Table 20.1.

When monitoring fluid intake and output in a ward it is usually fluids in the form of water and beverages which are calculated, whatever the route they are given by. Similarly, in measuring output it is usually urine which is measured and, when appropriate, vomitus, loose stools and drainage are

Table 20.1 Daily fluid balance.

Fluid sources	ml	Fluid losses	ml
Ingested water	1200 – 1500	Urine	1200 – 1700
Ingested food	700 – 1000	Faeces	100 – 250
Metabolic oxidation	200 – 400	Perspiration	100 – 150
		Insensible losses	
		Skin	350 – 400
		Lungs	350 – 400
TOTAL	2100 – 2900		2100 – 2900

estimated. Fluids ingested in food or lost as insensible loss are often ignored, as it is almost impossible to estimate them accurately, and for nearly all practical purposes it is unnecessary. Solid food varies enormously in its fluid content ranging from 4% to 98%. In the course of metabolism each gram of carbohydrate yields 0.6 ml of water, each gram of fat 1.07 ml and each gram of protein 0.41 ml. The sort of food eaten is, therefore important in fluid balance especially in some pathological states such as renal failure. A useful guide for estimating daily water requirements is to allow 1 ml of water for each calorie consumed, the amount of water produced from beverages, solid food and metabolism being included.

Intake of fluids is largely governed by thirst. However, thirst is a subjective phenomenon, with both physical and psychological influences, and is very poorly understood.

As far as output is concerned, the ambient conditions, person's temperature and activity levels are important influences as can be seen in Table 20.2.

It can be seen from the table that elevations of temperature and prolonged active exercise lead to a marked increase in the loss of body fluids.

Table 20.2 Daily fluid losses in ml under different conditions.

Exit route	Normal body temperature	Elevated body temperature	Prolonged increased physical exercise
Urine	1400	1200	500
Faeces	200	200	200
Perspiration	100	1400	5000
Insensible loss			
Skin	350	350	350
Lungs	350	250	650
TOTAL	2400	3400	6700

Another important consideration in fluid balance is the changing ratio of solids to fluids in the body as people get older. Table 20.3 shows that the average percentages of water in relation to bodyweight in persons of different ages vary within the various water compartments of the body.

Table 20.3   Variations in fluids as a percentage of body weight by age.

	Ages			
			Adult	
Water compartment	Infant	Male	Female	Elderly
Extracellular				
(intravascular)	4	4	5	5
Interstitial	25	11	10	15
Intracellular	48	45	35	25
TOTAL (%)	77	60	50	45

It can be be seen from Table 20.3 that the young and the old are both extremely vulnerable to changes in fluid balance. The amount of water in the body as a percentage of bodyweight is low in people who are obese, so that in calculations of body fluids, 'lean body weight' is used.

The Effects of Ageing on Homeostasis

Early in adult life in both animals and in man there is a steady decline in homeostasis and organ reserve in many vital systems. This is very evident in the kidney and not much can be done about it. It is one of those non-modifiable aspects of ageing like greying hair and skin wrinkles. However, because we start off with such an enormous reserve kidney function, the ageing kidney can maintain homeostasis. There is, however, decreasing capacity for adaptation and decreasing ability to maintain homeostasis especially in the face of internal and/or external stress.

At birth, the kidneys are not fully mature and have not the capacity to handle excess loads of fluids, or salts in particular. The kidneys, however, grow rapidly and by early adult life reach their maximum size. Each kidney has in the region of one million nephrons. Anatomical studies show that the kidney loses mass at a fairly steady rate, a rate that increases markedly after the age of 50 years. The studies show that whole nephron units are lost. Other changes include the development of longitudinal muscle in the renal veins, which is generally accepted as a marker of ageing. There are also changes in the basement membrane which becomes thickened. From 40 years of age onwards, there is also an increase in the quantity of connective tissue. These, along with other changes, account for the very significant loss of concentrating ability in the old kidney.

Kidney weight remains stable up to the age of about 40 years and then progressively decreases. By the age of 80 years the renal mass is 30% less than the adult volume. Also, and perhaps more significantly, renal perfusion is only some 50% of that of the young adult.

In older persons, levels of ADH are normal or may even be slightly increased. However, the nephron tubules are less responsive to ADH so that the old kidney can no longer concentrate the urine to the same extent as the young. The old person can only concentrate urine to less than three times that of plasma, instead of the usual four times. This means the elderly are slower to adapt to the need to conserve fluid whatever the reason may be. The old person is also less able to deal with the challenge of excess water. The old kidney is less able to dilute urine, compared with the young kidney and minimum osmolality remains near that of plasma. This is because the kidney is less able to recover salts from the filtrate. Excretion of a water load is therefore slow, because of the low glomerular filtration, whilst also expensive in terms of salt lost. As a rule it takes the older person more time to restore the balance to normal, though given time, the kidneys will do that. Levels of aldosterone are slightly lower in older people, perhaps accounting for some of the failure adequately to recover electrolytes.

There is no real evidence that the sensation of thirst in the old person is lessened. The problem is more often physical such as difficulty in obtaining and drinking fluids. Also, some elderly people who are troubled by incontinence may deliberately restrict their fluid intake in the mistaken belief that it will alleviate the problem. Others may be troubled by vomiting or dysphagia for varied reasons. The older person's acuity for salt is often reduced, as are taste sensations in general, they then increase their salt intake in an effort to satisfy their taste. An increased salt intake without a corresponding intake in water leads to dehydration and hyperosmolarity as opposed to salt depletion and hypotonicity. In conditions such as congestive heart failure, poor renal perfusion causes as increase in renin-angiotensin aldosterone activity, so that more salt and water is absorbed, resulting in oedema, especially oedema of the lungs and dependent oedema.

PRINCIPLES OF CARE

Creating the Right Climate

It often requires considerable ingenuity and patience on the part of nursing staff to persuade the elderly person to drink enough. The emphasis should always be on 'drinking' enough. Letting the patient drink the fluids he requires by himself is by far the best approach; it gives the patient some say in the choice of fluids, and even how much he wants to drink at a particular time.

Fluids need to be varied; find out the patient's likes and dislikes. Many elderly people are fond of tea and less fond of coffee, however, avoid giving too much beverage of this kind as it does tend to keep people awake at night so that there may then be a tendency to sleep during the day. Once this tendency develops, day and night seem to become somewhat confused. Encourage the patient's relatives to bring in drinks the patient likes. Lemonade can be made more enticing by adding a slice of fresh lemon and a few ice cubes, as can many other drinks such as cola. A glass of stout, beer or a lemonade shandy in the company of others over a game of dominoes or cards can aid communication and hydration. Eating and drinking are both very social activities and every opportunity should be taken to make the taking of fluids interesting and enjoyable.

Several foods contain a lot of fluid and can be a very good source of this. Many elderly people will enjoy a fresh fruit salad but be reluctant to eat fruit otherwise. In the ward situation patients will usually agree, if approached, to share their fruit in a fruit salad: very refreshing in the mid-afternoon after some activity! Jellies, ice-cream, junket and so on are all good sources of fluid and may be far more acceptable than yet another drink of fruit squash. When making up fruit squash drinks, use *fresh, cold* water. In hot weather a few ice cubes will help to keep the drink cool longer. A few slices of fresh orange add a bit of flavour and interest. Most people, including the elderly, prefer aerated soft drinks; they need not be all that expensive if a home dispenser is used, such as the Soda Stream. They are easy to use and, if placed strategically, patients can make up their own drinks whenever possible. Wards should also have other convenient outlets so that drinks are readily available and not simply supplied as part of the routine. Bedfast patients require a fresh supply of water 3 or 4 times per day, and the assistance to ensure they actually drink it; it is of little value decorating a locker top.

Should the person, in spite of every effort being made, not be able to drink enough fluid then some alternative means has to be devised. If possible the gastrointestinal tract should be used, the usual method being a nasogastric tube. Few elderly people like this method of giving fluids and it should only be used when attempts to persuade the patient to drink have failed. If the patient is unconscious, or unable to swallow for some other reason, then fluids and food via a nasogastric tube are often the only alternative.

If the gastrointestinal tract is not serviceable, then fluids will have to be given by intravenous infusion. This requires very great care in the elderly as fluid overload can be most serious, resulting in cardiac failure and pulmonary oedema. On many occasions giving fluid by the intravenous route is unavoidable. Provided care is taken, however, this can be life saving. The introduction of intravenous pumps of various kinds has made this procedure much safer for the elderly.

PATIENT PROFILE

Mrs Maria Pelosi, a 74-year-old lady of Italian origin, had been receiving treatment for heart failure for many years. She generally visited her doctor every three months for a check-up and renewal of her prescription. Her usual medication was digoxin 0.25 mg daily (Mon. to Fri.), frusemide 40 mg daily (Mon., Wed. and Fri.), Slow K (potassium 1200 mg Tues., Thurs. and Sat.). For reasons which are completely unknown Mrs Pelosi mixed her medications up completely . She consumed an excess of frusemide over what was thought to be a three-week period, without taking her potassium or digoxin.

Mrs Pelosi lived alone and was normally visited each week by her daughter. The daughter, for personal reasons, had to miss her visit one week and on her next visit found her mother far from well and called the doctor. The doctor suspected Mrs Pelosi had suffered a stroke and arranged for immediate admission to hospital. He was unaware at this time that she had mixed up her medication. On admission to hospital Mrs Pelosi was noted to be very thin and her skin and mucous membranes were very dry. Her muscles were very flaccid and she was virtually unable to move. She had difficulty in speaking, her speech being slurred. Her pulse was rapid, thready and irregular, suggestive of atrial fibrillation. This was confirmed by the electrocardiogram which showed inversion of the 'T' waves. The admitting doctor made a provisional diagnosis of hypokalaemia and atrial fibrillation due to wrong drug therapy. The hypokalaemia was confirmed by blood analysis. As she was elderly and in heart failure the doctor decided against an i.v. infusion and prescribed oral effervescent potassium and suggested a minimum of 150 ml of fluid hourly. He also prescribed therapy for her cardiac condition. The doctor's main concern was whether Mrs Pelosi had a degree of paralytic ileus. He asked to be kept informed if she complained of nausea and/or vomiting.

ORGANIZATION OF NURSING CARE

Subjective Evidence (What the Patient Says)

- 'I feel so weak.'
- 'Nurse, I am very thirsty.'
- 'My tongue feels like a piece of cork.'

Objective Evidence (What the Nurse and Others Observe)

- Skin and mucous membranes very dry.
- Urinary output scanty; 30 ml per hour.
- Pulse 120 beats per minute and irregular.

Assessment (Nursing Diagnosis)

- Extreme dehydration due to a mistake in taking her medication.

Plan of Nursing Care

GENERAL AIM

- To restore body fluid to normal.

NURSING ACTIONS

- Encourage patient to take at least 150 ml of fluids hourly.
- Give potassium supplement and other medication as prescribed.
- Weigh patient at start of therapy if possible and then 24-hourly until weight regained.
- Monitor urinary output hourly, if less than 30 ml/hour inform medical staff.
- Four-hourly temperature, pulse respirations and blood pressure.
- Two- to four-hourly oral hygiene.
- All general nursing care.

Expected Outcome

- Patients urinary output at least 60 ml/h within 48 h.
- Patient's skin and mucous membranes pink and moist.
- Patient able to perform basic activities of daily living.

POSTSCRIPT

Mrs Pelosi recovered within 48 h and, although still weak, was able to be up and caring for herself once more. Her drug regimen was simplified before her discharge in the hope that she would not get it mixed up in future. Had her daughter not visited on the day she did, the outcome might have been very different.

NURSING CARE OF A PATIENT WITH A
HYDRATION PROBLEM* (EXAMPLE)

06.30 hours	Early morning cup of tea (150-210 ml).
07.30	Encourage patient to take more fluid (100-150 ml).
08.30	Add up intake and output over previous 24 h. On the basis of this, calculate amount of fluid the patient will require over the next 24 h. If intake and output are below target set for previous 24 h, try to establish why. Discuss with patient and set new target. Calculate hourly fluids to be given over a 16 h period; for example, a 2000 ml intake calls for 125 ml/h. Arrange for 100-150 ml/h, or more.

08.00	Breakfast —Fruit juice 100 ml
	            —Milk in cereal 100 ml
	            —Tea or coffee 150 ml

09.00	Encourage patient to take fluid of choice (100–150 ml).
10.00	Mid–morning break. Bovril or other beverage (100–150ml).
11.00	Encourage to take fluid of choice (100–150ml).
12.00	Lunch—Soup 150 ml —Milk 150 ml Also if desired, ensure foods high in fluids, e.g. jellies and junkets.
13.00	Encourage fluid of choice (100–150 ml).
14.00	Mid–afternoon break. Tea (100–150 ml).
15.00	Encourage fluid of choice (100–150 ml).
16.00	Encourage fluid of choice (100–150 ml).
18.00	Dinner—Fruit juices (150 ml).
19.00	Fluid of choice—lemonade shandy in company of others enjoying the same (300 ml).
21.00	Nightcap. Drinking chocolate, Ovaltine, Horlicks (150 ml).
22.00	Encourage last drink before settling (100–150 ml). The patient need not be disturbed during the night to take fluids. Should the patient waken encourage him to take fluid if desired. (100 ml). Add up totals at same time each day. Total over 24 h = 2150–2550 ml

Once fully hydrated the urinary output should equal the fluid intake, more or less. It will never, or rarely, match exactly each day but should average out.

---

*Before and after discharge this patient was involved in an intensive and long-term educational/monitoring programme which minimized the possibility of a recurrence of the accidental medication errors.

ASSESSMENT OF HYDRATION STATUS

A perusal of many of the standard nursing and medical textbooks often presents the reader with formidable lists of clinical features which may be expected in fluid and electrolyte imbalance. Apart from being difficult to memorize they are often not very realistic when assessing the elderly person. Where the variation from normal is severe, there is usually not much of a problem; for example, extreme dehydration is evidenced by dryness of the skin and mucous membranes, scanty viscous saliva, sunken eyes, poor cell turgor as evidenced by slow recovery to normal when the skin is pinched, scanty output of dark-coloured urine, constipation and possible mental confusion. At the other extreme, gross oedema may be evident especially in the dependent parts: ankles; sacrum, scrotum; and also, sometimes, in the fingers and eyelids. It is worth remembering that dependent oedema does not become evident until the person has retained up to 5 l of fluid. However, in between it may be much more difficult to detect disturbances, and no one single feature or symptom in itself is necessarily indicative of fluid imbalance. It is important not to rely too much on a single observation. It is far better to observe the person over a period of days and look for changes which have taken place. Be as objective as possible, that is, whenever possible make measurements.

Tissue Characteristics

- Dryness of skin and mucous membranes.
- Little or no saliva which may be viscous.
- Sunken eyes.
- Turgor—when skin is pinched it only very slowly returns to normal.
- Excess fluids—pitting oedema.
- Poor muscle tone.

Behavioural Changes

These vary extensively but include:
- disorientation;
- confusion;
- irritability;
- hallucinations;
- lethargy;
- changes in conscious level;
- personality changes;
- extreme thirst;

- reserved, withdrawn;
- hyperactive, talkative.

Any change in behaviour is significant, with the emphasis on change. Of course, fluid and electrolyte imbalance may not be the only cause; beware of urinary tract infections, fever, transient ischaemic attacks and so on.

Specific Measurements (Nursing)

- Temperature—hyper-, or hypo-thermia.
- Respiration—rate and depth.
- Pulse—rate, rhythm.
- Blood pressure—hyper, or hypo-tension.
- Weight loss—any sudden loss or gain (a 1 kg weight gain is equal to 1 l of fluid).
- Peripheral vein filling.
- Intake/output chart.

Laboratory

- Urinalysis—including specific gravity.
- Osmolality of urine and blood.
- Haematocrit.
- Blood urea and electrolytes.
- Plasma proteins.

Questions to Ask

- Has the patient stopped taking fluids?
- Have there been any restrictions on the patient's intake for any reason?
- Has the patient been losing fluids abnormally, for example diarrhoea, vomiting or fistula?
- What is the patient's fluid intake and output?
- Has anyone reported that they have found a change in the person?

Nurses who are in contact with the patient each day may not notice slow insidious changes. Being alert to changes is a very important part of monitoring the patient's fluid status. This is especially so with the elderly whose normal physiological functioning is not as efficient as in younger persons.

Elderly Patients Particularly at Risk

Although all the elderly are at risk of dehydration, some are more so than others. These include elderly persons who:

- are undergoing surgery;
- have dysphagia;
- are nauseated and/or vomiting;
- have been injured; are pyrexial;
- have heart disease/failure;
- have respiratory disease/failure;
- have a stoma;
- are confused;
- are depressed;
- are demented;
- have impaired consciousness;
- are physically handicapped;
- have diabetes;
- are bedfast.

These are some of the main patients who are especially at risk and for whom extra vigilance is required.

FURTHER READING

Bowles L., Portnoi V. & Kenny R. (1981) Wear and tear: Common biologic changes of aging, *Geriatrics* **36,** 77–80.

Howells E.M. (1977) Managing fluids and electrolytes in surgical patients. *Geriatrics* **32,** 100–1.

Kenny R.A. (1982) *Physiology of Aging,* Year book Medical Publishers, Chicago.

Luker K. (1980) The elderly. *Nursing (Oxford)* 1st series, No. 13 May.

Maxwell M.B. (1982) Pedal oedema in the cancer patient. *American Journal of Nursing* **82,** (8), 1225–8.

Parsons V. (1976) What decreasing renal function means to ageing patients. *Geriatrics* **32,** 93.

Ramos L. Y. (1981) Oral hygiene for the elderly. *American Journal of Nursing* **81,** 1468–9.

Travenol Laboratories, Inc. (1967) *The Fundamentals of Body Water and Elecrolytes.* Deerfield, Illinois.

Wear J.B. (1975) Solving selected problems of the ageing urinary tract. *Postgraduate Medicine* **58,** 179–86.

Chapter 21
Nutrition

Nutrition is the term used to describe the whole process of taking in and using food, with all body cells requiring nourishment. An essential substance is water by which the fluid balance is maintained. Indeed, one suffers more acutely more quickly from lack of fluid than food. It is commonly held that 2 l is needed in 24 h, with very few elderly people, however, taking this amount. (See Chapter 20 for a full discussion of hydration.)

The problems of nutrition are varied and generally have interrelated causes. The major difficulty in the Third World, which is shared by those in the affluent West who are poverty stricken, is that of insufficient protein and calories. Conversely, where there is affluence, then the major problem is of an over-abundance of calories, and choosing a truly nutritiously balanced diet that does not provide too many calories is a real difficulty. Additionally, eating is a highly symbolic activity which is influenced by ethnic, religious and family habits.

Water, and also carbohydrates, proteins, fats, vitamins and minerals, are needed to give energy, build and repair tissue and play an important part in the production of enzymes and hormones. By ingestion and digestion, the blood and lymphatic system can absorb the nutrients in an appropriate form and carry them to the various parts of the body. Digestion involves breaking down the food mechanically by chewing, by intestinal movement and by being mixed with secretions in the mouth and gastrointestinal tract. Along the whole length of the gastrointestinal tract nutrients are absorbed, leaving waste products to be eliminated. This property of the gastrointestinal tract has been exploited by drug companies so that drugs are put inside various coatings which can determine how long after ingestion the drug will be released.

Research has shown that there are many nutritional needs, though this is still a young science; for example, vitamins are still being discovered. It is known what number of calories are needed for our energy requirements, though these vary with individuals according to their size, shape, age, activity and the weather. The various constituents found in food which a person requires to keep healthy have been cited and will be discussed below. However, as a rule of thumb, though unscientific since an individual view of a serving can vary, the following servings from the major food groups would supply a balanced diet: milk and milk products, two servings; meat or fish, poultry, eggs and cheese, two servings; vegetables and fruit, four servings; and bread and cereals, four servings.

Calories

A calorie is the amount of heat necessary to raise the temperature of 1 g of water 1°C. Foods can provide a specific amount of heat to the body and therefore a stated amount of that food will 'contain' a certain number of calories. Some nutritionists use the kiloJoule (kJ; heat units) as a measurement of food intake but since the public is more accustomed to talk of calories, it is probably an easier unit to use, both for nurse and patient.

The lowest level of bodily activity and biochemistry is called the basal metabolic rate. Naturally, with the general activities undertaken for much of the day the body operates at a level well above the basal metabolic rate (BMR). Therefore, the intake of calories must take account of this, as well as height, weight and sex of the individual, but this intake diminishes with age.

Protein

Compounds like haemoglobin, hormones, enzymes, as well as albumin, globulin and fibrinogen, the proteins in plasma, all necessary for repairing tissue require protein for their composition or maintenance. Protein is broken down into amino acids during digestion and is thus available to become human protein in the body. The ability of people to recover after suffering from a protein deficiency is poor—the perennial problem of the Third World. Since 1 g of protein supplies four calories, it can be an important factor in planning a balanced diet, that is not using too many calories. However, one of the problems for an elderly person buying protein in the form of meat can be the inability to find a butcher who will sell small portions to suit a single person. Additionally, meat, fish, poultry, eggs and cheese are expensive and many old people do not have the financial resources to buy such food without much thought about the cost. These are elements that must be kept in mind when giving advice to elderly people about diet. Bread contains some protein and it is claimed that some elderly people obtain about 20% of their protein intake from bread.

SOURCES OF PROTEIN

Animal protein such as meat, fish, cheese, eggs and milk; vegetable protein such as green peas, lentils, peanuts, baked beans.

Fat

Each gram of fat provides nine calories and so is the body's most concentrated form of energy. Fat is the source of fatty acids and carries fat-soluble vitamins; it also prevents the skin from allowing excessive evaporation or absorption of water as well as being important in the formation of hormones. However, perhaps its most important function is making a large part of our diet palatable. Most people find trying to adopt and persevere with a fat-free diet very difficult. As far as cost goes, fats fall between proteins and carbohydrates. Though adipose tissue provides insulation to the body and protection for internal organs, it is the accessibility, the high calorie content and the pleasure that fat provides which is a disadvantage to those who tend to be overweight.

SOURCES OF FAT

Butter, meat, milk, some fish, lard, vegetable oils and nut oils when converted into margarine.

Carbohydrates

Like protein, each gram of carbohydrate provides four calories. Cellulose consists of large molecules of carbohydrate which cannot be split and pass unaltered into the alimentary tract to provide bulk for digestion and elimination. Without the presence of carbohydrate, fat cannot be metabolized because its by-products accumulate: hence we put butter on bread and fry potatoes. From milk, we are provided with lactose which promotes bacterial growth in the intestines; without bacteria, digestion and elimination would be interfered with.

Granulated sugar is pure carbohydrate. When the body is provided with extra carbohydrate, it can be stored and used later. Indeed, it can be changed into body fat, that is to say, adipose tissue. This explains why, in common thinking, carbohydrate is associated with being overweight. However, it is the cheapest form of food and so the primary source of calorie intake. It is readily accessible, often does not need to be cooked and is easily served.

SOURCES OF CARBOHYDRATE

Fruit, sugar, potatoes, flour, bread, rice.

Vitamins

Vitamins, though not important in the calorie count, are fundamental to various processes which keep the body healthy. They must be ingested since they cannot be manufactured by the body. The only exception is vitamin D, which is formed in the skin by being exposed to sunlight. Table 21.1 shows the vitamins, their sources and main functions. It should be noted that vitamin C is the most readily destroyed, for example by overcooking vegetables. Flour is an example of a range of foods which have vitamins added to them.

Table 21.1   Vitamins: their sources and main functions.

Vitamin	Main functions	Sources
A—fat-soluble	Growth of body cells Vision, hair and skin, and integrity of epithelial membranes	Butter, cheese Fish liver oil and liver Fish
B_1 (thiamine)—water-soluble	Carbohydrate metabolism Functioning of nervous system Normal digestion	Lean meat and poulty Milk Whole grain cereals
B_2 (riboflavin)—water-soluble	Formation of certain enzymes Normal growth Light adaptation in the eyes	Eggs Liver, kidneys Milk
B_3 (niacin)—water-soluble	Carbohydrate, fat and protein metabolism Enzyme component Prevents appetite loss	Lean meat and liver Whole grain cereals Yeast
B_6 (pyridoxine)—water-soluble	Healthy gums and teeth Red blood cell formation Carbohydrate, fat and protein metabolism	Whole grain cereals and wheat germ Yeast Meat
B_{12} (cyanocobalamin)—water-soluble	Protein metabolism Red blood cell formation Healthy nervous system tissues Prevents pernicious anaemia	Liver and kidney Dairy products, cheese Lean meat Milk Fish

Vitamin	Main functions	Sources
B$_c$ (folic acid)	Protein metabolism Red blood cell formation Normal intestinal tract functioning	Green leafy vegetables
C (ascorbic acid)—water-soluble	Healthy bones, teeth and gums Formation of blood vessels and capillary walls Proper tissue and bone healing Facilitates iron and folic acid absorption	Citrus fruits and juices Tomato Soft fruit Cabbage Green vegetables Potatoes
D—fat-soluble	Absorption of calcium and phosphorus	Fish Milk Eggs Margarine Formed in the skin by exposure to sunlight
E (alpha tocopherol)—fat-soluble	Red blood cell formation Protects essential fatty acids	Green leafy vegetables Wheat germ oil Margarine Rice
H (biotin)—water-soluble	Enzyme activity Metabolism of carbohydrates, fats, and proteins	Egg yolk Green vegetables Milk Liver and kidney
K—fat-soluble	Production of prothrombin	Green leafy vegetables

Minerals

The well-balanced diet will provide a goodly supply of minerals. Perhaps the most commonly known mineral is calcium which occurs generally in the body since it is a structural component of bone. In the elderly, its deficiency, osteoporosis, is fairly common, which results in the bones being brittle with changes occurring that are detectable radiologically. In this country, salt has iodine added since there are areas where iodine does not occur naturally; for example, enlarged thyroid used to be called 'Derby Neck' because the low incidence of iodine occurring naturally in Derbyshire meant that the incidence of the condition in the population was abnormally high. Table 21.2 shows the minerals, their sources and main functions. A variety of sources which give much fuller information about various foods, their contents and their value are available, see, for example, the *Manual of Nutrition* (MAFF 1981).

Table 21.2 Minerals: Their sources and main functions.

Mineral	Main functions	Sources
Calcium	Formation of teeth and bones Neuromuscular activity Blood coagulation Cell wall permeability	Milk products Cheese
Phosphorus	Buffering action Formation of bones and teeth	Eggs Meat Milk
Iodine	Regulation of body metabolism Promotes normal growth	Seafoods Iodized salt
Iron	Component of haemoglobin Assists cellular oxidation	Liver Eggs Meat Green leafy vegetables Fish Wholemeal flour and bread
Magnesium	Neuromuscular activity Activation of enzymes	Whole grains Milk Meat
Zinc	Constituent of enzymes and insulin	Seafoods Liver

Clearly, how the elderly fit into all this has been a matter of concern for a long time, see, for example, DHSS (1972). In the White Paper presented to Parliament in 1981, the Secretaries of State felt that there was need to draw the attention of the community at large and the elderly, in particular, to the possibilities and remedies of malnutrition (DHSS 1981).In Copp (1981) the fact that very little research has been done into the effects of early eating habits on old age is bemoaned. Indeed, this may be a sensible approach for further investigation.

FACTORS RELATED TO NUTRITION

Social Factors

For almost all people, retirement brings with it a drop in income. With increasing age this can be a particularly sensitive subject. There are many old people on fixed incomes who are much too proud to take, for example, Supplementary Benefit, thinking of it as charity. This has implications on what they can afford to buy and for the quality of their nutrition, and is allied, at present, with the difficulty of finding grocers and butchers who will sell small portions.

With increasing years there are often changes in marital status, such as widowhood, or perhaps where one partner requires long-term care. This situation may mean that a man may be left to cope on his own without ever having cooked for himself, or the pleasure derived from cooking will have gone if food is being prepared for only one person. Many people will never have learned what a balanced diet is, or the temptation to spend a lot of time in the pub for company may also result in a lot of 'empty' calories being taken in as well as a diminished appetite.

Factors Related to Eating

Many older people experience a diminution in the sense of smell and taste, which, of course, makes food insipid. The tendency to add excessive salt is a real one which can cause fluid imbalance and hypertension. (See Chapter 20 for a discussion of hydration.)

Older people seem to experience the feeling of being 'full' at a much earlier stage than in their younger years, so that the cycle of feeling empty which is responded to by eating comes sooner. This, in effect, means that the elderly like little and often.

The gut in the elderly tends to be less active, causing persistent constipation which many sufferers respond to with the constant use of aperients. In fact, an increase in the intake of fluids and/or cellulose in fruit and vegetables or bran would solve this problem more appropriately.

It is important to remember the action of drugs; some, for example, lead to dryness in the mouth, while others are not absorbed from the gut in the presence of bran. Obesity in the elderly can make them predisposed to diabetes.

PRINCIPLES OF CARE

Strategies to Ensure Nutrition

The district nurse or health visitor may have one of the most important roles to play in ensuring good nutrition, namely that of education. Work on the nutritional education required by the elderly is described by Holdsworth and Davies (1982) and, contrary to popular opinion, it is possible to persuade elderly people to alter their dietary habits as shown by Barr *et al.* (1982). It may well fall to the community nurse to ensure that the newly diagnosed diabetic person understands the basis of his new regimen, or to encourage the obese older person to follow his restricted diet closely. The housebound person with severe problems of constipation for whom the district nurse is caring will also be given advice about increasing the fluid and/or cellulose content of the diet.

The community nursing service will almost certainly get to know about these patients by having them referred by the GP; there will be occasions where they will be 'collected' from a systematic check of the age-sex register. However, there are some patients who come to the attention of the community services because they have been in hospital for an acute episode of illness. This mechanism was described by Melia and Macmillan (1983) as a need felt by the hospital nurses that 'an eye be kept' on the patient. The community staff may be instrumental not only in educating the patient, but also in persuading neighbours or members of the family to help in the vital task of making sure that the patient is being nurtured.

Of course, there are occasions when the patient is isolated either socially or geographically and cannot personally provide the major nutrition needed each day. In this event, the nurse will utilize the meals-on-wheels service or organize a home help. Sadly, as Johnson *et al.* (1981) demonstrate, there are problems with all the community services designed to provide nutritional services for the elderly. It is very difficult to provide exactly the correct 'match' for a particular individual. One of the greatest problems is to produce a hot meal for a patient every day. Often it is possible for a home help to call on three days and meals-on-wheels on two days but no one appears to know what happens on Saturday and Sunday.

The other commonly used community service is the Luncheon Club. Of course, this service presupposes that the patient is fairly mobile and, as reported by the London Borough of Hounslow Social Services Department (1981), the social contact is as important as the nutritional content of the meal for this group of elderly people.

If the group of professionals involved decided to take an aged person into long-term care, one of the major criteria would be the knowledge that the patient could no longer look after his own nutrition, even with community help. Of course, this would not be the only reason but it does come high on the list. If it were the major difficulty, then a short period in hospital might be sufficient to rectify malnutrition and then return to the community might be possible if suitable provision to protect and ensure continued nutritional care could be made in the community.

Strategies to Enhance Nutrition

The enhancement of nutrition is one of the prime objects in drawing up a detailed patient profile. At this time, it is possible to find out what sorts of food the patient prefers and, possibly more importantly, what he usually eats since it is possible for there to be a divergence between these. The ethnic or geographical origins are important; for example, a person from the Western Isles of Scotland might grow up eating very few green vegetables. Religious persuasion may have a marked influence on diet; for example, the Jews' dislike of pork and the way in which food may be handled and cooked.

Providing what the patient would like may be a way of beginning a return to good eating habits. Sometimes people have very idiosyncratic names for food; for example velvet steak for liver. In such an instance it is important not only to ask the patient, but to ask members of the family or friends so that the dish can be supplied. On the other hand, providing this favourite dish can be one of the ways of caring for the terminally ill, as Willans (1980) has pointed out.

Great care must be taken to present a diet with variety. It is easy to forget with changes in staffing patterns that the patient might be offered an identical meal several times in a week and, indeed, a 'light' diet may consist of baked fish followed by custard each day till the patient progresses to a more robust diet.

The elderly patient feels hungry but is soon satiated, so the golden rule should be little and often. Large helpings look unappetizing to such a patient and may result in him only eating a mouthful or, indeed, refusing the food altogether.

Ensuring proper consistency of the food is another strategy that nurses ought to be careful about. The consistency may be spoiled by food being kept hot for too long which, for example, can put a skin on the top, for example with fish, or conversely by making it soggy, for example with buttered toast. Either state is equally unappetizing and should be a disappointment to the cook, patient and nurse alike.

Well-presented food can make the difference between it being eaten and the patient consuming nothing. It is said that orange on a tray is attractive; this might be achieved by the use of a traycloth. Though patients frequently have a choice of food, all too often the decision is made by nurses without reference to the patient. Involving the patient in selecting his menu, and making the tray individualized by using a name card can greatly enhance the enjoyment of food. It is possible that an ill or forgetful patient will not remember what he chose and seeing a tray 'hawked' around the ward till it arrives at the correct bed can be upsetting for patients. Eating is an important social *and* nutritional experience for our patients, we clearly have a key role to play in making it successful from both viewpoints.

Strategies of Providing Nutrition

Clearly, if the patient is unconscious, the most urgent need is to maintain fluid intake and balance. To this end, intravenous feeding will be introduced and it may need to be continued for some time because those patients cannot take food in any other way. It is both expensive and also very irritable to the vein and so is used only in extreme cases. Carbohydrate is given as fructose or glucose (the most common in use is 30% sorbitol), fat emulsion can be given and protein is provided in the form of amino acids.

In some cases where the patient is unconscious, intragastric feeding may be possible. This form of feeding is used where there are problems with the swallowing reflex, or where there is obstruction in the oesophagus, or sometimes brain dysfunction results in the loss of the swallowing ability. Where intragastric feeding is called for, a tube of suitable dimension is passed, taking great care that it has not entered the bronchus. When it is properly *in situ* it will be secured in position with adhesive tape and spigotted. Liquidized or proprietary foods can be used, taking care that fluid or food is at room temperature; it should not be too cold to avoid the patient being chilled, or conversely too hot so as not to burn the patient. Too much food should not be given at one time, to prevent distention. After completing the feed, a little water should be passed to prevent blocking of the tube.

From a conference paper (still in press), the author understands that in Scandinavia there are centres where, when caring for patients who are suffering from advanced senile dementia, the practice is to bottlefeed such patients. The rationale for this practice is that the sucking reflex is retained, and remains unimpaired, and that this method is much less damaging than attempting to use spoons. However, it raises interesting and disturbing questions, such as regarding the aesthetic feelings of both staff and relatives seeing elderly patients being treated as infants. Such treatment may be alarming for other patients and increase their fear about their future treatment. One would wish to consider the point at which it is proper to introduce such treatment; would one feel it right to treat young adults suffering the results of head injuries in a similar manner?

For patients who are conscious but require help to eat because of disability, the nurse has a range of responsibilities. The first is to ensure that the patient is clean and comfortable with special attention being given to a clean mouth and well-fitting dentures. Religious practice should be observed; for example, some people habitually say grace before eating. If this is so, then, when the first course is served, the nurse ought to wait quietly while the religious observance is carried out. In the instance of a nurse who shared such a conviction, it would be appropriate for her to be as involved in the observance as the patient wished.

In the area of feeding, enormous thought and sensitivity must be used to preserve the patient's dignity. Nurses should not attempt to feed several patients at the same time, and only small amounts of food should be offered at a time. It should be made clear by some agreed sign that the patient is ready for the next mouthful. Though obviously it is convenient for nursing staff to use children's bibs (with troughs attached), careful thought should be given as to how the patient feels about this. Such patients often have problems with drinking and a variety of feeding cups are used, though a straw might be more comely. Non-slip traycloths do help with the management of food, as do lipped dishes and specially designed cutlery. Food should be served course by course, otherwise hot food will be cold and the cold food, like ice cream, will be warm and altogether very unappetizing.

PATIENT PROFILE

Mrs Kennedy, a 75-year-old widow, was found unconscious by her neighbour who had noticed the uncollected milk and newspaper. The ambulance took Mrs Kennedy to the local hospital where she was diagnosed as having suffered a cerebrovascular accident (CVA). During the second day after admission she recovered consciousness but continued to suffer complete paralysis of her left arm and leg. Mrs Kennedy experienced frustration at her unresponsive left arm. Although she suffered a degree of dysarthria, she was able to express why. She grew cross appropriately, for example, about her inability to control food and at other times, equally appropriately, when unable to replace her clothing after going to the toilet. Frequently she asked, 'Can you lift me?' as she slumped to the left. When chewing, Mrs Kennedy would not notice that food dropped from the drooping corner of her mouth. After coughing and choking slightly, she became weepy and asked, 'Can I just have tea?' She became very reluctant to eat foods of solid consistency, partly because she could not control it on the plate and partly because it tended to make her choke. Hemianopia was diagnosed, a condition describing the loss of some part of the visual field in both eyes. This explained why Mrs Kennedy was unable to gauge distance, asking, 'Where is the plate?'. During the next three weeks she underwent active rehabilitation by physiotherapist, occupational therapist and speech therapist, whose efforts the nurse supported. Eventually, Mrs Kennedy, though regaining only paritial use of her arm, by learning to cope with her disability and regaining reasonable mobility, returned home.

ORGANIZATION OF NURSING CARE

Subjective Evidence (What the Patient Says)

Mrs Kennedy suffers emotional lability which is often expression of frustration at things being unmanageable by saying:
- 'Can I just have tea?'
- 'Please lift me up?' — this request may be repeated several times during a meal when she slumps to the left.
- 'I can't see the plate' — if, during helping Mrs Kennedy, a side plate is moved out of vision.

Objective Evidence (What the Nurse and Others Observe)

- Mrs Kennedy suffered paralysis of her left leg and arm, which made manipulation of food, cutlery and dishes difficult.
- She experienced choking and was therefore reluctant to take a varied diet.
- The drooping corner of her mouth made for untidy eating, of which Mrs Kennedy was unaware.
- Hemianopia was present which made judgement of where things were a problem.
- Emotional lability called for patience and perserverance from Mrs Kennedy and staff.
- Mrs Kennedy was weighed and, in conjunction with an assessment of her activity, her calorie intake was calculated.

Assessment (Nursing Diagnosis)

- Nutritional deficit (general).

Plan of Nursing Care

- Choose a balanced diet.
- Diversify the consistency of food.
- Help patient to manage eating without diminishing respect for the person.

- Introduce the patient to equipment that will allow return to food preparation and cooking as well as serving and eating.
- Arrange a home help to help with shopping, cleaning and other chores.

Expected Outcome

- Will be willing to choose a variety of foods.
- Ability to place things accurately, as well as an ability to cope with manipulation of utensils and food, will enable her to eat unaided.
- A diminution in the emotional instability.
- Patient's acceptance of a home help will enable a rapid return to the community.
- Patient's weight and mobility will be monitored and used as a basis for regulating calorie intake.

NURSING CARE OF PATIENT WITH NUTRITIONAL PROBLEM (EXAMPLE)

07.00 hours   Tea.

08.00   Help with washing and dressing, which provides an opportunity to discuss how the patient feels about her condition, how she will learn to dress herself with the use of aids. Demonstrate the use of dressing aids and encourage their use, slowly building up confidence and ability.

09.00   Breakfast: scrambled egg, toast and tea—use rimmed plate on non-slip traycloth, demonstrate then guide the use of suitably adapted cutlery. all help being given without rush.

10.00   Dietician to help with choice of menu/speech therapist to help with speech difficulty.

10.30   Physiotherapist to help progress of rehabilitation of limbs.

11.00   Coffee with digestive biscuit; again spend time giving guidance and help with the biscuit, making allowance for visual problems. This time might usefully be used not only teaching manipulative skills but discussing what other professionals have taught, either to reinforce or to clarify and encourage the patient.

12.30   Lunch: soup, pork cutlet with potato, carrots and onion boiled together and mashed, rice pudding with peach segments. Meal served with water followed by tea or coffee. Nurse helping with use of adapted cutlery: demonstrating, guiding and encouraging while not overtaxing the patient.

14.30   Occupational therapist to give advice about equipment; for example, various aids and adaptations to cookers, toilets, stairs at home, which would promote early discharge.

15.00   Tea with a slice of cake—served to visitors if present, showing them what help is needed as well as discussing the aid the patient will require while not doing everything for her but rather encouraging independence.

18.00   Supper: baked smoked haddock with peas and mashed potato if desired, biscuits and cheese with a piece of fresh fruit. Meal served with water followed by tea. Nurse giving as much help as necessary, remembering that the patient will be tired.

19.30   Reinforce something taught by one of the other members of the intraprofessional team, or talking about the patient's fears and worries about her condition, prognosis and her return home and the support she will need and what is available.

21.30   Hot drink with a biscuit if desired. Spend time encouraging speech. Also, with few implements needed, closely demonstrating for the patient the edges of the visual acuity and showing what measures the patient can take to prevent accidents.

23.00   Give a milky drink which may obviate the need for sleeping pills.

ASSESSMENT OF NUTRITION

- Height: overweight/underweight.
- Weight.
- Estimated/calorie intake.

Specific Deficiences

Examples are:
- specific vitamins;
- calcium;
- iron;
- fluids;
- protein.

Eating Habits

- Regular meals.
- 'Junk food'.
- Financial constraints.
- Hot/well-cooked food.

Nutrition Skills

- Ability to budget.
- Ability to select 'best buys'.
- Ability to prepare/serve attractively.
- Ability to cook.

Diet

- Well-balanced.
- Nutritional.
- Varied.

Social Factors

- Enjoys cooking/eating.
- Can/cannot enjoy meals alone.
- Opportunities to eat with others.
- Food enjoyed/disliked.

Allergies

- State specific items.

REFERENCES

Barr M.L., Milbank J.E. & Gibbs D. (1982) The nutritional status of the elderly. *Age and Ageing* **11**, 89–96.

Copp L.A. (ed.) (1981) *Care of the Aging—Recent Advances in Nursing, 2.* Churchill Livingstone, Edinburgh.

DHSS (1972) *A Nutritional Survey of the Elderly.* Report by the Panel on Nutrition of the Elderly. HMSO, London.

DHSS (1981) *Growing Older.* A White Paper. HMSO, London.

Holdsworth D. & Davies L. (1982) Nutrition education for the elderly. *Human Nutrition* **36**, 22–7.

Johnson M.K. with Di Gregorio & Harrison B. *Ageing, Needs and Nutrition.* Report for DHSS, Policy Studies Institute, London.

London Borough of Hounslow Social Services Department. Research and Planning Section (1981) Survey of Meals-on-Wheels and Luncheon Club Recipients in Hounslow, in *Clearing House for Local Authority Social Services Research,* No. 2, 45–113. Research and Planning Section, Clearing House for Local Authority Social Services Research, Birmingham.

Melia K.M. & Macmillan M.S. (1983) *Nurses and the Elderly in Hospital and the Community: A Study of Communication.* Report for SHHD, Nursing Studies Research Unit, University of Edinburgh.

MAFF (Ministry of Agriculture, Fisheries and Food) (1981) *Manual of Nutrition,* 8th edn. HMSO, London.
Willans J.H. (1980) Appetite in the terminally ill patient: A little of what the patient fancies is the secret of a hospice success in restoring the patient's appetite. *Nursing Times* **76**, (20), 875−6.

FURTHER READING

Bozian M. (1976) Nutrition for the aged or aged nutrition? *Nursing Clinics of North America* **11**, 169−77.
Ching N. (1979) Nutritional deficiencies and nutritional support therapy in geriatric cancer patients. *Journal of the American Geriatrics Society* **27**, 491−4.
Exton-Smith A.N. & Caird F.I. (Eds.) (1980) *Metabolic and Nutritional Disorders in the Elderly.* John Wright and Son, Bristol.
Greene M.L. (1979) Nutritional care considerations of older Americans. *Journal of the national medical Association* **71**, 791−3.
Iseminger M. & Hardy P. (1982) Bran works. *Geriatric Nursing* **3**, 402−4.
Lichtenstein V. (1982) Nutritional management. *Geriatric Nursing* **3**, 386−91.
Norberg A., Norberg B. & Bexell G. (1980) Ethical problems in feeding patients with advanced dementia. *British medical Journal* **281**, 847−8.
Tinker A. (1981). *The Elderly in Modern Society.* Longman, Harlow.
Williams H., McDonald E., Daggett M., Schut B. & Buckwalter K.C. (1983). Treating dysphagia. *Journal of gerontological Nursing* **9**, 638−47.
Yen P.K. (1983) Nurse−dietician teamwork. *Geriatric Nursing* **4**, 49, 57.
Yen P.K. (1983) Nutrition. Special help with eating problems. *Geriatric Nursing* **4**, 257−8.

Chapter 22
Pain

Pain is a protective mechanism of the body which can occur whenever there are interferences with physical, physiological or psychosocial processes. The process is not by any means fully understood and remains almost as much of an enigma today as it did in the past. Indeed the more that is learned about it, the more complex the phenomenon seems to become. Pain and its intensity are totally subjective phenomena which exist whenever and however the person perceives them. Past experience does not make the individual more immune to pain, so that the older person dreads pain every bit as much as the younger person. Also, as people grow older, they tend to suffer more from chronic disorders, many of which cause pain. For many an elderly person pain is a constant companion.

FACTORS RELATING TO PAIN

What is Pain?

There is as yet, no universally accepted definition of pain. The sensation we feel when our urinary bladder is full, is pain! Usually the pain is mild and we take steps to 'relieve' this form of pain whenever it is socially convenient. If, however, the individual is unable to empty his bladder because of an urethral obstruction, he soon experiences very severe pain which will cause him to seek help urgently. The pain in this circumstance would seem to be caused by stretching of, or pressure on, nerve endings, from the expanding volume of fluid. In the same way obstruction in the lumen of the ureter, bile duct or bowel will cause an accumulation of fluid or gas so giving rise to some of the worst pains man can experience. Another common cause of pain is inadequate oxygen supply to the tissues — ischaemic pain. Any physical or chemical damage internally or externally will result in pain. Pain warns the individual that some type of damage is occurring and gives him the opportunity to avoid its source or take action to reduce it. The relationship between cause and effect is not always, and indeed seldom, very obvious. Often noxious smells or sights or anything the individual perceives as a threat to well-being can result in him experiencing pain. There need not be any direct physical or chemical insult. The 'pain' experienced on the loss of a loved one, or the loss of his love, is perhaps different qualitatively from the pain of acute urinary retention but it is a form of pain nevertheless. Severe pain, whatever its source, tends to blunt or negate all other sensations so that the individual becomes totally preoccupied with it and in trying to relieve it.

Manifestations of Pain

Pain is a personal and realistic experience for the individual, although he may show little evidence of his suffering. Much depends on the intensity of the pain, its duration, past experience, culture, sex and so on. Individuals experiencing pain exhibit both verbal and non-verbal clues. There are three main responses the individual makes: voluntary, involuntary and emotional.

Voluntary responses include screaming, crying and verbal claims that the individual is in pain. Non-verbal clues include extreme restlessness; for example, the patient with biliary or renal colic will be restless and adopt all sorts of positions or get up and pace about in an attempt to relieve the pain. Others suffering from peritonitis will usually be lying in bed very still as any movement causes their pain to increase. Patients who have gangrene of the toes and feet may sit holding their leg, constantly shifting it around, lifting it off the ground. The pain being so intense that it draws attention to itself, so much so that one can almost see the patient thinking about his pain. Other patients will be irritable and angry and say things which they may later regret deeply. Who is to say whether their response was voluntary or involuntary?

Involuntary responses vary depending on whether the pain is acute or chronic, its duration and intensity. Acute pain usually causes the most obvious involuntary responses which include increased perspiration, increased pulse and respiratory rate, elevated blood pressure, muscular tension, dilated pupils and expressions of anxiety. Pain is not just a terrible physical feeling, it can also be frightening. The responses just listed are due to increased levels of adrenalin from activation of the sympathetic system, the 'fight or flight' response. The sympathetic manifestations are less apparent in patients with chronic pain showing some adaptation to pain or the effects of fatigue and exhaustion. Both acute and chronic pain give rise to emotional responses.

Emotional responses to pain are complex and at times, inexplicable. They can only be appreciated if one considers the individual's personality, race, religion, culture, state of health, past experiences and so on. These responses are so complex, in fact, that it is impossible to say with any certainty whether one variable is more important than another. Personality has a great bearing on his response to pain. Personality is of course shaped by many factors, and influences how the individual responds to any situation, including pain.

Individuals who typically react to events with stoicism and fortitude are more likely to react to pain in a similar fashion, whilst those who typically react to events with cries of anguish and despair are likely to do the same when experiencing pain. This of course is a gross oversimplification and many people experiencing pain respond in ways which surprise even themselves, as well as those near and dear to them.

Societal and cultural expectations and attitudes towards pain help to determine, to some extent, the individual's response. Generally, in Western culture, men are expected to show less response to pain than women or children. Overt displays of anguish may be seen as a sign of weakness, so that patients at times deny or cover up the fact that they are in pain. As nurses, we should be wary of cultural, racial and religious stereotyping with regard to pain. Pain assessment, as we shall see later, is a very subjective sort of exercise. It behoves nurses and others concerned with pain assessment to keep cultural, racial and religious aspects of the individual's background in perspective.

Other influences on how people experience pain depend on the state of their health, level of anxiety, knowledge of their illness, its cause and prognosis, as well as expectations of how much pain a particular operation or treatment should reasonably produce. Suffice it to say that each individual reacts to pain in a unique fashion. His response may not always be the same each time but may depend, as we have seen, on a variety of factors.

The Pain Experience

It is perhaps reasonable to assume that the majority of individuals have similar thresholds for pain, but differ in their reactions to the pain experience. Pain threshold is the point where the person has the sensation of pain: perception of pain. Pain tolerance refers to the manner by which the individual deals with pain: emotional response to pain. Drugs and alcohol tend to raise the pain threshold, whilst fatigue, anger, boredom, apprehension and weakness lower it. Pain can be either acute or chronic. Acute pain is usually the result of some insult to the tissues and can be from trauma, ischaemia, inflammation, obstruction, stress and tension. This form of pain can be very intense and is usually unexpected, that is, it comes on suddenly; most people realise that it is not going to last forever. On the whole it can be relieved without too much difficulty by various means. The most common form of relief being from analgesics. However, the use of potent analgesics in treating the elderly is not without risk as discussed later.

Chronic pain, on the other hand, is a very different experience for the individual. By definition it is long-standing, persistent and, unlike acute pain, does not seem to serve any particular function; because it is prolonged and usually unremitting it tends to absorb the entire person. It demands total attention and may even preclude the individual from meaningful interaction with his fellow man. It saps the individual's resources so that even matters of daily living become a burden. In short, it is physically and emotionally exhausting so that irritability and chronic fatigue are common accompaniments.

The elderly experience both sorts of pain but are more likely to suffer from chronic pain than the young person. Table 22.1 lists the common causes of chronic pain experienced by the elderly. Some causes are poorly understood but all can severely limit the elderly person's enjoyment of life.

Table 22.1   Causes of pain in the elderly.

Rheumatic diseases
Headache
Terminal illness
Temporal arteritis
Herpes zoster
Trigeminal neuralgia
Ischaemia
Surgery
Gout
Psychogenic origin

Rheumatic diseases cause perhaps more pain and misery than any other disease process, including cancer. Almost any part of the body can be involved and, combined with the normal ageing of the musculoskeletal system, can severely limit the elderly person's mobility and independence. Pain is often the most limiting factor in these disorders, along with stiffness and limitation of movement; pain precludes movement, joints become stiff, more pain ensues and so on. A vicious cycle of pain and loss of mobility is set up. When the large joints are involved, for example the hip, the individual is severely restricted and the pain unremitting. Pain is relieved permanently by hip replacement operation. This also gives more or less a full range of movement so that the patient feels like a 'new person'. Involvement of small joints, wrist, fingers, vertebral column, can be equally distressing. Unfortunately, surgery on the small joints is not so successful. More resources need to be allocated for this type of surgical rehabilitation.

Headache is a very common complaint of the elderly. The cause is not usually very obvious though cerebral ischaemia, hypertension and lying too long in bed may be contributing factors. Migraine headaches are not common among the elderly. Treatment of the underlying cause, if known or treatable, may help. Most headaches are relieved by simple analgesics such as aspirin and paracetamol.

Terminal illness is not always painful and indeed with good control, can be painless. However, what people fear more than anything if they have a terminal illness such as cancer, is dying in pain. Many people still associate death from cancer with a painful death. The pain, however, can be controlled by skilled and dedicated staff. The pain is often from secondary deposits in the bones and central nervous system. It is often a very severe pain made worse by the debilitated state of the patient (see also Chapter 16). Pain from secondary deposits in the bones may, on many occasions, be relieved by radiotherapy which shrinks the tumour mass and so relieves pressure.

Temporal arteritis (sometimes called cerebral arteritis) is a self-limiting non-specific inflammatory condition of the temporal and other arteries. It is a very painful disorder causing severe throbbing headaches. The condition is treated by steroids such as prednisolone 10 mg four times/day initially, then on a reducing dose. The prednisolone brings relief from the pain in a few days. The disorder usually clears up completely in about two years.

Herpes zoster is a viral infection involving the peripheral nerves. It often seems to arise concurrently with some other illness which has lowered the individual's resistance. It is a very painful condition in the acute phase, the pain usually being present for a few days before the typical lesions take place along the nerve routes. The lesions are usually self-limiting and clear away in a few weeks. However, many people contine to experience pain for months or years after the lesions have gone — post-herpetic neuralgia. This type of pain often responds poorly to conventional analgesia, but may respond to transcutaneous stimulus (see Patient profile pp. 272–3).

Trigeminal neuralgia is pain of unknown aetiology which affects the tri-geminal nerves. It is usually unilateral and may involve only one branch of the trigeminal nerve. It is one of the most excruciating pains suffered by human beings. It can sometimes be relieved by anticonvulsant drugs such as carbamazepine, or by surgical intervention.

Ischaemia, or the lack of tissue oxygen, causes very severe pain. The pain is usually brought on by exercise and disappears with rest (angina and intermittent claudication). However, because of its appearance every time the individual takes exercise it can be wearying. In many cases the blood supply fails completely and the individual has a myocardial infarction or, if in the lower limb, it becomes gangrenous. This is a very tiring pain often worst at night. The treatment of lower-limb gangrene is usually amputation, which the patient may even welcome in some ways to obtain relief. Occasionally an unusual type of pain following amputation, phantom-limb pain, is a problem. It is a poorly understood phenomenon and often fails to respond to analgesics though it may diminish over a period of time.

Surgery always results in some pain. Its effect can be minimized by good pre-operative teaching, This can mean less analgesia being required — an important consideration in the elderly, in view of their response to drugs such as morphine.

Gout is a metabolic disorder in which there is an accumulation of uric acid in the tissues. If the uric acid collects in a joint, it gives rise to excruciating pain. Drugs are available which reduce the levels of uric acid in the blood. Gout is exquisitely painful. One colleague who developed gout claimed that if he had had a gun he would have shot his toe off! Humour can, on occasion, be very effective in giving relief from pain!

Psychogenic pain is a sensation of pain with no recognized physiological stimulation. It is a form of pain for which the medical and nursing professions have little tolerance. However, given the subjective nature of pain it is not wise to arrive at a diagnosis of psychogenic pain without a very thorough evaluation of the patient's story. Psychogenic pain is used by patients as a means of fulfilling some need; giving it up is threatening. Patients are often able to modify the pain to a degree that is more tolerable. Pain, in itself, is seldom life threatening which is perhaps one of the reasons why nurses and doctors do not always give it the attention it deserves.

This brief review of the common causes of pain in the elderly highlights the complexity of the pain experience and the diverse ways in which it can be treated.

PRINCIPLES OF CARE

Many patients have their own strategies to relieve pain. This must be respected and can be of great benefit in helping the patient to cope with his pain.

Talking to the person, hearing his story in a sympathetic fashion and providing simple comfort measures, will often be nearly all that is required. You should approach the patient in an unhurried fashion and reassure him that the pain will subside. Handle him gently, and position him comfortably in whatever way the patient finds gives most relief, provided this is compatible with safety. Discuss pain-relieving measures with the patient and reassure him that if one method fails there are others. Encourage, or enforce if necessary, adequate rest; rest generally assists recovery from pain. One way to encourage adequate therapeutic rest is to use positive relaxation techniques; for these to be effective the patient should be lying or sitting comfortably in a quiet environment. The aim is to reduce the effects of stress and anxiety. It is best to use a technique the patient already knows. If the patient has not practised relaxation techniques before, he may be sceptical, so that some discussion of the technique and expected outcome is desirable. One technique is to encourage the patient to breathe deeply and to clench his fists; he should then breathe out and at the same time go as limp as a rag doll. This routine should be repeated rhythmically for several minutes. The patient should also start yawning. If successful, muscle tension should be alleviated and the patient should feel relaxed and may even go to sleep. The technique enhances the effectiveness of other pain-relief measures, and is particularly useful between medication doses. With appropriate experience and training the basic relaxation technique can be extended using meditation, yoga or hypnosis. It should be stressed that these techniques require special skills and should not be used without adequate training and supervision (see Further Reading p. 277).

Analgesics

There is a wide range of analgesics available for the treatment of pain. Given the complexity of the pain phenomenon it is not in the least surprising that there is no one single analgesic which is suitable for all types of pain. In the treatment of acute and chronic pain the selection of the most appropriate analgesic is essential if optimal pain relief is to be obtained. However, the use of analgesics in the elderly has risks, especially some of the medium-range drugs such as pentazozine which may cause a toxic psychosis (Pfeiffer 1982). Also, some of the anti-inflammatory agents such at phenylbutazone cause gastric and other upsets whilst some of the psychoactive drugs such as imipramine may cause tremor, cardiotoxicity and postural hypotension. The narcotic drugs depress the respiratory system, causing serious consequences in an already hypoxic patient.

It is now generally accepted that analgesia is best given on a regular basis rather than on demand (p.r.n.). This prevents severe pain 'breakthrough', minimizes the risk of addiction and usually means less analgesia is required. If the drug is given on a p.r.n. basis, the patient will experience regular predictable periods of pain which will take from 20-30 min to ease while the analgesic takes effect. If the patient expects pain, this heightens his anxiety and lowers his pain threshold; the experience of pain is increased and harder to ease. Analgesia given on a regular basis, before the pain returns, erases the memory of the pain and decreases anxiety and fear whilst increasing trust and understanding (Waterhouse 1982).

Whenever possible, analgesics should be given orally; this is certainly the easiest method when the patient is at home. Elderly patients dislike injections and, if patients are very thin and cachexic, the injections are often painful in themselves.

Analgesia then should be given with enough frequency to ensure pain relief without causing drowsiness or euphoria. In severe pain, especially in terminal illness due to cancer, a well-tried and proven agent is Brompton's cocktail (see Chapter 16).

PATIENT PROFILE

John Laidlaw's health had been deteriorating for about four years. Aged 80 years old, he had enjoyed good health with only the occasional bout of influenza or injury to upset his routine. A keen golfer and painter, he had kept himself fully active during his retirement. At 76 years old, he had required vascular surgery and then, two years later, gastric surgery. These operations left him weak and generally debilitated, and as often happens in these circumstances, he suffered a serious attack of herpes zoster, involving his shoulder and neck. The lesions cleared slowly after about six weeks but Mr Laidlaw continued to experience severe post-herpetic neuralgia. The pain made his life a misery. His neck and shoulder muscles became tense and stiff. Analgesics gave little relief, and in addition, caused gastric upsets. Heat pads made the pain worse. His own doctor referred him to the local pain clinic where he was supplied with a transcutaneous stimulator. The clinic nurse showed Mr Laidlaw how to use the stimulator and after a few lessons he was soon able to operate the stimulator by himself. Being mechanically minded and basically inquisitive, he soon mastered the use of the stimulator's three controls to obtain good pain relief. Initially, he used the stimulator up to three times during the day, but after a few weeks could keep the pain at bay by two applications per day. The pain clinic nurse called once a week to provide support and ensure all was well. Mr Laidlaw required no additional analgesia and after three months' use of the stimulator, the pain had almost completely gone except for short periods which were bearable. Mr Laidlaw had to be careful not to sit in draughts and to take regular exercise to keep the muscles of his neck and shoulder from going into spasm. The nurse instructed Mr Laidlaw how to do basic stretching, extension and flexion exercises and a series of range of motion activities for the affected body parts, as suggested by Miller and Lelieuvre (1982). These were especially important in view of Mr Laidlaw's intolerance of analgesics. The exercises also helped to restore Mr Laidlaw's general fitness, enabling him to play five or six holes of golf and to sketch and paint once more.

ORGANIZATION OF NURSING CARE

Subjective Evidence (What the Patient Says)

- 'I have a constant boring type pain in my neck and shoulder.'
- 'My neck is stiff and feels seized-up.'
- 'It has been this way since I had the shingles.'

Objective Evidence (What the Nurse and Others Observe)

- Patient has to turn whole body when he wishes to look to his right or left.
- Patient attempts to ease pain by rubbing his shoulder.
- Evidence of post-herpetic scarring over shoulder/scapular area.

Assessment (Nursing Diagnosis)

- Severe unremitting post-herpetic neuralgia.

Plan of Nursing Care

GENERAL AIM

- To assist patient to overcome his chronic pain problem by teaching him appropriate stretching, flexion and extension exercises.
- Teaching patient how to use a transcutaneous stimulator to relieve pain and muscle spasm.
- Advise patient to keep warm and to avoid draughts.
- Advise of need to maintain reasonable level of physical activity.
- Encourage patient to participate in social activities such as at his golf club.

Expected Outcome

- Patient will experience diminished, and less frequently complain of, pain, be free of muscle spasm and able to enjoy life more fully in two to three weeks.

NURSING CARE OF PATIENT WITH A PAIN PROBLEM (EXAMPLE)

07.30 hours	On waking up commence gentle exercises to help relieve muscle spasm and stiffness. If pain severe use transcutaneous stimulator. Avoid chills.
08.00	Wash and dress prior to breakfast.
08.30	Read daily paper.
09.00	Participate in household chores helping with cleaning, etc.
10.00	Morning coffee.
10.15	Exercises as prescribed.
10.30	Walk or other activity.
12.00	Lunch.
13.00	Pain relief using transcutaneous stimulator. Exercises as prescribed.
14.00	Social activity — meet friends in club or on visits.
16.00	Afternoon tea with friends.
17.00	Pain relief and exercises as prescribed.
18.00	Evening meal.
19.00–21.00	Watch television or pursue other recreation as desired.
21.00–22.00	Prepare for bed. Pain relief and exercises as prescribed to induce muscle relaxation and minimal pain so that sleep will be possible. Night sedative as required.

An essential feature of the nursing care of a patient who is experiencing pain is giving ample opportunity for discussion of the pain experience, of treatment strategies, and of what the future holds in store. These opportunities would form an integral part of the activities described above.

ASSESSMENT OF PAIN

From what has already been said, it should perhaps be obvious that assessing pain is far from easy. Pain is a subjective personal experience that cannot be seen or touched, consequently it is impossible to measure it in any objective fashion. In a sense, it is the patient who makes the diagnosis, and in this respect he is the only real authority about the pain he is experiencing. It is important for nurses and doctors to realize their prejudices when assessing whether a patient has pain. Yet, in daily clinical practice nurses are constantly being called upon to assess if a patient is in pain, and whether or not it is of such an intensity as to require therapy. The first essential is to believe the patient; if he says he is in pain, then he is in pain. Being in pain can produce a profound feeling of vulnerability, of being exposed to the mercy of others. The patient needs to be able to trust those caring for him, and can easily perceive when someone doubts he is in pain. Listen to the patient. Question the patient, 'What is the location of your pain?' The patient will usually be able to indicate where it hurts and so give clues as to the cause of the pain. 'What is the intensity of your pain?' This is very difficult to assess but is vital if proper therapy is to be given. The use of a 'pain ruler' as suggested by Bourbonnais (Fig. 22.1) may be useful. This is only one of several rating scales which have been devised. No one claims any of them to be perfect but they are better than nothing at all. It might be useful to use the same one over a period of time so that experience in its use is gained. The answers to other questions such as, 'When did the pain begin?', 'How long have you had pain?, 'Do you know what brought on the pain?', 'Does the pain keep you awake at night?', 'Does the pain get worse when you take exercise, or prevent you from taking exercise?', 'Is the pain related to eating?', 'Does the pain cause difficulty in feeding or drinking?', can help in the evaluation of the patient's pain.

To complete the assessment, the patient's skeletal muscle and autonomic nervous system response should be noted. Remember, patients with chronic pain usually do not display the intensive musculoskeletal and autonomic nervous system responses.

Skeletal Muscle Response

BODY MOVEMENTS

- Immobility.
- Purposeless or inaccurate body movements.
- Protective movements including withdrawal reflex.
- Rhythmic or rubbing movements.

FACIAL EXPRESSION

- Clenched teeth.
- Wrinkled forehead.
- Biting lower lip.
- Widely opened or tightly shut eyes.

Autonomic Nervous System Response

SYMPATHETIC NERVOUS SYSTEM ACTIVATION

- Increased pulse.
- Increased respirations.

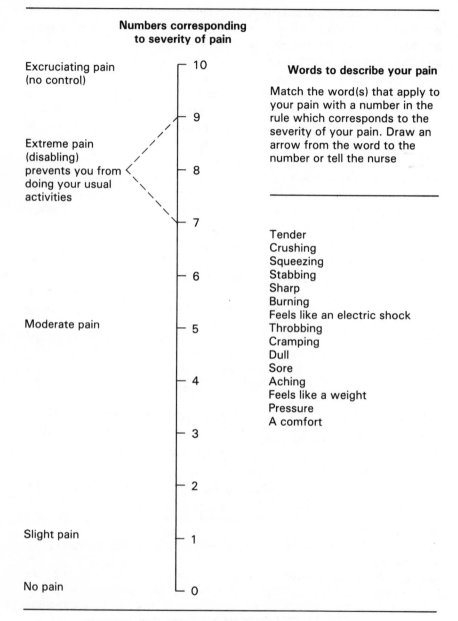

Fig 22.1 The painruler devised by Bourbonnais (1981).

- Increased diastolic and systolic blood pressure.
- Cold perspiration.
- Pallor.
- Dilated pupils.
- Nausea.
- Muscles tension.

PARASYMPATHETIC ACTIVATION IN SOME VISCERAL PAIN

- Low blood pressure.
- Slow pulse.

REFERENCES

Bourbonnais F. (1981) Pain assessment: development of a tool for the nurse and the patient. *Journal of advanced Nursing* **6**, 277–82.

Miller C. & Lelieuvre R.B. (1982) A method to reduce chronic pain in elderly nursing home residents. *Gerontologist* **22**, 314–17.

Pfeiffer R.F. (1982) Drugs for pain in the elderly. *Geriatrics* **37** (2), 67–76.

Waterhouse M. (1982) Don't despair — dying can be painless. *The Australian Nurses Journal* **11**, 40–2, 53.

FURTHER READING

Collins J.A. (1982) 'Cocktails' for relief of cancer pain. *Geriatrics* **37**, 136–43.

Heidrich G. & Perry S. (1982) The patient in pain. *American Journal of Nursing* **82**, 1228–33.

Johnston M. (1976) Pain, how do you know it's there and what do you do? *Nursing 76 (USA)* **1**, 48–50.

McCaffery M. (1980) Understanding your patient's pain. *Nursing 80 (USA)* **10**, 26–31,

McCaffery M. (1980) Relieving pain with non-invasive techniques. *Nursing 80 (USA)* **10**, 55–7.

McCaffery M. (1980) How to relieve your patient's pain. *Nursing 80 (USA)* **10**, 58–63.

Zahourek R.P. (1982) Hypnosis in nursing practice — Emphasis on the 'Problem Patient' who has pain — Part I. *Journal of psychosocial Nursing* **20**, 13–17.

Zahourek R.P. (1982) Hypnosis in nursing practice — Emphasis on the 'Problem Patient' who has pain — Part II. *Journal of psychosocial Nursing* **20**, 21–4.

Chapter 23
Reality (Orientation)

Orientation is the self-awareness of one's position in relation to time, person and place. It enables an individual to be aware of *when* it is: of the present time, day of the week and time of the year. It enables him to know *who* he is, and to identify others in the environment. It enables him to know *where* he is, and to find his way to other locations. It should be noted, of course, that 'normal' disorientation is an experience which we all have from time to time; when we lose our way in a strange town, for example. Thus, disorientation is only abnormal and pathological if it relates to items which the person could reasonably be expected to know. A person who 'gets lost' during his first day in a hospital would not be labelled 'disorientated'. However, if the same person is unable to find the toilet, *having been shown it's location several times,* he might be considered to be disorientated. It is essential that we recognize that not all aspects of disorientation are pathological, and that we take full account of additional features which may compound existing (often minimal) disorientation. Wolanin (1980, pp.7-8) expressed this concern as follows:

'. . . disorientation cannot be assessed unless the total situation is taken into account: the sterility of the environment, the sensorioperceptual apparatus of the patient, the anxiety created by the assessment process and the relevance of the questions to the life and the world of the patient. I have found that many older people do not have access to information on which we base our standard mental status examinations. If this were a course examination in a school, we would cry "Foul". Instead we put the elderly person at a severe disadvantage in an artificial situation with our tests.'

What is being suggested by Wolanin is that the *apparent* disorientation of an elderly person may result from his limited access to information, and be caused by his environment. The following should be borne in mind when caring for a person with an orientation problem. First, the problem will generally get worse as the disease process continues. The disorientation, which may range from relatively mild to very severe, is a term which must be qualified and be accompanied by a description of its severity in terms of how it affects the patient's ability to function. Second, measurement of the patient's orientation should relate to useful and potentially therapeutic questions and factors; for example, it may be less relevant to establish whether or not the patient knows the name of his hospital, and more relevant to establish if he knows how to find his way to the toilet. The ability to measure and describe disorientation is extremely important in relation to the provision of nursing care. Third, disorientation is a problem which can be positively influenced by appropriate nursing care, and by other care givers under the direction of nursing staff. Indeed, nurses have a far greater role to play than any other staff group in relation to this problem.

Orientation is closely related to memory, particularly short-term memory. The reason we are able to remember where we are, the time of day, and the identity of people we meet, is that we have a relatively effective short-term memory. All disease processes which affect an individual's short-term memory, will result in a greater or lesser degree of disorientation. The most common disease processes which cause disorientation are those affecting the function of the brain; the dementias and the acute confusional states, for example. It is not being suggested that disorientation is only associated with these illnesses, but that they always result in some degree of disorientation.

FACTORS AND PRINCIPLES OF CARE RELATING TO DISORIENTATION*

A number of closely related factors are important in relation to the cause, prevention and resolution of patient orientation problems. It is recognized that these factors are *not* independent nor do they represent the full range of such factors. Rather, the discussion is designed to illustrate the fact that a range of relevant factors exist, and to illustrate how these relate to the role of the nurse.

Orientation Cues and Uses

Every contact with disorientated patients should be used as an opportunity for giving orientation for time, person and place. Although this may seem pedantic, even unnecessary, at times it must be regarded as an important and integral part of nursing care. You should prescribe and, if necessary, *insist,* that all who come into contact with the patient introduce themselves by name and give frequent orientation cues.

---

*Because the therapeutic input of the nurse in dealing with this problem (disorientation) is closely related to the factors which relate to (cause) it, both of these aspects of the discussion will be dealt with together in this chapter.

Whenever possible, opportunities should be sought whereby patients can demonstrate their orientation skills rather than be given orientation by others. Patients must be encouraged to find their own way to the toilet, only being given assistance when it is certain that they are not going to succeed. This withholding of care 'until the last minute' is something which many nurses are unused to doing, but which must be learned in order to maximize the patient's personal orientation.

In the early stages of diseases which cause progressive disorientation, patients are aware of, and frequently able to discuss, their feelings about this very distressing problem. Indeed, this personal awareness is often largely responsible for the anxiety and hostility which may accompany disorientation.

The use of sociotherapeutic groups to optimize the patient's existing orientation skills, and to minimize the progressive nature of the problem, can achieve considerable success. Such a 'reality orientation group', although more easily formed in an institutional setting, could just as easily be arranged in private homes, community care settings, day hospitals and the like.

Experience and Education of Care Givers

There can be no doubt that the elderly person who experiences orientation problems requires to be cared for by those who have a high level of experience and education relating to that area of care. It is *not* the case that such patients, particularly those in institutions, can easily be cared for by a group of relatively inexperienced and poorly educated care givers, *even* if they are supervised by a well-trained nurse. Whether the person is cared for at home, or in some form of institution, the trained nurse has a crucial role to play in assessing the patient's nursing needs, planning and delivering care, and evaluating its outcome.

Where the major amount of care is given by unqualified persons, relatives for example, the experience, the expertise and education of a trained nurse must be used to enable the relatives to optimize their quality of care. In this instance, you will have a very important role to play in terms of teaching others how to care for the patient with an orientation problem.

Disorientation problems can be positively influenced by well-trained, experienced and motivated nursing staff. If the care of such patients is relegated to relatively inexperienced and poorly trained (even untrained) staff, the outcome will be a failure to positively influence the problem. In many instances it will result in the problem being significantly increased by the very staff who are expected to decrease it. *Iatrogenesis,* the term used to describe those problems which are caused by the very people who are responsible for preventing or resolving them, will continue to occur in the form of increased disorientation for as long as inexperienced and poorly educated staff care for the disorientated elderly person.

Physical Environment

The physical environment in which the disorientated person is nursed can do much to decrease his disorientation, or to increase it. There can be no doubt that an iatrogenic increase in disorientation levels frequently results from a failure to view the physical environment as having a very strong therapeutic potential. To some extent, this problem is related to the experience and the education of the staff.

The environment in which such patients are cared for, at home or elsewhere, should be safe. Attention to such detail as the state and type of floor covering, the location of occasional tables, and the location of steps leading from and to the environment are obvious examples. In some instances, particularly in psychogeriatric wards which contain a number of disorientated patients, it might be necessary to lock the ward doors. In recent years it has become fashionable to unlock all ward doors, resulting in the loss, and occasional death, of some patients and resulting in extremely high anxiety levels, and frequent guilt, on the part of nursing staff.

Bed spaces should be personalized, with bed and covers being as individualized as possible; for example, a photograph of the person and/or his family should be on the locker, bed covers should be in individualized colours, and changes in the location of the patient's bed should be kept to an absolute minimum for obvious reasons. In wards where items are liable to be removed from lockers, there is no reason why the patient's name should not be firmly fixed on to the locker and, when necessary, appropriate photographs fixed on to the locker by way of a special frame. All name labels, whether they be on the bed, locker or personal wardrobe, *must* be at a height no greater than eye level for the average elderly patient, and should be in letters of no less than half an inch tall.

All areas which are used by patients, whether at home or in an institution, must have distinctive colours or markings on the walls, doors or floors. These orientation aids, like all others, may not be of use to all patients in every circumstance. However, all of them will be of some benefit to some patients on some occasions. In one ward with which the author is familiar, containing 17 patients, 5 were able to find the toilet by following the bright floor marking which had been placed between the toilet door and the sitting room. Three other patients were able to find the toilet by recognizing its pink door.

Orientation aids in the form of a Big Ben clock, a large letter calendar and an 'orientation board' with the name of the hospital, ward number, day of the week and information about events for that day should be a feature of all wards with disorientated patients. Similar arrangements should also be made for persons living at home. Current newspapers, magazines and other news items should be available and drawn to the person's attention. Television and radio newscasts could be used as the basis of group discussions.

Staff Expectations

To a large extent the expectations of staff and other care givers will influence the extent to which orientation problems are made better or worse. If care givers wrongly assume that a person is unable to find his own seat in the dining room, for example, they will repeatedly show him to his seat. In a very short period of time any ability which he did have to find his own seat in the dining room will be lost. It is essential that care givers assume that patients have orientation skills, until experience proves otherwise.

Disorientation exists on a continuum which will range from the mild to the severe, thus all patients with a disorientation problem will only be partly disorientated during the initial phases of the illness. It is best that care givers encourage and expect patients to make optimum use of their orientation facilities for as long as possible.

Physical Health

The extent to which a person's physical health can influence his orientation status has been well documented. This may take two forms and relate to the development of an acute confusional state in a person in any age group, it can also cause the orientation problems being experienced by a demented patient to become considerably worse. Areas of particular importance relating to physical health include hydration, nutrition, infection, temperature increases, use of sedatives and tranquillizers, and constipation. Any such changes in the patient's physical health dramatically result in the person becoming very much more disorientated than he was previously.

The role of the nurse in preventing these physical health problems occurring is both obvious and crucial. However, it is important to realize that, on some occasions, the actions (or inactions) of nursing staff or other care givers can cause these problems. They can be said to have an iatrogenic cause when nursing staff, or other care givers, cause them; for example, it is not unusual for demented patients to be nursed in dayrooms from which they have no easy access to water or other fluids. This particular problem is made much worse if the person happens to be confined to a 'geriatric chair'. There is no reason why, as is the case in some wards, a drinking fountain or some other means of obtaining fluids, should not be available in all dayrooms of all hospitals. Another common example of iatrogenic disorientation is that caused by the overprescription of sedatives and tranquillizers. Although nursing staff do not make these prescriptions personally, they can easily obtain them by making appropriate representations to medical staff.

The role of the nurse in monitoring the patient's physical status, and in preventing deterioration in physical health is of extreme importance. Failure to do so may result in the symptoms of physical illness, dehydration for example, causing an increase in the level of disorientation which may be misdiagnosed as a 'normal' increase.

Routine

In many contemporary health care settings it has become fashionable to criticize the delivery of 'routine' nursing care. However, the existence of a recognizable, predictable and familiar routine is of considerable value to the person with an orientation problem. It is not being suggested that such a routine be blindly followed for all patients in all circumstances, rather it is being proposed that the therapeutic potential of the routine be given full recognition; for example, the practice of unnecessarily changing the bedspace or the eating-space of a patient should be recognized as compounding the orientation problem. Similarly, rapid staff turnover and the overuse of 'relief' staff who spend short periods in that particular ward will undoubtedly aggravate the orientation problem.

PATIENT PROFILE

Mr Black is aged 84 years old and lives with his daughter in a groundfloor flat on the outskirts of a small town. He has a medical diagnosis of 'senile dementia'.

At 02.00 hours on Wednesday Miss Black was awakened by the noise of movement coming from her father's room. Mr Black then knocked on his daughter's door and called, 'Aren't you up yet? We've slept in for church, we'll miss the 10 o'clock service.' Mr Black had dressed himself and was wearing his 'Sunday suit' and was carrying his bible (disorientation for time). Miss Black persuaded her father to go back to bed where he slept soundly until 07.30 hours.

On awakening, Mr Black put on a bathrobe and *attempted* to find the bathroom which was next door to his bedroom. Miss Black found him leaving the house via the back door and pointing to a nearby house. She asked where he was going, he replied, 'I'm going to the toilet. Is that it over there?' (disorientation for place). Miss Black led her father back into the house towards the bathroom.

On entering the bathroom, Mr Black said to his daughter, 'Who are you? What are you doing here?' (disorientation for person).

ORGANIZATION OF NURSING CARE (DISORIENTATION FOR TIME)

Subject Evidence (What the Patient Says)

- Says to daughter at 02.00 hours on Wednesday, 'Aren't you up yet? We've slept in for church, we'll miss the 10 o'clock service.'

Objective Evidence (What the Nurse and Others Observe)

- Dresses for church at 02.00 hours.

Assessment (Nursing Diagnosis)

- Disorientation for time.

Plan of Nursing Care

- Place a large letter/number calendar in room.
- Encourage use of personal diary.
- Use large-number 24-hour clock.
- Use personal (daily) timetable of personal events/activities.
- Discuss orientation problem with Mr Black.
- Give orientation cues at all opportunities.

Expected Outcome

- Will be aware of time of day and night.
- Will be aware of day and month.
- Will not dress before 07.00–07.30 hours.

NURSING CARE OF PATIENT WITH DISORIENTATION PROBLEM (EXAMPLE)

The actual form which the nursing care may take during any given 24 hour period will vary according to the patient's particular circumstances. In the case of Mr Black it will be assumed that he attends a geriatric day hospital from Monday to Friday (09.30−13.30 hours), and is visited by the district nurse two afternoons per week. His daughter does not work and has considerable help from her brother in caring for her father. Her brother lives nearby and visits most evenings.

07.30 hours Waken Mr Black, if he is not already awake. Remind him of who you are, where he is, and of the time. Do this slowly and repeat information if required: 'Good morning, Dad, it's half past seven', or, 'It's Monday. Dad, shall I fry your bacon and egg?'

07.45 Help with selecting clothes and dressing *only if absolutely necessary*. Talk about plans for the rest of the day. Discuss memory and memory problems.

08.00 Wait and see if Mr Black manages to wash, shave and use toilet without help. Give help *only if absolutely necessary*. Toilet items should be left in the same place each night. If necessary, the toilet door should be clearly marked or distinctively coloured.

08.30 Discuss yesterday's activities over breakfast. Make plans for rest of the day. Fill in diary with times, activities, people's names, etc. Mr Black should make diary entries personally.

09.30 Driven to the day hospital by his daughter and personally introduced to the nurse who looks after him on each visit to the hospital. Each day, the first half hour at the hospital is spent on informal social chat, giving Mr Black the opportunity to reorient himself to the hospital, the staff, and the other patients.

10.00 Mr Black attends an orientation therapy group along with six other patients and 'his' nurse. The purpose of the group is to encourage members to talk about their orientation problems and to discuss the tactics which they are using to minimize these problems. Clearly, some individuals will be more able to participate in this group than others. However, the nurse is able to use her knowledge of individual patients and their problems to encourage and enable them to participate as fully as possible. Those patients who use a diary as a memory aid discuss its contents and usefulness.

11.00 The next hour is spent practising and rehearsing a small number of daily living skills which Mr Black and two other patients are currently having problems with. In Mr Black's case these skills relate to shaving, making tea and cleaning his false teeth. The nurse who takes this group is known to Mr

Black and encourages him, and other patients, to make full use of their orientation abilities as they relate to time, person and place. There is also opportunity for informal discussion about the anxieties and frustrations which they experience in relation to their orientation problem.

12.00   During the lunch hour all patients are encouraged to do as much as possible for themselves, to find their own way to their personal eating place and to clear their own table when the meal is over.

13.00   The final half hour is used as 'free time' in which patients can relax and chat to each other.

13.30   Mr Black is collected by his daughter and accompanies her on a shopping trip to the local supermarket. During the shopping trip every opportunity is taken to encourage Mr Black to recognize and identify common items and experiences; for example, he is involved in choosing and finding the items which will be bought. The shop which is used by Mr Black and his daughter, and which is visited weekly, is a place with which he is quite familiar and in which he feels comfortable.

15.30   On returning home Mr Black has his daily half hour nap.

16.00   On awakening he begins to prepare the evening meal which they usually have at 17.30 hours. The arrangements for the meal, which were discussed earlier in the day, have been noted in his diary. Although requiring some help with the arrangements, weighing one of the ingredients for example, he successfully manages to prepare the meal in the one and a half hours available to him.

17.30   Mr Black and his daughter discuss the earlier events of the day and plans for the evening. They discuss the fact that Miss Black will be going out for the evening and her brother will be coming over to visit and generally look after her father. The arrangements are that her brother (John) will arrive at 19.00 hours when she will leave to go out for the evening. John will stay in the house until Miss Black returns at around 23.00 hours. They discuss the television programmes which will be available for that evening and make decisions about those which Mr Black will watch.

18.30   Mr Black washes up the dishes while his daughter prepares for going out.

19.00   John arrives and his sister leaves for the evening. John and his father talk about the day's events and the plans for the evening. John reminds his father that he will be there until his sister returns home at 23.00 hours. During the evening Mr Black and his son watch television and talk about the rest of the family who live elsewhere in the town. John is careful to give his father full information about others in the family, without 'overloading' his father with detail.

22.00 John helps his father to write his diary which he has kept since boyhood. Although requiring some assistance with detail and with remembering the sequence of events for the day Mr Black is still capable of keeping a meaningful diary. He refers to plans and notes of events which he has prepared earlier in the day.

23.00 Mr Black's daughter returns home and his son returns to his family. Mr Black and his daughter discuss how they both spent their evening and they also spend some time reminiscing. The subject of the conversation on this particular occasion is Mr Black's wife who died ten years ago.

24.00 Mr Black prepares for bed and is encouraged to do so as independently as possible. He sleeps with a nightlight which, although it is not sufficiently bright to affect his sleep, enables him to find his way to the toilet should he waken. The nightlight is situated near his bedroom door and, if necessary, helps him to find his way to the toilet which is in the lobby nearby.

Most nights Mr Black sleeps soundly until 04.00 or 05.00 hours when he rises and goes to the toilet. The toilet door is clearly marked and can be seen with the help of the nightlight. Should he need assistance from his daughter, Mr. Black has learned that he can get this by either knocking on the bathroom wall or by knocking on his daughter's bedroom door.

07.30 Mr Black is awakened by his daughter if he is not already awake.

Although the visiting community nurse has not been directly involved in Mr Black's care for that particular day, or has not visited, she will play a central supportive, advisory and direct care role generally. Indeed, many of the strategies which are used by Mr Black, his relatives and other care givers will be prescribed, monitored and evaluated by the community nurse. Her job will be to coordinate the care which is given to him in relation to his orientation and other problems.

ASSESSMENT OF ORIENTATION

Orientation for Time

- Is aware of:
  year;
  season;
  month;
  day;
  time.
- Can identify:
  day and night;
  approximate times of meals;
  time for appointment/activities.
- Uses/has access to:
  watch/clock;
  newspapers;
  calendar.

Orientation for Person

- Can identify:
  own name;
  name/s of close relatives;
  names of some/all staff;
  other patients by name.
- Uses/has access to:
  written name 'labels' of others;
  photographs of close relatives.

Orientation for Place

- Can locate:
  own house/ward;
  rooms/kitchen/toilet/bathroom, own bed, locker.
- Uses/has access to:
  labels/indicators on doors;
  directions to toilet/bathroom;
  name indicators on dining-room tables.

REFERENCE

Wolanin M. O. (1980) Mental health assessment as part of the physiological status. Unpublished paper presented at the American Nurses Association, Houston.

FURTHER READING

Burton M. (1982) Reality orientation for the elderly: A critique. *Journal of advanced Nursing* 7, 427–33.

Campos R. G. (1984) Does reality orientation work? *Journal of gerontological Nursing* 10, 53–64.

Chenitz W. C. (1983) The nurse's aide and the confused person. *Geriatric Nursing* 4, 238–41.

Chisholm S. H., Deniston O. L., Igrisan R.M. & Barbus A. J. (1982) Prevalence of confusion in elderly hospitalized patients. *Journal of gerontological Nursing* 8, 87–96.

Drummond L., Kirchoff L. & Scarbrough D. (1978) A practical guide to reality orientation. *Gerontologist* 18, 568–73.

Hayter J. (1981) Nursing care of the severely confused patient. *Nursing Homes* 30, 30–7.

Hogstel M. O. (1979) Use of reality orientation with aging confused patients. *Nursing Research* 28, 161–5.

Langston N. F. (1981) Reality orientation and effective reinforcement. *Journal of gerontological Nursing* 7, 224–7.

Levine N. B., Dastoor D. P. & Gendron C. E. (1983) Coping with dementia. *Journal of the American Geriatrics Society* 31, 12–18.

Mulchax N. & Rose N. (1981) Reality orientation in a general hospital. *Geriatric Nursing* 2, 264–8.

Nodhturft V. L. & Sweeney N. (1982) Reality orientation therapy for the institutionalized elderly. *Journal of gerontological Nursing* 8, 396–401.

Parker C. & Sommors C. (1983) Reality orientation on a geropsychiatric unit. *Geriatric Nursing* 4, 163–5.

Rabins P. V., Mace N. L. & Lucas M. J. (1982) The impact of dementia on the family. *Journal of the American medical Association* 248, 333–5.

Seymour D. G., Henschke P. J. & Cape R. D. T. (1980) Acute confusional states and dementia in the elderly: The role of dehydration/volume depletion, physical illness and age. *Age and Aging* 9, 137–46.

Voelkel D. (1978) A study of reality orientation and resocialization groups with confused elderly. *Journal of gerontological Nursing* 4, 13–18.

Woods R. T. (1979) Reality orientation and staff attention: A controlled study. *British Journal of Psychiatry* 134, 502–7.

Zepelin H., Wolfe C. S. & Kleinplatz F. (1981) Evaluation of a yearlong reality orientation programme. *Journal of Gerontology* 36, 70–7.

Chapter 24
Reality (Perception)

The way in which we correctly (or incorrectly) perceive the world in which we live is influenced by, and influences, the input we receive from our five senses. We know there is a chair in the room because we can *see* it; we know we are eating mint sweets because we can *taste* them; we know a friend has been eating garlic because we can *smell* it on his breath; we know a patient is calling us because we can *hear* him; and we know there is a fly on our ear because we can *feel* it. Thus, there is a stimulus, a chair or a fly, for example, and our brain correctly interprets the stimulus as a chair and a fly respectively.

HALLUCINATIONS

Imagine a situation where our brain 'sees' a chair or 'feels' a fly when, in reality, there is no chair and no fly. In such a circumstance, the individual is said to be hallucinating and has a 'reality' (perception) problem. Hallucinations can be visual (seeing), tactile (feeling), auditory (hearing), olfactory (smelling) and gustatory (tasting).

A hallucination is false sensory perception which occurs in the absence of any external stimulus.

DELUSIONS

Another way in which we correctly (or incorrectly) perceive the world in which we live is by forming reasonably accurate beliefs about our circumstances, environment and relationships. Although these beliefs often fall short of being 100% accurate, we might believe we can run a mile in five minutes when in reality it would take us six minutes, they are relatively accurate and realistic. However, if we believe we can run a mile in five seconds, this is certain to be totally inaccurate and unrealistic; this is a delusion.

A delusion is a false and fixed idea or belief which is not in keeping with the person's social, educational, cultural or religious background. The false idea or belief is *not* amenable to persuasion, reason or logical argument.

In deciding whether or not a false idea or belief is a delusion, it is essential that you take full account of the person's social, educational, cultural and religious background. By doing so, you might find that such a belief might be delusional for one person, but not for another; for example, if a well-educated and socially sophisticated man who has lived all his life in a 'western' society began to believe that his neighbour was harming his business success by using her 'evil eye' to influence him, you might suspect he was deluded. On the other hand, such a belief would certainly not be regarded as delusional if expressed by inhabitants of many rural areas of Africa or South American countries.

As with hallucinations, there are different types of delusions which include the following.

Delusions of unworthiness occur in which the person experiences great guilt and low self-esteem. He may say 'It's all my fault', or, 'I have caused the sins of the world' or, 'Don't come near me; I'm dirty; I'm contaminated'.

Delusions of persecution make the person feel that people generally, or specific individuals are 'against him'. He might say, 'Why are you torturing me?', or, 'MI5 is trying to poison me', or, 'My food is being tampered with'.

Delusions of grandeur are when the person wrongly feels that he is extremely wealthy, a figure of national importance, or that he has the power to control and manipulate people and events. He might say, 'I have the power', or, 'I am the real king', or, 'This year, I will allow President X to be returned to office', or, 'Just order a yacht for yourself; I'll pay the bill'.

Nihilistic delusions are those when the person believes he does not exist or that part of his body is missing. He might say, 'I have no brain; my head is full of concrete', or, 'My body is gone; what you see is my ghost' or, 'I have no bones, only plastic plates and rods'.

ILLUSIONS

Illusions, which are very different from delusions and hallucinations, are false perceptions which *do* occur in the presence of external stimuli. Illusions, which are not necessarily features of illness, are something we all experience; for example, the moving shadow of a bush in poor light (external stimulus) may be misinterpreted as a person or animal. Background sounds in a hospital, the television and staff conversation for example, might be misinterpreted as the voice of a friend.

The reason for including this brief reference to illusions is not because of their importance in terms of illness and pathology; it is included to demonstrate the differences between illusions, hallucinations and delusions, these differences being the cause of some confusion to those who are not fully familiar with them. Illusions are normal experiences which we all have and are invariably *not* associated with illness processes.

FACTORS RELATING TO REALITY (PERCEPTION)

Hallucination/Delusion Overlap

Traditionally delusions (false beliefs) and hallucinations (false perceptions) have been treated as two very different experiences for the ill person. This difference is probably more apparent than real in that both delusions and hallucinations cause the person to believe something which, in reality, is not true; for example, one 'sees' something which, in reality, does not exist and consequently believes that it is there. The other person believes something is present when in reality it is not, although he may be unable to see, hear, smell, taste or touch it.

In practice both hallucinations and delusions often occur simultaneously, and require near identical nursing interventions, A person might believe that his food is being poisoned (a delusion), and also be able to smell the poison (a hallucination). Both are found in a wide range of illness processes experienced by the elderly; examples include psychotic depression, acute confusional states and dementia (see Chapter 8).

Duration

In some illnesses such as acute confusional states, these perceptual problems can be of very short duration, one week for example. As the cause of the acute confusional state is treated, all symptoms, including the hallucinations and delusions, disappear.

In longer term illnesses such as dementia, schizophrenia and paranoid psychosis the symptoms may be ever present and lifelong.

Role of Anxiety

Although the mechanisms which cause perceptual symptoms are poorly understood, it is widely believed that they develop, in part, as a defence against anxiety. As psychotic illnesses such as schizophrenia develop, the ability of the person to cope with the 'reality' of normal daily experiences decreases, consequently he develops his own 'reality' which is made possible by, and takes the form of, delusions and hallucinations. Any situation that increases the anxiety level, will increase the delusions and hallucinations as the person seeks to escape from the anxiety (reality).

In the course of time the manufactured reality of delusions and hallucinations becomes preferable to the reality of the 'real world', with more and more time being spent in the former. Any attempt to bring the person back to actual reality will be strongly resisted because of the anxiety which it causes.

Finally, the individual virtually loses any ability which he may once have had to control the hallucinations and delusions, they are now in control of him and are frequently terrifying and hostile.

Environmental Cues

Much of our knowledge of reality comes from the environment in which we live, particularly the people in it. Those who are at risk, including the hard of hearing, blind, psychotic and isolated person, need to be given clear and specific 'messages' about the real world by those of us who can interpret it correctly.

PRINCIPLES OF CARE

Patient Experience

Those who have hallucinations and delusions regard them as accurate and factual representations of reality, *they are real to the person who experiences them*. As nurses, we have a duty to recognize this and to try and understand what the patient is experiencing and feeling; we must empathize with him. Because of our difficulty in understanding this concept, it is often easy to believe that the problem is being 'faked' by the patient, or to reject him. Equally, we need to realize that there is much that we as nurses can do to minimize delusions and hallucinations or, alternatively, make them less difficult for the patient to live with.

Accept the Person

Irrespective of the nature and content of the delusions and hallucinations, you must maintain a positive attitude toward the patient, and 'keep in touch' with him. This can be difficult if you become part of his misrepresentation of reality, he may believe that you are trying to poison him or that you are one of his disciples. Maintaining an objective and therapeutic position is essential, as is the need to ensure that you do not take personally insults prompted by delusions and hallucinations. If you are accused of theft by the person experiencing paranoid delusions, this should remain the patient's problem and not become your personal problem.

Accept the Problem

In general terms, you must accept the reality as experienced by the deluded or hallucinating person. That reality cannot (by definition) be changed by argument, logic or presentation of evidence to the contrary. It is not being suggested that you should agree with the patient, but that you do not disagree to the point of coming into conflict with him; for example, if he says, 'I have two heads', you might reply, 'I see only one head Mr X'. If he says, 'I smell poison gas; they are trying to kill me', you might reply, 'I do not smell it Mr X'. Remember, *he is expressing what he believes to be reality,* do not make value judgements about what he feels is real.

Focus on Reality

A major part of the nurse's role, and that of others close to the patient, is to focus him on reality. Reality takes many forms, most of which are part of our daily living experiences and result from our interactions with others. Such experiences and interactions include eating, playing games, social talk, being in a room with others, watching television and reading newspapers. Anything which exposes the patient to the real world and the feeling of real people has an important therapeutic potential,

With this patient, your job will be to focus his attention and time on real (as opposed to delusional and hallucinatory) experiences.

Estimate Level of Insight

Insight might be defined as the level of self-understanding which the individual has about himself, his circumstances, abilities, illness and so on. In health care terms, insight must be seen as relating to all aspects of physical, mental and social factors, and existing on a continuum ranging from full to no insight.

Although many textbooks imply that the person suffering from a psychotic illness and the accompanying reality perception problems has no insight, this is not quite true. While it is true that many such patients are severely lacking in insight (perhaps suggesting that, 'No, I'm not ill, they really have borrowed my real head for the experiments), others have retained or recovered a considerable level of insight; for example, a person who suffered from chronic schizophrenia said to me: 'I'm keeping quite well on the whole. The voices (hallucinations) were quite bad at Christmas time but they didn't bother me too much', and, 'The doctor thinks I might be suffering from the early effects of senile dementia. I know my short-term memory is failing; it makes me so angry'.

In monitoring insight levels, *talk* to patients about their hallucinations and delusions, establish how aware they are of the fact that they are unreal. Knowing this, will tell you how much work has to be done to help him 'get in touch with' reality. Additionally, you can establish what makes the experiences better or worse, and how he feels about them. Your conversation with a patient might be as portrayed in the following example (note the way in which you could confirm that he is indeed hallucinating).

You have been talking to a patient for a few minutes and notice that he is preoccupied and occasionally looks over his shoulder and talks, although there is nobody behind him.

Nurse: 'I notice you looked over your shoulder and talked.'
Patient: 'Yes, yes, yes.'
Nurse: 'Who did you talk to?'
Patient: 'Him, the policeman. He spoke to me first.'
Nurse: 'Can you tell me what you were talking about?' (Patient describes the conversation he has had with the non-existent policeman.)
Nurse: 'I don't see a policeman there, this experience may be part of your illness."
Patient: 'So they tell me. Maybe.'
Nurse: 'I've noticed you talking in this way quite a lot in the past few days.'
Patient: 'Yes, I've been hearing the voices since before I was admitted.'
Nurse: 'Can you think of any times when they get worse?'
Patient: 'No, not really. Well, maybe they get worse when I have to do something.'
Nurse: 'Do something?'
Patient: 'Yes, like go to therapy or wait for the doctor coming round.'
Nurse: 'Do the voices bother you?'
Patient: 'Yes.'
Nurse: 'In what way?'
Patient: 'They tell me to do things, to take my clothes off.'

This example demonstrates the need to encourage patients to talk about these experiences when we know little about them. This is an important part of the assessment phase and will give direction to your future nursing strategies.

Minimize Use of Delusions/Hallucinations

These are important, and often serious, features of psychiatric illness and, as such, must be fully recorded and reported on. Initially, it is appropriate to encourage the patient to describe these experiences in detail and to continue to do so until their nature and content are well understood and documented.

In due course, the pathological nature of these experiences needs to be made known, and you must discuss relevant nursing and other strategies with the patient. Subsequently you will want to avoid 'feeding' these experiences and encourage him to spend more time in reality. From time to time it will be necessary to discuss the delusions and hallucinations in order to determine changes in their content and nature. Your conversation with him might be like this:

Nurse: 'Hello Mr Smith. How are things today?'
Mr Smith: 'They have taken my head.'
Nurse: 'We talked about this yesterday; I still see your head on your shoulders.'
Mr Smith: 'No, it's a mirage you see. My head has been taken for the experiment.'
Nurse: 'Have you made plans for the weekend?'
Mr Smith: 'My head is ...'
Nurse: (interrupting) 'Could we talk about the weekend Mr Smith. Have you made any plans?'
Mr Smith: 'My head ...'
Nurse: (interrupting) 'The weekend Mr Smith. Any plans?'
Mr Smith: 'The weekend? Yes, I'm going to town with my friend.'

Controlling Anxiety

As your patient is moved closer to reality and has to leave behind his manufactured reality, he will experience increasing levels of anxiety. This position goes some way towards explaining the resistance to accepting reality which is presented by many patients.

At this time, you or some other person will have to act as an 'emotional crutch' to enable him to cope with the increased anxiety. This is best done via the development of a planned and structured one-to-one relationship between the patient and nurse.

Recognize Danger to Patient and Others

People who are deluded and hallucinated frequently respond to these experiences and behave in a way which is potentially very dangerous to themselves and others; for example, he might leap out of a high window to avoid capture, kill himself to avoid torture, kill his family to prevent their suffering or harm a neighbour who is allegedly trying to poison his food. We must, therefore, take these experiences seriously and learn as much about their nature and content as possible.

PATIENT PROFILE

Mrs Franks is aged 74 years and lives at home with her husband. She recently visited her family doctor at the insistence of her husband who reported that she was refusing to sleep during the night, preferring to sleep during the day-time.

This lady informed her doctor that she was in good health, which she indeed was from a physical viewpoint. On being asked why she did not sleep during the night, she replied, 'If I try to sleep at night, the whispers keep me awake'. She further explained, 'The Chinese Embassy has moved into my neighbour's flat next door. They do their work in secret at night-time. I can sleep in my room during the daytime because they also sleep at this time.' It was reported by her husband that she occasionally knocked on the wall to indicate her annoyance.

The family doctor subsequently diagnosed paranoid psychosis, a recurring illness which Mrs Franks had previously been treated for on two occasions. As before, she experienced a number of delusions and hallucinations of the persecutory/paranoid type. On this occasion, these problems apparently all related to the alleged use of the neighbour's flat by the Chinese Embassy.

As on previous occasions, the family doctor decided to treat Mrs Franks conservatively (without medication) and arrange that she be visited by a community psychiatric nurse (CPN) following consultation with a psychiatrist.

The first CPN visit took place the next day, she met with Mrs and Mr Franks and both freely discussed the current problem generally, the delusions and hallucinations in particular. Mr Franks fully understood the pathological nature of his wife's experiences; *she* was fully convinced of their 'reality' and suggested that only she 'understood the full picture'. A further visit was arranged and the visits continued weekly for four months when, as on previous occasions, the symptoms disappeared.

ORGANIZATION OF NURSING CARE

Subjective Evidence (What the Patient Says)

- 'If I try to sleep at night the whispers keep me awake.'
- 'The Chinese Embassy has moved into my neighbour's flat next door.'
- 'They do their work in secret at night-time.'

Objective Evidence (What the Nurse and Others Observe)

- Refuses to sleep in own room at night.
- Knocks on the wall to indicate her annoyance.

Assessment (Nursing Diagnosis)

- Reality (perception), delusions and hallucinations.

Plan of Nursing Care

- Establish interpersonal contact via structured one-to-one relationship.
- Discuss problem, encourage patient to recognize and verbalize.
- Having established nature/content of delusions and hallucinations, discourage her attempts to talk about them.
- Focus on reality, provide and encourage 'reality' experiences, conversation, social activities and so on.
- Provide opportunities for discussing the problem, discussions which will lead to improved insight.
- Be alert to possible danger to patient and/or others resulting from delusions and hallucinations.

Expected Outcome

- Reduced frequency of complaints about 'whispers' and night-time noise in neighbour's flat.
- Increased ability to focus on reality as opposed to delusions and hallucinations, e.g. can interact for half hour without referring to them.
- Spends more time in bedroom during the night (for example, goes to bed at 02.00 instead of 02.30).
- Spends less time asleep during the daytime (for example, 1½ h instead of 2 h).

NURSING CARE OF A PATIENT WITH A REALITY (PERCEPTION) PROBLEM (EXAMPLE)

This example is taken from a period halfway through the illness, a time when Mrs Franks was spending *part* of the night in bed.

07.30 hours   Awakens her husband with morning tea, she says, 'There was quite a bit of activity last night; they were sending messages'. As arranged, Mr Franks replies in a way which indicates that *he* did not hear these activities.

08.00   Breakfast. Mrs Franks attempts to engage her husband in conversation about the Chinese. He ignores such requests and *only* replies when she is in touch with reality, for example:

Mrs Franks: 'They were at it last night.'

Mr Franks: (No reply.)

Mrs Franks: 'The noise was awful.'

Mr Franks: (No reply.)

Mrs Franks: 'I don't know what I'm going to do.'

Mr Franks: (No reply.)

Mrs Franks: 'What are we having for lunch?'

Mr Franks: 'Why don't we have a walk down to the butcher's shop and see what we fancy?'

Alternatively, Mr Franks could have replied to his wife's first statement ('They were at it last night') by saying, 'Are you enjoying your breakfast'.

09.00   Housework with Mr Franks focusing attention and conversation on reality.

10.30   CPN visits and meets with Mr and Mrs Franks. The purpose of the meeting is to:

    (i)   Discuss progress to date (particularly changes in sleep patterns).

    (ii)   Monitor Mrs Franks' delusional and hallucinatory levels, and her feelings about them.

    (iii)   Reinforce reality and the pathological nature of the delusions and hallucinations.

    (iv)   Monitor the extent to which Mr Franks is coping with this situation and provide a supportive therapy for him.

    (v)   Discuss all activities which the couple have undertaken in the past week.

    (vi)   Set new goals if those which were set last week have been reached; for example, 'Will now get to bed at 02.00 instead of 02.30'.

11.30   Visiting the local Old Folks Club and interacting, with the help and support of her husband, with others who are attending.

12.30   Lunch at the club.

14.00   Returns home and sleeps for two hours, a practice which is strongly discouraged by CPN, husband and close relatives.

16.00   At home and preparing for evening meal. Interactions between Mr and Mrs Franks will take the same form throughout the day in terms of focusing on reality (see 08.00).

17.00   Evening meal.

18.30	Visiting married daughter who lives nearby. The daughter and her husband, who have both met the CPN, play an important part in the interventions planned with and for Mrs Franks. Typically, they will allow her to mention 'the problem' (which she invariably does) and encourage her to talk about it for two to three minutes. They will then use the technique described above (see 08.00) to focus her on reality.
20.00	Returns home, reads newspapers and watches television.
21.30	Supper.
22.30	Mr Franks prepares for bed. Before retiring he indicates that he expects his wife to join him at 02.00 or earlier.
23.00	Mr Franks retires. Mrs Franks, now 'disturbed' by the activities of the Chinese in the flat next door waits and listens. By prior arrangement with the CPN she plays recordings of her favourite music which apparently reduces the stress which the activities cause her.
02.00	Mrs Franks joins her husband in bed.

ASSESSMENT OF REALITY (PERCEPTION)

Concentration

- Distractible, preoccupied, e.g. mutters to self, looks over shoulder.
- Good/poor concentration.

Anxiety

- Tense/relaxed.
- Accepts/rejects being focused on reality.

Verbalizing/Recognizing

- Describes/denies having hallucinatory, delusional experiences.
- Recognizes/denies that these experiences are pathological (level of insight).

Concept of Reality

- Responds to hallucinations/delusions.
- Realistic, obviously disturbed.

● Deluded (state type): ....

....

....

● Hallucinated (state type): ....

....

....

FURTHER READING

Buckley M. (1983) Tormented by delusions. *Nursing Mirror* **157**, 43–6.

Clack J. (1962) An Interpersonal technique for handling hallucinations in Monograph No.13 *Nursing Care Of The Disoriented Patient,* p.16–26. American Nurses Association, New York.

Donner G. (1969) Treatment of a delusional patient. *American Journal of Nursing* **69**, 2642–4.

Field W.E. & Ruelke W. (1973) Hallucinations and how to deal with them. *American Journal of Nursing* **73**, 638–40.

Grosicki J.P. & Harmonson M. (1969) Nursing action guide: Hallucinations. *Journal of psychiatric Nursing and Mental Health Services* **vii**, 133–5.

Hare E.H. (1973) A short note on pseudo–hallucinations. *British Journal of Psychiatry* **122**, 469–76.

McIvor D. (1976) Myopia, hallucinations and delusions. *Psychiatric Nursing* **xvii**, 7–8.

Schwartzman S.T. (1975) The hallucinating patient and nursing intervention. *Journal of psychiatric Nursing and Mental Health Services* Nov.–Dec., 23–36.

Chapter 25
Respiration

Respiration is the process of supplying oxygen to the tissues and removing carbon dioxide, oxygen being essential for normal cell function and hence for life. Tissues, in particular the brain cells, can survive for only three to four minutes before being irreversibly damaged if deprived of oxygen. To be deprived of air for even a few moments causes extreme anxiety and panic in everyone. For these reasons acute respiratory distress is always an emergency and needs to be treated quickly and efficiently. Chronic respiratory problems are also very common and are a major cause of morbidity and death amongst the elderly. 'Breathlessness' is perhaps second only to pain as a symptom complained of to doctors. 'Shortness of breath' is, of course, a symptom of many non-respiratory diseases, such as heart failure, anaemia, thyroid disease and kidney failure. 'Dyspnoea' or 'difficulty in breathing' is a feature of chronic airway disease and disorders such as pulmonary oedema. Whether young or old, poor respiratory function seriously affects the quality of life the individual can lead.

FACTORS RELATING TO RESPIRATION

Normal Respiration

The ability to acquire and deliver oxygen to the tissues is a complex phenomenon. It depends on a network of organs and tissues that effects exchange of gases between the individual and the environment. The activity of the tissues and organs must be matched in such a way that oxygen is delivered to the venous blood in exchange for carbon dioxide. Therefore, the ventilation of the lungs, the pumping action of the heart, the oxygen-carrying capacity of the red blood corpuscles and the ability of the tissues to utilize the oxygen have all to be considered. Respiration then includes two processes: external respiration, the absorption of oxygen and removal of carbon dioxide through the lungs, and internal respiration, the exchanges of these gases between the cells and the blood.

The respiratory system is remarkably efficient in health at acquiring all the oxygen the body tissues need. The lungs have an enormous reserve capacity and are highly efficient at gas exchange. The exchange of gases is dependent on the alveoli (the functional units of the lungs) being ventilated and the capillaries supplying the alveoli being perfused with blood. When alveoli are both ventilated and perfused, gaseous exchange proceeds normally and ventilation and perfusion are said to be in balance.

On inspiration the size of the chest cavity increases. This causes the pressure inside the chest to become lower and air is sucked in, or, to put it another way, moves from an area of high pressure to an area of low pressure. On expiration the size of the cavity is decreased and the air is exhaled passively.

Respiratory Control

The control of respiration is mediated through chemoreceptors located in the carotid artery and aortic arch. These chemoreceptors detect changes in the pH, P_{CO_2} and P_{O_2} levels (see Table 25.1) and relay this information to the respiratory centre in the medulla oblongata. Of the three, changes in carbon dioxide and pH levels have the greatest effect on the respiratory centre. The respiratory centre in the medulla oblongata relays information to the muscles of respiration which either stimulates them to increase or decrease their activity, depending on circumstances. In addition to the chemoreceptors there are stretch receptors (Hering-Breuer reflex) within the lungs which prevent their overexpansion. This control system is very efficient and if, for example, carbon dioxide levels rise, the rate of ventilation can be increased many times to restore normal levels. Campbell and Lefrak (1978) report studies in young normal individuals which show a striking linear increase in minute ventilation* when arterial P_{CO_2} is increased by increasing the P_{CO_2} of inspired air, so that a minute volume of 60 l/min (about 10 times normal) can be reached. The elderly person's performance contrasts poorly with this as we shall see later.

Table 25.1 Normal blood gas values.

Symbol		Normal value
pH	= hydrogen ion concentration	7.35 – 7.45
P_{O_2}	= arterial oxygen tension	100 mmHg (13.3 kPa)
P_{CO_2}	= arterial carbon dioxide tension	40 mmHg (5.3 kPa)

*Minute ventilation = Tidal volume (volume of air per breath) × Respiratory rate (number of breaths per min).

Respiratory Defences

The alveoli provide an enormous surface area for gaseous exchange within the restricted and confined space of the lungs. Given also that this surface is in direct contact with the external environment, it follows that some means of protection and defence are essential. The lungs are protected by various means. First, incoming air is warmed and moistened by the upper air passages. Dust and other larger particulate matter are filtered out by the vibrissae or hairs in the nostrils. However, the main defences consist of the ciliated epithelium and goblet cells lining the trachea, bronchi and bronchioles, and by large numbers of macrophages supplied by the haemopoietic system. Mucus produced by the goblet cells traps inhaled dust, bacteria, spores and so on. The ciliated epithelium wafts the mucus, dust, etc., towards the larynx where it is then swallowed, if in large quantities, the cough reflex will be activated and this is also protective. The macrophages are scavenger cells capable of ingesting and destroying invading bacteria. In addition, the lungs have a generous amount of lymphatic tissue which gives added protection against pathogens. As people get older, cilia are lost from the airways whilst the vigour of those remaining declines. This means inhaled material, bacteria and mucus are less easily cleared from the lungs; the process is often made worse by environmental pollutants. The macrophages are also impaired over the years by pollutants so that the older person is at much greater risk from pathogenic bacteria, viruses and fungi as well as general anaesthesia. The decline in the effectiveness of the lung defences, plus the many other age-related changes which take place, leaves elderly subjects with decreased compensatory mechanisms for dealing with even moderate stress.

Effects of Ageing on the Respiratory System

Often the first time people realize they are growing older is when everyday tasks once performed with ease require greater effort. They discover that they can no longer sustain physical activity as they once used to. Part of this increased effort and decreased endurance comes about because of changes to the musculoskeletal system (see Chapter 12). It is not only skeletal muscle strength that declines with age, the muscles of the respiratory apparatus are similarly affected. This results in significant decreases in both maximal inspiratory and maximal expiratory pressures in comparison with younger persons. The chest also stiffens with advancing age. This decrease in chest wall compliance presumably follows structural changes such as calcification of the articulations of the rib cage. If other skeletal deformities, such as kyphoscoliosis, develop, chest wall compliance will be further decreased.

There is reduced ability to elevate the rib cage on inhalation because of weaker muscles of respiration and a chest which has grown stiffer and, therefore, harder to move. In short, the work of ventilating the lungs becomes greater as we grow older.

Like most other systems in the body the respiratory system has a considerable reserve capacity. At 20 years of age the alveolar surface area is in the region of 80 m^2. The number of alveoli has been estimated at 300×10^{16}. In the normal ageing process the alveoli become smaller and more shallow which has the effect of reducing the alveolar surface area to perhaps 65 – 70 m^2. The total lung volume remains virtually constant throughout life but the vital capacity falls at a steady rate from young adulthood. As much as a litre of capacity is lost between the ages of 20 and 60 years (Kenny 1982). There are age-related changes in all timed ventilatory functions, such as forced expiratory volume in one second (FEV$_1$) and maximal breathing capacity both showing a significant decrease in the aged individual who is free of lung disease (Kenny 1982). These changes are at least partly due to changes in the large and small airways which become more 'floppy' with age. Hence during a forced expiration, the more compliant airways may be more prone to collapse, contributing to the decrease in maximal expiratory flow rates and also to the increase in residual volume seen with ageing (Campbell & Lefrak 1978).

One way to appreciate this more fully is to consider the lung as a balloon. The lung has elastic properties like a balloon so that when it is inflated it is always trying to expel its gaseous contents. If you keep blowing up a balloon, it begins to lose its elastic properties and can be inflated more easily; it also expels the air less forcefully. The ageing lung also loses some of its elasticity and so can be blown up to much larger volumes and is also less able to expel its gaseous contents as efficiently and completely as previously.

Another observation which has been made in elderly people is their reponsiveness to changes in Po_2. It has been found that the decrease in Po_2 in the elderly person has to be much greater than that in the younger person to bring about equal change in the minute ventilation; for example, in the young person an arterial Po_2 of 40 mmHg would result in the minute ventilation increasing to as much as five times the basal level. Also, in the young person low Po_2 would result in a greatly increased heart rate compared with the minor increase exhibited by the older individuals. Therefore, the older individual's response to decreased oxygen content of the arterial blood is less vigorous. One might conclude, therefore, that the older individual's oxygen delivery to the tissues may be inadequate if subjected to stress.

This is but a brief resumé of the more significant changes that occur with ageing. However, the majority of elderly persons have enough respiratory capacity to function adequately provided they are not put under stress. Stress of course produces multi-system failure, and collapse of other systems may be of equal or greater significance in some circumstances. The elderly are also subject to many respiratory disorders which exacerbate the effects of the ageing process.

Hypoxia and Emphysema

Hypoxia signifies a reduced amount of oxygen either in the lungs or in the tissues, whilst hypoxaemia is a reduced amount of oxygen in the arterial blood. There are various types of hypoxia, as can be deduced from an understanding of external and internal respiration. At rest the normal adult breathes about 15 times per minute, air is breathed in and mixes with air in the air passages and alveoli. Oxygen in the air then passes across the alveolar walls into the pulmonary capilliaries, at the same time carbon dioxide passes out and is exhaled. The pressure (or partial pressure, Po_2) of the oxygen in the inspired air must be sufficient to force it to dissolve in the thin layer of fluid that lines the alveoli and to propel it into the pulmonary capillaries. Should anything obstruct the passage of oxygen across the alveolar membrane, hypoxia will ensue. This type of hypoxia is called 'obstructive' hypoxia and is caused by primary lung diseases such as chronic bronchitis, emphysema and pneumonias, and also by pulmonary oedema secondary to heart failure or other cause.

Another type of hypoxia is called 'stagnant' hypoxia and , as the name implies, results from failure of cardiac function in which blood flow is reduced. Anaemia hypoxia is the name given to the hypoxia which occurs when the person is anaemic. A fourth rarer type of hypoxia, histoxic, occurs when the tissues are unable to utilize the oxygen, as occurs in cyanide poisoning! Some conditions increase the cell's oxygen requirements; for example, thyrotoxicosis and pyrexia, both of which increase the metabolic rate. This increased metabolic rate can be quite critical in the elderly, especially in those who have conditions such as emphysema.

Emphysema is defined as the permanent enlargement of the gas-exchanging part of the lung, the alveoli. The condition is characterized by the destruction of the alveolar wall. This lesion results in a number of functional consequences which are primarily due to the effect on the mechanical properties of the lung. The physiological changes observed in patients with emphysema are much the same as those seen in the normal old person in certain respects, as are the anatomical changes (Campbell & Lefrak, 1978). The same authors have compared the normal aged person's lung and emphysema as is shown in Table 25.2.

Emphysema is a complex disease process and largely preventable. It

Table 25.2 Comparison of changes in lung function due to ageing and emphysema.

Parameter	Advanced age	Emphysema
Static recoil pressure	↓	↓↓↓
Airway closure	↑	↑↑↑
VC	↓	↓↓
RV	↑	↑↑↑
FEV$_1$	↓	↓↓↓
P_{O_2}	↓	↓

VC   = Vital capacity.
RV   = Residual volume.
FEV$_1$ = Forced expiratory volume in one second.
P_{O_2} = Arterial oxygen tension.

Table 25.3 Typical progression of emphysema (after Fries & Crapo 1981).

Age (years)	Change
20	Starts smoking
30	Mild airway obstruction
40	X-ray hyperinflation
50	Shortness of breath
60	Recurrent hospitalization
70	Intractable oxygen debt

rarely occurs in non-smokers and Fries and Crapo (1981) suggest the pattern as shown in Table 25.3 as being a fairly typical course for the disorder.

It can be seen from this that the damage to the lungs begins early, though overt clinical symptoms may not appear for 20 or 30 years. Emphysema is without doubt the most serious and most common of all chronic repiratory disorders. Like others, such as chronic bronchitis and lung cancer, the incidence could be reduced if people were to stop smoking and if environmental pollution was better controlled.

PRINCIPLES OF CARE

Reduced Activity Tolerance

Chronic respiratory problems such as chronic bronchitis and emphysema affect the individual in many ways; if severe, the sufferer may have such a reduced activity tolerance that he is unable to perform any physical task without experiencing dyspnoea. Even the thought of activity such as having to get up out of bed and get dressed may make the dyspnoea worse. As the dyspnoea worsens over the years he becomes less and less able to perform the activities of daily living and becomes dependent on others. He may come to rely on oxygen therapy and this, combined with the fear that he may not be able to take in enough air, increases his anxiety thus further reducing activity tolerance.

Improving Respiratory Function

Efforts then have to be made to break the vicious cycle of events. The patient's activity level must be increased. This can only be done gradually; the first step being to teach breathing exercises, which will maximize breathing capacity. The patient's problem is that he is unable to breathe out; his residual volume remains high and so the amount of gaseous exchange between the atmosphere and the alveoli is reduced. In some patients this may be as low as 100 ml, or less, instead of the normal 400−500 ml. Teaching of breathing exercises should concentrate on breathing out. The patient needs to learn how to use his abdominal muscles to raise his diaphragm on expiration and to co-ordinate the work of the chest and the diaphragm. Breathing out through 'pursed lips' can also prolong the exhalation period and so reduce carbon dioxide retention.

It is also important that the patient learns to cough properly, since retained secretions will also interfere with breathing capacity and, of course, may lead to serious infection. Breathing exercises are often linked to specific medical therapy and/or postural drainage. In hospital, a physiotherapist will be required to assist the patient in clearing his bronchial secretions, which are often copious and tenacious. In severe cases this will be required three or four times per day or more often. Breathing exercises should be performed for 2-3 minutes, four or five times per day.

In addition to breathing exercises, the patient should be encouraged to do as much as he can for himself. Generally most patients are worst in the morning and improve a little as the day goes on. Smoking should be discouraged as it only makes the condition worse, though many will claim a cigarette helps to mobilize the bronchial secretions. However, when dealing with people in their 70s and 80s who have smoked for a lifetime, perhaps they should be left to decide whether or not to continue. Often a smoke and a few hours watching television is about all they have to look forward to, and by that age the damage is done. It is easy to be critical, but when they started smoking the dangers were not recognized. Also, control of industrial pollutants in many work areas was non-existent or very poor compared with modern standards. The patient with extreme chronic respiratory distress is a sorry sight, he deserves whatever help we can give. He does not need to be reminded of his plight, it is with him every waking minute of the day and often at night as well.

Disturbed Sleep Pattern

Many patients with chronic obstructive lung disease experience drastic changes in their sleep pattern. Yet, for them rest and sleep are critical. The work of breathing is greatly increased so that instead of only 1 or 2% of the oxygen intake going towards it, up to 20% may be used. The disturbed sleep may be related to changes in the breathing pattern. During sleep, the rate and depth of respiration decreases and carbon dioxide levels increase whilst oxygen levels decrease. These changes possibly trigger a mechanism which awakens the patient to correct hypoventilation. In these circumstances the acute dyspnoea experienced causes intense anxiety. The patient may also fear that he will not wake up and may, consciously or unconsciously, sleep lightly. Some patients do indeed become unconscious due to carbon dioxide retention, so that the fear is a real one.

Some drugs used to treat the disorder may also prevent sleep because of their adrenergic effect, that is their stimulant effect, for example aminophylline.

Social and Environmental Factors

For anyone, the environment for sleep and rest is important. Extreme dyspnoea may force the person to change his sleeping place; for example, he may no longer be able to climb stairs and will have to sleep in the living room. People who are seriously handicapped by chronic respiratory distress need to prepare themselves for bed in much the same way as anyone else. They should avoid undue exercise near their bedtime, or other activities which lead to increased alertness. They should be strongly discouraged from sleeping during the day except perhaps for a short period of rest after lunch. Instead of trying to get back to sleep once awoken in the night, it may be better for them to get up and read a book or watch a late night movie on television. This sort of thing is likely to be frowned on in most hospitals, yet it is easily arranged and should inconvience no-one. Once the patient feels sleepy again he can return to bed. A hot drink and a biscuit will also be helpful to many patients. Sedatives must be used with great care in any patient who has a severe respiratory disorder. This is even more so in the elderly in whom drug metabolism may be less efficient. Drugs such as diazepam, chlordiazepoxide, meprobamate and chloral hydrate can be given safely if insomnia is a major problem.

Effects of Chronic Illness

After years of suffering, most patients will have their own routines and often please themselves anyway. Indeed poor compliances with drug regimens and recommendations is very common in many patients who have chronic illness. As nurses we tend to be fairly glib in our advice to stop smoking, lose weight, change your life style, take more exercise, sleep sitting upright, eat more fibre in your diet, and so on. For the individual with chronic illness it is seldom quite as simple. Adjustment to any chronic illness is very difficult after a lifetime of normal human activity. Not only does it affect the individual but also his family, especially those nearest to him. Some families become overprotective which may lead to almost total isolation and very low self-esteem. The individual feels guilty and worthless and becomes depressed. In this state he is unlikely to comply with any therapeutic regimen, further increasing his dependence on others. Chronic illness can disrupt even the most loving families so that family members also need much support and help; for them also there is often no escape.

Other Causes of Respiratory Disorder

There are, of course, many other forms of chronic respiratory disorder. Many of them are caused by exposure to industrial pollutants, especially amongst coal miners and quarry workers. In addition to the effect of industrial pollutants, many workers in these areas also suffered from tuberculosis which often left permanent scarring with lowered efficiency of the lungs. Disorders of the central nervous system often cause respiratory difficulties. However, chronic obstructive airways diseases, chronic bronchitis, emphysema and asthma, are by far the most common and serious disorders, and the basic principles in caring for them are equally applicable to all forms of chronic respiratory distress. Acute respiratory distress is managed in much the same way regardless of age, though one must bear in mind that the elderly person is always more at risk, whether the stress be internal or external.

PATIENT PROFILE

Mr Andrew Begg, aged 68 years, was forced to retire at 55, when no longer able to carry out his job. Mr Begg's history is very typical. He started smoking when 13 or 14 years old and at one time smoked up to 80 cigarettes per day. He started work in a jute factory at 14 and gradually worked his way up to works manager. His only break from the jute industry was a four year spell in the Royal Air Force during the Second World War. Many of the jobs Mr Begg did in the jute mill were very dusty and little was done to combat it. By the time Mr Begg was aged 40 years he already had a productive cough and had reduced activity tolerance. To a certain extent he was able to mitigate the worst effects for many years as he moved from mainly manual work to more supervisory type of work. In the last five years that he did work, Mr Begg required hospital treatment for 2-3 months each year. At 55 years old he was forced to accept the fact that he was no longer able to work. Since his retirement Mr Begg has become progressively more handicapped, rarely able to leave his own home. He has spells of up to 4 or 5 months in hospital each year. Chronic airways obstruction for 30 years has also inevitably affected his heart which is now failing badly (cor pulmonale).

Mr Begg is cared for mainly by his wife, assisted by a district nurse who calls three or four times a week. Mr Begg has been prescribed a range of drugs for his respiratory and cardiac disorders. He requires oxygen therapy most of the time, this is given to him via nasal catheters; the nasal catheters being attached to the oxygen cylinder via a long tube which gives him some scope for mobility around the living room.

ORGANIZATION OF NURSING CARE

Subjective Evidence (What the Patient Says)

- 'I haven't the energy to drink a cup of tea nowadays.'
- 'I couldn't blow out a candle.'
- 'I am tethered to this damn thing.' (Referring to his oxygen.)

Objective Evidence (What the Nurse and Others Observe)

- Patient requires up to two hours each day to dress.
- Respirations obviously laboured, breathes out through pursed lips.
- Respiratory rate 36 per minute, heart rate 110, peak expiratory flow rate (PEFR) 1.5 l/min.

Assessment (Nursing Diagnosis)

- Chronic respiratory distress with low activity tolerance.

Plan of Nursing Care

GENERAL AIM

To improve on respiratory function and activity tolerance.
- Encourage Mr Begg to do breathing exercises as instructed.
- Encourage him to cough and expectorate to clear bronchial tree.
- Encourage good fluid intake — up to 2000 ml/day at least.
- Encourage him gradually to increase his level of activity each day.
- Ensure good compliance with prescribed drug therapy.
- Set patient goals to attain, e.g. increase in PEFR/min.

Expected Outcome

- Patient's respiratory rate will be down to <24 breaths/min at rest.
- PEFR >2 l/min.
- Patient activity level will increase.

Postscript

Mr Begg continues to be nursed mainly at home by his wife with assistance from the district nurse. Any little improvements gained seem just as quickly lost. In the long-term Mr Begg's prospects remain gloomy. Little can be done other than therapy for symptomatic relief and maintaining general well-being at the best possible level compatible with his poor respiratory status.

NURSING CARE OF PATIENT WITH A RESPIRATION PROBLEM (EXAMPLE)

07.00 hours	Early morning tea, assist if necessary.
07.30	Breathing exercises, coughing and expectoration combined with prescribed drug therapy.
08.00	Breakfast of choice. Sit well up, give time to enjoy meal.
08.30	Start to get up and dressed. Encouraged to do as much as possible for himself.
10.00	Mid-morning drink. If possible in company of others.
10.30	Visit by district nurse. Skin and hair care. Breathing exercises.

Lung function tests to assess progress (PEFR).

12.00   Lunch, food of choice. Food should be prepared which does not demand a lot of chewing, which will increase breathlessness. Whenever possible meals should be taken in company of others.

13.00   Rest for one hour. Patient should rest in position he finds most comfortable, preferably should have legs elevated for this period to assist venous return and minimize oedema formation.

14.00   Recreational activity depending on what the patient feels up to; for example, a table game such as cards or dominoes, or, if able, something more strenuous such as weaving on a hand-loom will encourage chest expansion.

15.00   Mid-afternoon tea.

16.00   Breathing exercises. Three to five minutes duration as taught.

17.00   Recreational activity depending on what the patient feels up to. Preferrably in company of others to encourage social intercourse.

18.00   Evening meal of choice. Ensure patient is getting a balanced diet. (See note for lunch.)

19.00   Breathing exercises as taught for three to five minutes.

19.30–21.00 Watch television or participate in family activities, e.g. card games, monopoly, jigsaw puzzles, scrabble, etc.

21.00   Prepare for bed. Patient should be encouraged to do as much as possible for himself. Oral hygiene. Late night drink such as drinking chocolate.

22.00   Bed. Medication as prescribed.

22.00–07.00 Allowed to rest throughout the night undisturbed if possible. Leave adequate fresh fluids for drinking during the night. Ensure adequate oxygen supply. Patient should sleep in whatever position he finds most comfortable.

Each day should be varied as much as possible. Try to introduce something new or novel from time to time, especially activities which will help to maintain or improve respiratory function.

ASSESSMENT OF RESPIRATION

General Observations

- Skin colour — lips, mucous membranes, nail beds.
- Body posture.

- Chest deformity.
- Mental status.

Respiratory Pattern (Expected)

- Rate: 16–18/min.
- Rhythm: regular, even.
- Depth: moderate, neither shallow or deep.
- Effort: no conscious awareness.
- Sounds: no overt sounds.

Common Symptoms

- Cough: nature of.
- Sputum: nature of (bacterial culture).
- Pain: nature of.
- Haemoptysis: frequency.
- Weight loss: recent, rapid, insidious.
- Dyspnoea: (see below).

Exercise Tolerance in Relation to Activities of Daily Living

Partridge (1984) suggests the following five-grade system for recording the patient's exercise tolerance.

- Normal.
- Able to walk with healthy people his own age and sex on the level but unable to keep up on hills and stairs.
- Unable to keep up with healthy people on the level but can walk long distances at his own pace.
- Unable to walk more than 100 metres on the level before being stopped by breathlessness.
- Unable to walk more than a few steps without dyspnoea, becomes breathless on washing and dressing.

Respiratory Function Tests

- Forced vital capacity (FVC; measure of the rate at which a person can expel air). The normal individual can expel 75% of their FVC in one second, that is the forced expiratory volume in one second (FEV_1). This measure can be easily recorded on a Vitalograph.

Peak Expiratory Flow Rate (PEFR)

● Recorded using a Wright's Peak Flow Meter. This measures the maximum rate of flow of air during a forced expiration. The result is expressed in litres of air per minute — normal 4 – 6 l/min.

Blood Gases

● These tests are not done routinely but are essential in some situations where the respiratory system is seriously compromised, and failure is a possibility.

REFERENCES

Campbell E.J. & Lefrak S.S. (1978) How aging affects the structure and function of the respiratory system. *Geriatrics* **33**, 68 – 74.

Fries J.F. & Crapo L.M. (1981) *Vitality and Aging*. W. H. Freeman and Co, San Francisco.

Kenny R.A. (1982) *Physiology of Aging*. Yearbook Medical Publishers, Chicago.

Partridge M. (1984) Difficulty in Breathing. *British Journal of Hospital Medicine* **31**, 288 – 91.

FURTHER READING

Block E.R. (1979) Pitfalls in diagnosing and managing pulmonary diseases. *Geriatrics* **34**, 70 – 80.

Bowles L.T., Portnoi V. & Kenney R. (1981) Wear and tear; Common biologic changes of aging. *Geriatrics* **36**, 77 – 86.

Ghory A.C. & Patterson R. (1982) Treating asthma in the elderly. *Geriatrics* **37**, 32 – 8.

Grenville – Mathers R. (1983) *The Respiratory System,* 2nd edn. Churchill Livingstone, Edinburgh.

McDonald G.J. & Hudson L.D. (1982) Important aspects of pulmonary rehabilitation. *Geriatrics* **37**, 127 – 34.

Perry J.A. (1981) Effectiveness of teaching in rehabilitation of patients with chronic bronchitis and emphysema. *Nursing Research* **30**, 219 – 22.

Saul K. (1978) The aging lung. Part 1. Loss of elasticity. *Geriatrics* **33**, 124 – 32.

Sjoberg E.L. (1983) Nursing diagnosis and the COPD patient. *American Journal of Nursing* **83**, 245 – 8.

Thomas S. (1979) Pulse, Respiration and Blood Pressure. *Nursing Mirror* **148**, 24 – 7.

Wheeler H.H. (1980) A patient with chronic bronchitis, emphysema cor pulmonale and pulmonary embolism. *Nursing Times* **76**, 1339 – 45.

Chapter 26
Self-esteem

Self-esteem is the value that the individual places on his own worth, for example, if an individual feels that he is unimportant, worthless, and a poor father or employee, his level of self-esteem is low. Conversely, if a person feels that he is of some importance, and that he is a good father and employee, his self-esteem is high. In reality, self-esteem is more global and more all encompassing than I have just suggested; if a person's self-esteem is low, he or she tends to have negative feelings about all aspects of himself or herself. Conversely if a person's self-esteem is high then he or she tends to have positive feelings about all aspects of himself or herself.

In order to fully understand self-esteem it is necessary to realize that it relates to the person's *perception* of himself or herself. It might be suggested that no one can make your self-esteem low 'without your permission'. For example, if I am told that my ability to play golf is terrible, that it will never improve, and that I am wasting my time with the game, this may or may not negatively affect my perception of myself as a golfer. Even if the statements are all true, made by a golf professional for instance, if I feel good at my golf game then I will continue to have a positive perception of it. More generally, the way in which an individual *interprets* information from his environment, and the people in it is as important, if not more important, than the actual content of that information.

It is also necessary to appreciate that an individual's level of self-esteem is only partially related to his material, economic and social circumstances. It would be just as possible to find a 'down and out' who is generally impoverished and living rough with a high self-esteem, as it would be to find an apparently successful and economically secure person with a low level of self-esteem.

Thus, it must never be assumed that a person's level of self-esteem can be measured or determined by what he or she *appears* to be. Some years ago this author worked on a ward in which a socially successful, physically attractive and upper social class woman was a patient. The major reason for her hospitalization (in a psychiatric ward) was that she experienced uncontrollable outbursts of aggression towards other people. After she and a nurse had spent a considerable amount of time together as part of a psychotherapeutic process, it was determined that her problem was in fact low self-esteem. The basis of this lady's problem was that, when she saw other groups of people talking together, she (wrongly) assumed that they were talking about, and criticizing, her. Thus, her low self-esteem caused her (probably at an unconscious level) to attack those people whom she wrongly perceived as being threatening.

Maslow (1954), who ranked human needs in a hierarchy ranging from basic physical needs to self-actualization needs, included self-esteem as an important part of this hierarchy. Although it cannot be denied that basic physical needs, those upon which the physical existence of the person is dependent, are of prime importance, needs such as self-esteem are equally important and add a great deal to the quality of life.

SELF-ESTEEM IN THE ELDERLY

As with all adult groups, self-esteem is a necessary and important part of the make-up and needs of the elderly person. The author's view is that the self-esteem of the elderly person is both less 'brittle' than other groups, *and* is more prone to 'attack'.

The reason why self-esteem of the elderly person is less 'brittle' than for other groups is that the elderly person has had a longer time in which to develop, and become comfortable with himself. This proposition is best illustrated by comparing the well-developed self-esteem of the elderly with the poorly developed (and developing) self-esteem of the adolescent who, at the slightest provocation, will have his level of self-esteem seriously damaged by an *apparently* trivial event.

The circumstances which place the elderly person 'at risk' of having his self-esteem damaged include those that follow. First, the negative views of society and the individuals in it (see Chapter 4 which discusses ageism) do little to make the elderly in most Western societies feel good about themselves. Second, the physical, psychological and social decline which often accompanies the ageing process (resulting in death) is generally perceived as a negative phenomenon which does not enhance self-esteem. Similarly, the changes that result in wrinkles, baldness, toothlessness, facial hair on women, loss of strength and the many overt consequences of old age do *not* enhance self-esteem.

Thus, we need to build on the resilience and strength which the elderly have in relation to their well-developed and substantial reserves of self-esteem. Additionally, we need to work very hard to prevent and neutralize the many negative consequences of the ageing process, particularly as these relate to ageism.

FACTORS RELATING TO SELF-ESTEEM

Previous Personality

The normal range of self-esteem, which varies considerably between individuals, is such that some of us develop a relatively high self-esteem, whilst others have a relatively low self-esteem. We have all met individuals who seem constantly to feel good about themselves, happy with themselves and their lot, and who seem to be resilient and strong in the face of any attack on their self-esteem. Conversely we have all met individuals who seem to be perpetually unhappy about themselves and their performance, who are self-critical and who will readily agree that they and/or their performance is usually below average.

Although the development of self-esteem is outwith the scope of this chapter, remember that levels of self-esteem do vary between individuals and, vary within the same individual over a period of time. Clearly, if the elderly individual we are concerned with has a high level of self-esteem to begin with, he or she is better equipped to deal with the process of growing old and with the (unfortunate) negative consequences which that process results in.

Attitudes of Others

The attitudes of other individuals, including health care staff and other care givers, with which the elderly person comes into contact is a significant feature in relation to self-esteem. If other individuals are warm, supportive, encouraging, positive and enjoy the company of the older individual, this will have positive consequences for that older person's self-esteem. If the old person is perceived as being a burden or as 'someone I'd rather not care for or work with', then the negative attitude will, consciously or otherwise, be transferred to the old person who will feel worse rather than better about himself.

Physical Environment

The quality of the physical environment in which the elderly person is cared for will, undoubtedly, be reflected in his feelings about himself; for example, if we provide an environment which clearly reflects our positive feelings about the elderly person, that we value and care for him, and which is designed to increase his level of self-esteem we will reduce the possibility of a self-esteem problem developing (see Chapter 33 for a discussion of the therapeutic use of the environment).

Meaningful Life Routine

A meaningful, positive and active life routine for the elderly person will considerably add to his level of self-esteem, making him feel wanted and useful. Allowing each person to develop and participate in the planning of their own activity, and routine, requires a high level of staffing, with well-trained and understanding staff, it also requires that staff feel good about and want to work with the older person.

Opportunities for Personal Expression

All of us enjoy individuality and the opportunity to express ourselves in an individual and personal way. Although group activity and participation are, for most of us, highly enjoyable, all of us need to be able to identify those experiences which are 'ours'. This individuality for personal expression is reflected in personal possessions, personal clothing, personal events such as birthdays, personal choices, the ability to choose solitary or group activities, and generally to be in control of decisions about oneself.

PRINCIPLES OF CARE

The first general principle of care which relates specifically to self-esteem is the recognition of the worth and importance of the elderly person without which very little can be achieved in this area. A recognition that ageing is a normal and natural process which will (hopefully) be experienced by us all is essential as is the recognition that the elderly who require our help must be given it by staff of the highest quality and experience.

Opportunities for making therapeutic use of the environment are probably greater with the elderly than with almost any other group. Although they may not require sophisticated, expensive or ultra-modern equipment and/or facilities, they do require an environment in which every item (from the smallest to the largest) is seen as having some therapeutic or antitherapeutic potential. Nurses, as 'keepers' of the patient's environment, have an obligation to make use of that environment. If you feel that painting the toilet door pink, or giving *every* bed in the ward a bedcover of a different colour is therapeutic *then it must be done.*

The individuality of each older person must be preserved and encouraged while recognizing that group activities and considerations are of some value. The temptation to organize a bus trip for them (*all* patients in the ward) or a walk for *all* the patients who are mobile must be strongly resisted. Again, individual care demands adequate quantities and quality of staff, it is *your* job to ensure that this staffing requirement is made known to those who handle staffing resources.

Strong interpersonal relationships between older individuals, and between the older individual and the individual nurse are the foundation upon which much of the success in working with the elderly person depends. Many older people are, by nature, reserved and rather reluctant to express their feelings and concerns to a relative stranger. For this, and other reasons, it is necessary to make a special effort to get to know the individual patient and to gain his trust and respect. Finally, the recognition that a self-esteem problem can exist in exactly the same way as a dehydration or anxiety problem will help you to recognize it quickly and effectively. Similarly, the things which we as nurses can do in relation to a low self-esteem problem are just as specific and effective as those nursing actions which relate to a multitude of other physical and non-physical problems.

PATIENT PROFILE

Mrs Smith is an 85-year-old lady who was recently admitted to a nursing home following the death of her husband. She has no specific medical diagnosis but is physically frail and is experiencing some problems with short-term memory. She shares a room in the nursing home with one other lady who is about the same age. Mrs Smith has a house in town which is occupied by her granddaughter who is studying at the local university. Apart from her granddaughter, one other relative, a younger sister, lives in town.

Mrs Smith has settled well into the nursing home since admission and is fairly independent. She is reluctant to accept the time and attention which other residents and staff offer her, rejecting them with statements such as, 'I'm too old. Why don't you talk to the younger ones?' and, 'I don't have much hair left and it's very thin; I don't think a hairdo would do me any good' and, 'I'm on the scrap heap now. Why don't you just let me die in peace?'

Mrs Smith rarely initiates conversation with staff or other residents, believing it to be a waste of their time. Although of very well-groomed and smart appearance prior to admission to the nursing home she has 'let herself go' and is generally untidy, poorly made up and reluctant to make full use of her full wardrobe of clothes. On being invited by staff and other residents to visit the nearby restaurant for afternoon tea recently she replied, 'I'm a mess; I don't want anybody to see me'.

ORGANIZATION OF NURSING CARE

Subjective Evidence (What the Patient Says)

- 'I'm too old, why don't you talk to the younger ones.'
- 'I don't have much hair left and it's very thin; I don't think a hairdo would do me any good.'
- 'I'm on the scrap heap now. Why don't you just let me die in peace?'

Objective Evidence (What the Nurse and Others Observe)

- Rarely initiates conversation with staff or other residents.
- Generally untidy and poorly made up.
- Wears the same outer clothes each day of the week unless prompted to do otherwise.
- Refuses to visit public places outwith the nursing home because she feels unattractive and untidy.

Assessment (Nursing Diagnosis)

- Low self-esteem.

Plan of Nursing Care

- All staff to make a special effort to spend time with Mrs Smith.
- Selected staff member to form an intensive and close one-to-one relationship. The general purpose of the relationship will be to enable Mrs Smith to talk about and express her feelings about herself. More particularly it will be used to indicate to her that people in her environment do feel positive and warm towards her.
- Compliment her when her appearance is improved over the previous position.
- Give regular and consistent encouragement to improve appearance generally, clothing and make-up in particular.

Expected Outcome

- Will make less frequent negative remarks about self.
- Will play an active part in looking after personal appearance generally, make-up and clothing in particular.
- Will initiate conversations with staff and/or other residents at least once daily initially.

- Will agree to go outwith the nursing home at least once weekly in the first instance, e.g. to the local restaurant.
- Will take an interest in and make positive plans about the future.

NURSING CARE OF PATIENT WITH LOW SELF-ESTEEM PROBLEM (EXAMPLE)

07.30 hours   Waken, if not already wakened, with a genuinely warm and friendly tone. Address Mrs Smith by name and make some positive remark such as, 'How are you today?' or, 'I hope you slept well' or any other sort of conversation which indicates an interest in her, and a concern for her. Before leaving her make such comment as, 'I'll leave you to get washed and dressed now Mrs Smith; I wonder what you will be wearing today'.

08.00   Return and check on progress. If Mrs Smith has not done so, help and encourage her to wash, dress and make-up to look as well as she did before admission to the nursing home.

08.30   An appetizing breakfast is served in an attractive and socially stimulating dining room environment. She is encouraged, as far as is possible, to help herself and other patients. Mrs Smith sits at a table with three other patients, one of whom she is asked to help, the other two being generally socially supportive and stimulating.

09.30   Having been helped to make her own bed and tidy her room, Mrs Smith meets with her 'special' nurse and makes plans for the rest of the day.

10.30   Morning coffee/tea is served in a social environment which encourages maximum interaction between residents. Invite her to join a group consisting of two other residents and a nurse, the object of which is to stimulate and develop interactional skills.

11.15   The daily one-to-one meeting between Mrs Smith and her assigned nurse takes place. This meeting which lasts for 45 minutes has two major purposes: first, as a general indication of her worth and purpose within the nursing home environment; second, to enable and encourage Mrs Smith to identify and explore her general feelings about herself and, particularly, those negative feelings which result in low self-esteem.

12.00   The next hour is 'free time' in which Mrs Smith is helped and encouraged to relax in an informal way whilst interacting with and enjoying the company of other residents. General attention from, and genuine compliments by, other residents and staff are part of the continuous process of elevating Mrs Smith's level of self-esteem to a realistic point.

13.00   Lunch is served with the same general purposes and goals as for breakfast (see 08.30).

14.00   The weekly meeting of the residents committee of the nursing home takes place to discuss general matters and to function as a means by which the staff and residents of the home can share in the general decision-making process. Mrs Smith has, reluctantly, agreed to participate in a passive way in this meeting. It is intended that, in due course, she will participate more fully as her level of self-esteem increases.

15.00   Participates, with considerable help and encouragement from a nurse, in a game of bridge with three other residents. Mrs Smith had previously been a member of a local bridge club and a leading local expert in the game.

16.00   Free time in which Mrs Smith is expected and encouraged to participate in a meaningful activity; for example, reading, chatting, mending her clothes or tidying her room.

17.00   Tea time. See the general purposes and principles which apply to breakfast time at 08.30.

18.00   Free time. Mrs Smith is allowed to make personal arrangements for this time, these arrangements may well include 'doing nothing'.

19.00   Visiting time in the nursing home is 'open', visitors are free to come in, and residents are free to go out, at any time, Mrs Smith is visited by a granddaughter at this time.

21.00   Relaxing watching television in the company of two other residents. At this time, as at all other times, nursing staff are aware of what Mrs Smith is doing and ensure that the activity has some meaning and purpose for her.

23.00   Bed time. Before going to sleep Mrs Smith is visited by a nurse who spends 20–30 minutes chatting about things in general and the day in particular. It is essential that Mrs Smith be made to feel that staff are concerned about her, willing to spend time with her and, most importantly, wish to see her functioning at her optimum level.

During the night she has access to a call system which will enable her to summon help if required. Her room, in common with all other parts of the nursing home environment, is clean, comfortable, well repaired and as 'domestic' in style as possible.

Although physically frail, there is a real possibility that Mrs Smith may return to her own home in due course. Whether or not she does return is partly dependent on her own feelings about herself and her ability to cope. By diagnosing and working on a serious problem experienced by Mrs Smith, low self-esteem, nursing staff are maximizing the possibility that the quality of her life as a long-term resident in the nursing home or, alternatively, on her return to her own house will be much increased.

ASSESSMENT OF SELF-ESTEEM

General Appearance

- Tidy/untidy.
- Clean, well-shaven/dirty.
- Make up/hair styling.
- Variety of clothing used.

Posture

- Stooped/erect.
- Brisk/slow movement.
- Animated/little movement.

Interpersonal Skill

- Initiates/rejects conversation.
- Seeks company/isolated.
- Assertive/passive.
- Independent/dependent.
- Confident/lacking in confidence.

Decision Making

- Relies on others/makes own decisions.
- Questions/accepts health care decisions.
- Comments on/accepts decisions of others.

Feeling About Self

- Indicates feeling of self-worth.
- Negative/positive statements about self.
- Expects high/low quality of care.

Interest in Environment

- Interested/disinterested in environment.
- Uses/ignores television and radio.
- Reads/ignores newspapers.
- Visits/avoids shop, town, recreational facilities.

REFERENCE

Maslow A.H. (1954) *Motivation and Personality*. Harper and Row, New York.

FURTHER READING

Beaton S.R. (1980) Reminiscence in old age. *Nursing Forum* **19**, 271–83.
Benson E.R. (1982) Attitudes toward the elderly: A survey of recent literature. *Journal of gerontological Nursing* **8**, 279–81.
Brink C., Wells T. & Diokna A (1983) A continence clinic for the elderly. *Journal of gerontological Nursing* **9**, 651–5.
Burnside I.M. (1980) Why work with the aged? *Geriatric Nursing* **1**, 28–33.
Dimond M (1980) Caring: Nursing's promise to the elderly. *Geriatric Nursing* **1**, 196–8.
Epstein L.J. (1976) Depression in the elderly. *Journal of Gerontology* **31**, 278–82.
Gioilla E. (1978) The relationship between slowness of response, state anxiety, social isolation and self esteem and preferred personal space in the elderly. *Journal of gerontological Nursing* **4**, 40–3.
Harris R. (1981) Learning about aging from the aged. *Geriatric Nursing* **2**, 51–2.
Hirst S.P. & Metcalf B.J. (1984) Promoting self esteem. *Journal of gerontological Nursing* **10**, 72–7.
Hodgkinson P. (1982) Growing old gracefully. *Journal of District Nursing* **1**, 16–18.
Holzapel S. (1982) The importance of personal possessions in the lives of the institutionalized elderly. *Journal of gerontological Nursing* **8**, 156–8.
Keisel M. & Bininger C. (1979) An application of psycho-social role theory to the aging. *Nursing Forum* **18**, 80–91.
Kibbee P. & Lackey D (1982) The past as therapy: An experience in an acute setting. *Journal of practical Nursing* **32**, 29–31.
Lous M. (1981) Personal space boundary needs of elderly persons. *Journal of gerontological Nursing* **7**, 395–400.
Madrid M. (1984) Nurses can help turn the tide: Helping the elderly to regain self worth. *Journal of gerontological Nursing* **10**, 8–12.
Medley M.L. (1976) Satisfaction with life among persons sixty-five years and older: a causal model. *Journal of Gerontology* **31**, 448–55.
Miller P. (1980) Interrupting the depression cycle. *Geriatric Nursing* **1**, 133–5.
Myles J.F. (1978) Institutionalisation and sick role identification among the elderly. *American sociological Review* **43**, 508–20.
Neugarten B.L. (1961) The measurement of life satisfaction. *Journal of Gerontology* **16**, 134–43.

Palmer M.H. (1982) Assisting older women with cosmetics.*Journal of gerontological Nursing* **8**, 340–2.

Rodin J. & Langer E. (1980) Aging Labels. The decline of control and the loss of self esteem. *Journal of Social Issues* **36**, 12–29.

Roosa W.M. (1982) Territory and privacy; residents views. Findings of a survey. *Geriatric Nursing* **3**, 241–3.

Ryden M. (1981) Nursing intervention in support of reminiscence. *Journal of gerontological Nursing* **7**, 461–3.

Rynerson B.C. (1972) Need for self esteem in the aged. A literature review. *Journal of psychiatric Nursing* **10**, 22–5.

Schwirian P.M. (1982) Life satisfaction among nursing home residents. *Geriatric Nursing* **3**, 111–14.

Skeet M. (1982) Enhancing old age: The role of the nurse. *New Zealand Nursing Journal* **7**, 8–9.

Wysocki M.R. (1983) Life review for the elderly patient. *Nursing 83* **13**, 47–8.

Zarit S. (1979) Helping an aging patient to cope with memory problems. *Geriatrics* **34**, 82–90.

Chapter 27
Social Skills (Interpersonal)

Interpersonal social skills* are of fundamental importance to the business of living and surviving with other individuals. They have to do with participating in the give and take of life as it relates to having meaningful contact with other people. Interpersonal skills, if used constructively, help us to make use of, and contribute to the functioning of other individuals and groups.

The use of these skills enables us to enjoy the company and activities of others on a one-to-one or group basis. They help us to work with others towards common goals such as setting up a card game, going for a walk, raising a family, teaching, entertaining and informing. As with other concepts in this section, interpersonal skills are very much on a continuum. At the one extreme there is the shy, introverted and relatively isolated person who has some difficulty in relating to other people. At the other extreme is the extroverted gregarious type who has no difficulty whatever in meeting, mixing and communicating with other individuals or groups. It is not, of course, being suggested that individuals who are at one of these extremes are in any way 'abnormal'. Rather, it is being suggested that there is a very wide 'normal' variation in the extent to which individuals have and use interpersonal skills.

In our older patients we need to consider their present interpersonal skill functioning in the context of what is normal for *them*. Although it is unlikely that the lifetime habits of a shy and introverted elderly person should be, or need to be, changed we must be able to identify the individual whose level of interpersonal skills have recently changed as a result of an altered health care status. Such a change might take place in an individual who has been admitted to a nursing home or hospital and who has previously functioned with a high level of interpersonal skill. It is not uncommon for such a person to have difficulty in making the adjustment to institutionalization and have

*This chapter should be read and used in combination with Chapter 15 (Communication) which contains a considerable amount of material relevant to Social Skills (Interpersonal) — see pp. 172-81.

The reader is also referred to Chapter 26 (Self-esteem) and Chapter 33 (Therapeutic use of the Environment).

difficulty in relating to other patients and/or staff. For this reason it is essential that we have detailed information about the previous normal level of functioning for each individual patient.

FACTORS RELATING TO INTERPERSONAL SKILLS

In assessing our patients levels of interpersonal skills functioning, the starting point is always an examination of their levels of skills prior to the onset of this particular illness or hospitalization. Thus, the existing position can only be compared against the 'norm' for each patient and is thus relative in terms of whether the skills are adequate or inadequate. A number of factors are presented which may influence the skills level of our patient in the context of his present illness and/or hospitalization.

Opportunity to Practice Interpersonal Skills

As with all skills which the elderly person has, he must be given reasonable opportunity to practice them in order to maintain them. An environment which is stimulating and active and which prevents social isolation will offer opportunity for interpersonal skills practice. One which contains alert and responsive patients and staff can be supplemented by voluntary workers whose main task it is to engage patients in meaningful conversation.

The main ingredient in stimulating interpersonal skills usage is *time*. As nurses we must be willing to sit with individual patients, and patient groups, and enable them to engage in social chat. Additionally, we must develop the skill with which to stimulate patient groups to engage in group communication. The importance of all communication as a means of developing and sustaining interpersonal skills cannot be overemphasized.

The Environment

The environment can either be therapeutic or anti-therapeutic in terms of optimizing the patient's interpersonal skills. The obvious examples relate to noise levels, seating arrangements, environmental stimulation and the ability to move freely within the envionment and seek out opportunities for interpersonal skills use.

Self-esteem

The effect (positive or negative) of self-esteem on interpersonal skill is considerable. As self-esteem levels, which can be influenced by nursing staff, decrease then the ability of the patient to function well on an interpersonal basis is also decreased. A high level of self-esteem with a resultant high level of confidence and personal initiative will dramatically increase these abilities.

Pathology

As nurses, we must always be aware of the effect that a disease process may have on interpersonal skill. If the patient is depressed, hallucinating, deluded, in pain, dehydrated, hyperactive or unduly dependent, his interpersonal skills will almost certainly be diminished. Invariably, all disease processes have a greater or lesser influence on interpersonal skill and this effect must be fully taken into account when we deliver nursing care.

Expectations of Others

The extent to which others expect the individual to function poorly, or well, will strongly influence his level of interpersonal skill functioning. Although we should not overestimate our patients' abilities, we often underestimate the skills level of the elderly generally, and of the elderly patient in particular. The level of functioning which the elderly person has achieved by virtue of experience is, in reality, sophisticated and considerable. His resources, which can be utilized to adapt to new circumstances, death of a spouse for example, are considerable.

Communication Ability

Finally, our ability to communicate is closely linked to our level of interpersonal skills. The principle means by which we exercise them is through verbal and non-verbal communication. Any impediment, deafness being the classic example, to communication skills will seriously interfere with interpersonal skills.

PRINCIPLES OF CARE

Determining Interpersonal Skill Levels

Pre-morbid (pre-illness) levels of interpersonal skill functioning should be ascertained from information collected from relatives, the patient and others. Thus a picture of the 'norm' for this *particular* person can be built up and compared with his present level of functioning. Measurement of current interpersonal skills begins with an examination of how he functions in relation to individual nurses and groups of nurses. If the patient apparently does not have problems in this area, it should not be assumed that, because he functions well with nurses, no problem exists. Remember, nurses have acquired a high level of skill in this area and could, unwittingly, make adjustments for the patient's interpersonal skill deficits.

Careful observation of the person in terms of how often, when and for what reason he interacts with and relates to other patients will be necessary; for example, if he spends much of his time on his own, in his room for example, one might suspect that a problem exists. Similarly, if he rarely initiates conversations with, has difficulty getting on with, or frequently finds himself in disagreement with, others his interpersonal skill level may be suspect.

Although an elderly person may be skilled in using interpersonal skills in relation to nursing staff, it should not be assumed that he does not have a problem in this area. We must remember that, in our role as nurses, we are neither typical of the population generally, or of a patient's peer group. Careful observation, collection of information from others with whom he does/does not interact, and a detailed discussion with the patient himself must be done in order to assess whether or not a problem exists.

If it is thought that an interpersonal skill problem exists (that his personal level of functioning is significantly below his pre-morbid level of functioning), it will be necessary to discuss your observations and conclusions with the patient. Remember, not all individuals who have a problem in this area will be willing to admit that this is so. Statements such as, 'I see you spend most of your time on your own', and 'I hear you were arguing with Mr X this morning. How do you get along with the patients generally?' and, 'How are you settling in and getting along with the others?', may be useful opening phrases.

Encourage Interpersonal Skills Use

Any environment such as a private home, ward, social club and shopping mall which contains other *people* should be used as a therapeutic tool for encouraging and developing interpersonal skill use. Your job in these situations will be to assess the suitability of a particular situation, discuss participation in it with your patient, 'arrange' his participation in it, support his participation in it, and evaluate the outcome.

An example of such an intervention might be arranging that your patient participate in a walk in the hospital grounds with you and one fellow patient. The process might be:

1 previous identification of an interpersonal skill problem (difficulty in making friends with other individuals for example);

2 problem discussed with patient and possible strategies agreed (including that described below);

3 other individual patient identified and recruited to participate in this particular intervention — the person involved is known to interact easily and is viewed by your patient as being 'a fairly nice person';

4 you and both patients go for a walk in the hospital grounds — your role is, as far as possible, to play a passive/facilitative role in enabling the two patients to interact and use their interpersonal skills;

5 after the walk you will discuss the outcome with your patient, focussing on the success and problems experienced by him.

In institutional environments, there are an abundance of opportunities for encouraging interpersonal skills use; examples include playing cards, casual conversation, *all* nurse-patient contact, mealtimes, visiting times and meetings with casual visitors to the ward. For patients living at home, even on their own, a variety of opportunities also exist but will have to be organized differently; examples include contact with visiting nurses, home help, neighbours, relatives, others who attend social clubs and the day hospital.

Environmental Structure

The structure of the environment can do much to maximize *or* inhibit interpersonal skill use. The positioning of ward furniture and chairs should be used as a means of facilitating interpersonal contact: groups of four to six chairs in loose circles, for example. As many old people are hard of hearing, they rely heavily on facial expression and lip movement in order to communicate.

Background noise in the form of television, radio, record player and general ward activity and machinery is problematical for those trying to communicate with, and relate to, others.

The increasing use of single rooms for institutionalized patients is to be encouraged in terms of increased privacy. However, this development presents a very serious *potential* problem in relation to social isolation. As nurses, we have a heavy responsibility in terms of motivating socially isolated patients who may be 'imprisoned' in their single rooms; we must make them want to meet and interact with others; no easy task.

Finally, the environment must be relatively slow paced and relaxed; nurses and others need to demonstrate to patients that they have time to spend with them. One way of demonstrating this willingness is to sit and 'do nothing' in view of patients, this way they will not feel guilty about 'wasting your time' or taking you away from your 'real work'. This author believes that such time (sitting doing nothing) is a crucial feature of geriatric nursing and does much to encourage patients who would not otherwise initiate conversation, to do so.

Practice with Nurses

All interaction with nurses gives vital experience and confidence to patients who have problems with this skill, particularly those who have a speech impediment or some other communication deficit. This view of our role emphasizes the importance of casual social 'chat' with our patients; for many this should be regarded as a vital part of the nursing care.

Intensive, formal and structured one-to-one or group therapy are powerful tools in assisting appropriate patients in developing interpersonal skills. Behavioural approaches are also very effective and use systematic and specific reinforcement of interpersonal skill success (see Chapter 9).

PATIENT PROFILE

Mr Lopez is 82 years old. His wife, to whom he had been married for 61 years, died four months ago. He has lived in a 'sheltered housing' flat for five years and is described by the warden as 'keeping himself to himself'. Mr Lopez rarely interacts with other residents of the complex, and rarely leaves his flat except to collect his pension and weekly groceries.

The local health visitor recently visited Mr Lopez at the request of the warden who was concerned at his increasing self-imposed confinement to his flat. After four very short visits in which Mr Lopez insisted that he was 'OK' and, 'Doing very well', a fifth visit provided evidence of an interpersonal skill problem. During that visit, he became very tearful and described himself as being isolated and lonely since the death of his wife and explained the difficulty thus: 'When she was alive, we did everything together and never had any real friends; we felt we didn't need them. We were happy together and never seemed to be apart. I've accepted that she is gone, she suffered a lot before she died and it's probably a blessing in disguise.

I now realize how few people I *really* know. I want to make friends with some of the neighbours, but I just don't know what to do. Maybe they won't want to know me since I hardly ever spoke to them when my wife was alive. I'm really quite lonely now; I don't even go to the weekly bingo in the common-room.'

ORGANIZATION OF NURSING CARE

Subjective Evidence (What the Patient Says)

- 'I now realize how few people I *really* know.'
- 'I want to make friends with some of the neighbours, but I just don't know what to do.'
- 'Maybe they (the neighbours) won't want to know me . . .'
- 'I'm really quite lonely . . .'

Objective Evidence (What the Nurse and Others Observe)

- Keeps himself to himself, leaves the flat only once per week.
- Never initiates interaction with the warden or neighbours.
- Does not attend the weekly bingo session; had done so with his wife before her death.

Assessment (Nursing Diagnosis)

- Interpersonal skill deficit.
- Has difficulty in initiating interactions and making friends with others.

Plan of Nursing Care

- The health visitor (or a community psychiatric nurse) will develop a one-to-one relationship with Mr Lopez, via a number of pre-arranged meetings with him.
- Identify the specific nature of the problem and appropriate strategies to reduce it (e.g.).
- Use the contact and interaction to give him practice at interacting with others.
- Arrange a social meeting with a neighbour and the warden or nurse; purpose: to practice interpersonal skill in a relatively supportive environment.
- Identify other social contact/situations which he feels he could manage unaided.

Expected Outcome

- Will leave the house for purposes other than to collect groceries and pension.

- Will initiate contact with (for example, will visit or stop to speak to) one or more neighbours at least once daily.
- Will begin to form a longer-standing relationship with at least one other person.
- Will feel less lonely and isolated as evidenced by less frequent use of statements described in 'Subjective Evidence' section.

NURSING CARE OF A PATIENT WITH AN INTERPERSONAL SKILL PROBLEM (EXAMPLE)

In the following example a 'nurse', who could be a district nurse *or* health visitor *or* a community psychiatric nurse, plays a key role in organizing care, and a minor role in actually delivering it. Indeed, a major feature of nursing care delivered in a community setting is that it utilizes many non-nursing personnel, and depends considerably on everyday situations and experiences. However, these must be used and/or arranged by the nurse responsible for the elderly person in a specific and organized fashion; otherwise, the care is not *nursing* care.

07.45 hours   Mr Lopez gets up and washes, shaves, dresses and so forth, prepares for breakfast.

08.30   Eats breakfast and tidies up the flat.

09.30   Makes his *daily* visit to the local grocery shop. He has willingly agreed to shop daily for himself and for a housebound neighbour who is physically unable to leave the sheltered housing facility.

10.30   Returns from shopping and has morning coffee with his neighbour.

11.00   Daily housework.

12.00   Has lunch at the local 'Old Folks Social Club' to which he has been introduced by the nurse who accompanied him on his first two visits.

14.00   Visited by the community nurse who called weekly at first, now visits monthly. During the visit, progress is discussed, as are new goals and strategies.

14.30   Visited by nephew with whom he has recently renewed contact.

16.00   Afternoon 'nap'.

17.00   Prepares evening meal.

18.00   Evening walk to the local park, brief visit to the warden with whom an appointment has been made. The warden has agreed to help the nurse generally oversee and facilitate the

	programme which has been prepared in collaboration with Mr Lopez.
19.30	'Calls in' on the housebound neighbour, whom he now regards as a friend, and asks if he will need shopping done tomorrow.
20.00	'Settles in' for the evening, watches television and writes one letter.
21.30	Supper.
22.00	Bed.

Problems relating to 'interpersonal skills' can take any of a wide variety of forms. They can be serious and can seriously damage *all* facets of the health of the person who experiences them. As nurses, we have an interest in *all* aspects of health; physical, psychological and social. As such, we have an important role to play in preventing, detecting and reducing problems of this type and, in so doing, make considerable use of our *personal* attributes and skills.

ASSESSMENT OF INTERPERSONAL SOCIAL SKILLS

Interactions with Others

- Initiates interactions.
- Spends time with others.
- Positive/constructive input to interactions with others.
- Identifies some individuals as 'friends'.

Activities

- Enjoys *some* group activities, e.g. cards, bingo, bus rides.
- Finds the company of others pleasant and stimulating, seeks the company of others.
- Is alert to, and supportive of, the needs of others.

Feelings About Self

- Feels positive about self, confident in interactions with others.
- Feels others enjoy his company.
- Feels he has something to offer other individuals, and the group/s of which he is a part.

Communication

- Has no serious impediments to communication.
- Communicates freely and fluently.

See assessment of Communication skills in Chapter 15.

FURTHER READING

Alves E.A. (1981) The nursing contribution to social skills training for psychiatric in-patients. *Nursing Times* **77**, 1026–9.

Arnetz B.B. & Theorell T. (1983) Dateline: Sweden. Research on activation for the elderly. *Journal of gerontological Nursing* **9**, 614–19.

Arnetz B.B., Eyre M. & Theorell T (1982) Social activation of the elderly — a social experiment. *Social Science and Medicine* **16**, 1685–90.

Briggs K. (1983) Counselling skills for students. *Nursing Times* **79**, 41–3.

Briggs K. (1982) Interpersonal skills training for student nurses during introductory course. *Nurse Education Today* **2**, 22–4.

Brunning H. (1981) Social skills and personal effectiveness training for student nurses. *Nursing Times* **77**, 919–20.

Bryant B.M. (1976) A survey of social inadequacy among psychiatric outpatients. *Psychological Medicine* **6**, 101–12.

Crawford D.A. (1978) Social skills training for psychiatric patients. *Nursing Times* **74**, 1322–3.

Davies A.D.M. (1980) The social behaviour of geriatric patients at mealtimes. *Age and Ageing* **9**, 93–9.

Harris H., Lipman A. & Slater R. (1977) Architectural design: the spatial location and interactions in old people. *Gerontology* **23**, 390–400.

Le Lievere J. (1983) Social skills training. *Nursing Times* **79**, 46–8.

McCormack D. & Whitehead A. (1981) The effect of providing recreational activities on the engagement level of long stay geriatric patients. *Age and Ageing* **10**, 287–91.

Powell D (1982) *Learning To Relate*. Royal College of Nursing, London.

Powell L., Felce D., Jenkins J. & Lunt B. (1979) Increasing engagement in a home for the elderly by providing an indoor gardening activity. *Behaviour Research and Therapy* **17**, 127–35.

Chapter 28
Social Skills (Psychomotor)

Psychomotor social skills include all those activities by which we are aware of our environment, and our reactions to it. The environment, of course, does not just mean the rain or sun and our enjoying the feel of them on our skins. Accepting that total liberty to rush around with no clothes is not open to us most of the time unless, of course, we frequent an area set aside for naturists, we begin to see that we live in a social environment as well. Donne's oft-repeated adage that, 'no man is an island' applies even before birth. As we grow older, our social ambience expands and it matters that we please not only our parents, but their friends and society in general. The propriety of keeping ourselves covered is an activity that is impressed upon us at a very early age. However, there may be occasions when this can be flaunted; for example, the shapely girl wearing a low-cut evening dress. This licence does not extend to men going about with their trouser flies undone; indeed, if we do see someone in this state we tend to be embarrassed on the man's behalf if not on our own. Intriguingly, the man observed in the street in such a condition is quite likely to be referred to as a 'dirty old man', no matter what his age.

Social skills do not, of course, refer only to matters of dress, but also to meeting people and engaging them in conversation; they are about keeping ourselves and our surroundings in a state of cleanliness and tidiness so that others will want to meet us and spend time in our company; they mean being able to share mealtimes without being embarrassed or embarrassing others. It is also a social skill to be able to get about independently. Indeed, psychomotor skills are perhaps the best example of man acting upon his environment and modifying his subsequent actions as a result of his previous ones.

All these skills are probably learned, though there are some who would dispute this. How that learning happens has been the object of research for a very long time. These skills involve motor function, which is to say muscles contract and relax. As an example, let us imagine you want to pick up a glass; that mechanical act is complex. The intention to lift the glass starts the process, the eye sees the glass, the arm by nerve messages from the brain prepares to lift the glass, it moves through space and at the same time the hand is being prepared by similar mechanisms to lift the glass, adapting to its girth and weight. The lifting of drinking vessels is an activity we are taught in early childhood. Various steps, like using plastic or lidded drinking cups, are precautions against disaster for the child, which, if they occur frequently cause much distress. The process of learning the skill of drinking unaided with confidence and relatively little thought, is achieved with a great deal of practice. The activity of using a knife and fork takes children even longer.

A most important component then is one of intention, or response to sensory stimuli; for example, the process by which we experience the sensation of a full bladder: we rise from the chair on which we have been sitting watching television, walk to the toilet, undo our clothing, void, re-arrange our clothing, wash our hands (if that is our habit) return to the chair and recommence watching television. The number of components in that one cycle of activity is very complex indeed. The influences involved in the learning process are not simply a response to a full bladder, but include learning when and where it is proper to void, and all the myriad other muscular activities that allow that to be achieved successfully.

So far, this chapter has paid particular attention to children, but what of the elderly, since, if it is so that these activities are learned by repetition, one might assume that the difficulty lies only with the young? As we age, changes occur which sometimes affect our abilities. Though there is a widely held belief that memory diminishes with age and while many older people do, indeed, suffer malfunction of memory, there are very many others who have no difficulty whatever. Though, possibly, memory will be the most important factor which interferes with perhaps only one section of a very long complex series of activities; for example, the old man who successfully goes to the toilet but, in fact, forgets to close his trouser fly; or the older person who, instead of being able to carry on an animated conversation during a meal, needs to spend more time concentrating on getting the food to his mouth and loses the train of the conversation.

To return to the example of the man with the undone fly, if one asks why the fly was left undone the most common response will be one of forgetful-ness. On the other hand, if one asks the man to tell you in sequence exactly what he does when he goes to the toilet, then the rearrangement of clothing will be more that likely included, so that there are probably other explanations for the omission.

Clearly, the primary intention in either of the examples given, the intention to empty a full bladder or eat dinner, has been satisfied and presumably the feedback from the empty bladder or full stomach are entirely satisfactory. However, that is not quite the whole story since in one case the clothing is not suitable rearranged and, in the other, participation in the conversation has been minimal. In both these instances, the feedback from outsiders is likely to be less than satisfaction and might well be embarrassment. Either is liable to result in the labelling of the man as being confused or withdrawn.

The means which we rely on to provide our brains with stimuli often become less acute as we age. The eyesight of the elderly is frequently less good, for example, as a result of such conditions as cataract. Such difficulties can, in fact, cause elderly people to miss a table altogether when trying to put down a cup and saucer. Hearing, also often affected by age, can result in isolation or merely being withdrawn. However, there are times when older people give erroneous answers to questions which can result in their being labelled as confused when in fact, their 'confusion' would disappear with a hearing aid.

Also, with declining sensory acuity, there can be diminshed conduction velocities, that is to say the speed at which impulses travel neural pathways. Though there has been research on this, it must be remembered that the laboratory setting hardly mirrors performances in daily life. There may be extraneous environmental inputs; for example, a person goes upstairs to the bedroom to get a book, but having gone into the bedroom feels that the temperature has dropped, so proceeds to close the window and goes downstairs without the book. Or again, he may know that the dishes require to be washed but, knowing that he is not expecting any visitors, there is not a sufficiently strong motivation to commence the task.

In consideration of the elderly, it is often accepted that the old cannot learn — a view held for generations as the saying goes, 'You can't teach an old dog new tricks'. This, however, is fallacious; the elderly can and do learn. Part of the difficulty is that thinking of learning *only* in terms of memory tends to cloud the issue. Frequently, short-term recall seems to decay with age, it has been suggested that this is because of poorer sorting strategies. However, long-term memories of remote events do not seem to show similar changes. Often, elderly people can give you very detailed information about their childhood, while they appear to have great difficulty remembering what they had for lunch.

Perhaps one of the most important areas which affects the elderly and their ability to maintain a high level of psychomotor social skills is the environment. By environment, I mean how society thinks about older people, what is expected of them and how it treats them. We know that hospitals, nursing homes and, perhaps to a lesser extent eventide homes, tend to institutionalize people. Mealtimes are set by the hospital routine and do not give sufficient time, or perhaps a choice of menus. In such settings all the beds tend to look the same. There will be universal colour schemes which may make the toilets or dayroom difficult to identify. In a real sense, the patient is made to feel a visitor in someone else's home; he is hardly free to put on the light or turn off the television. Not only that, but these institutions tend to depersonalize the patients. In many of these 'homes', staff are guilty of calling elderly patients, 'Pop', 'Gran' or some other unpersonalized name. Such a message of incompetence can lead to an atrophy of psychomotor social skills. Kuypers and Bengston (1973) set this out graphically (see Fig. 28.1).

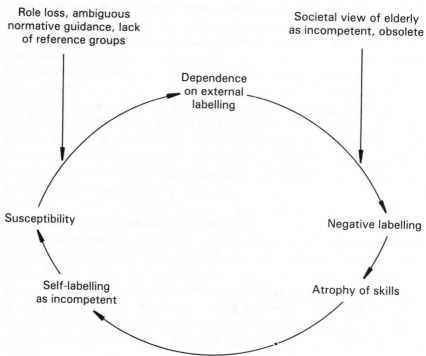

Fig. 28.1 The process of institutionalization and depersonalization as depicted by Kuypers and Bengston (1983).

FACTORS RELATING TO SOCIAL SKILLS (PSYCHOMOTOR)

The *environment* in which the old person has to operate is one of the most important factors which affects his ability to maintain his social skills. If an old man is removed from home and taken into long-term care, the degree of confusion which he will experience may be very marked. In a word, he has to learn where his bed is and, more important, be able to pick it out from a lot of others which look identical. The geography of the ward might involve him in longish walks, for example, to the toilet. He has to cope with a quite different routine, with lots of new people, some of whom he will not like. He has been made, in effect, a visitor and there are many inhibiting conventions that he has to observe in someone else's house.

Many of the difficulties that elderly people experience are related to *stress*. The old man who has been accustomed to spending 20 minutes in the toilet after breakfast, perhaps with a book, suddenly in a communal setting can no longer do so. He is harried to move since there is a queue. He is likely to be rushed at mealtimes because the trolleys have to be returned to the kitchen by a certain time. The old lady in the supermarket may well feel harassed by the volume of other customers and the looks of irritation on the faces of staff when she takes time to get through the checkout point. After all, this mode of shopping is one she may have had to learn in her seventies.

The prescribing of *drugs* to the elderly can be a very important factor. Often when they experience anxiety the immediate reaction on the part of the professional is to resort to chemical treatment. The elderly person may complain of not sleeping well and again the prescribing of sleeping pills is a quick and apparently effective response. The other difficulty that the elderly have to cope with unwittingly is sometimes the combinations of drugs that have been prescribed, often appropriately, over time, but the 'cocktail' can have profound effects. Once a patient has become dependent on pills it can be hard to persuade him to give them up. We often do not know exactly how particular drugs will affect individual patients and the elderly seem particularly vulnerable. Often, it is this factor which initially provokes professionals and relatives to consider the older patient confused.

There are many older people who become increasingly *isolated*. They may well have lost by death either a spouse or close friends. Sometimes after such an occurrence they have, perhaps, to be near their children or move to a smaller house. In these conditions, some old people have great difficulty in developing new social contacts. Such isolation can lead to people becoming more and more confused or merely increasingly strange, which becomes a never-ending vicious circle since such behaviour frightens neighbours and other members of the community from making overtures. Thus, the isolation increases.

Factors like the environment, stress, drugs and isolation can, singly or collectively, lead to *depression*. The profound sadness at the loss of a loved one can, at any age, lead to depression; in this the elderly are not so different. When an elderly person also has difficulty with *mobility* and *sensory abilities* like hearing and sight, he may well get very depressed. He may spend a lot of time wishing for the past or, indeed, for death. His general pose may be one of sitting about doing nothing but staring into space and speaking, when he does, in a low monotone. He may weep and generally be very difficult to interest in what is happening now. These patients present problems of diagnosis and treatment since the great skill is a matter of unpicking the signs and symptoms, defining the causes and then treating. Lack of motivation also produces great problems in trying to re-educate patients.

Disturbed sleep causes people, even when fit and young, problems of orientation. The attempt must be made to procure for an elderly patient undisturbed, peaceful sleep in a ward despite nurses and patients moving about during the night, not to mention snoring patients. The predetermined hospital night period may also not be conducive to patients getting to sleep.

PRINCIPLES OF CARE

The main principle that nurses ought to exercise is that of prevention. It seems that for many older people it is easier for them to accept what society says about them. If they are thought to be incompetent, slow, forgetful, or rather dotty, then it takes an enormous act of courage and determination to demonstrate to the world that personally they do not fit that picture. Nurses, both in the community and hospital setting, have plenty of opportunity to meet very many older patients who certainly do not fit that image. It is not good enough for them to dismiss these people as simply not being 'old'. Nurses, therefore, have a responsibility to look at each patient as an individual and forget generalized myths about the old and also to help dispel these myths.

The attempts that nurses can make in the general community would be enhanced if they could show that they had made serious efforts to put their own house in order. Sadly, this has not been shown and, in some cases, wards particularly set aside for the elderly have suffered badly as Bowder (1980) has pointed out. Of course, to care on an individual basis for these patients who are having difficulty with psychomotor social skills takes a lot of money in the form of staff as well as implementing imaginative schemes, like painting doors different colours, to give one example.

If it were possible to change the views of the public, more patients suffering from such problems would be able to return to the community. Slack and Simon (1980) have achieved good results in Buckinghamshire, as have Fottrell *et al.* (1980) in another setting. However, it must always be remembered by nurses that if patients with severe difficulties are being returned to the community and cared for there, sensitive support and help must be given to the relatives or others who are tackling the burden of support. Sheldon (1982) writes well of this.

However, the fact remains that most nurses in an acute ward will meet patients who have lost some of their social skills on a short-term basis, possibly as a result of infection or anoxia. The blanket term 'confusion' is hardly good enough. Generally, nurses consider one of their most important skills to be observation, most of them considering themselves to be good at it. That may well be, certainly any nursing textbook one picks up will have some reference to observation and its importance. My plea here is for nurses to make a very detailed examination of what is observed. It is too easy to accept as confused the old man who gives inappropriate answers to questions, who does not much want to walk about, who cannot dress properly because he has difficulty doing up buttons and so leaves most of them undone, or who has difficulty finding his bed. However, if one unpicks all these signs and examines them individually the story might be quite different. He might be deaf and need a hearing aid; his toe nails may need cutting; he may have arthritis; it may be that replacing zips and buttons with Velcro will solve a problem; it might be, finally, that his long distance sight is failing. It would, indeed, be wrong and very unkind to treat him as if he were confused.

There are, however, many patients who are, indeed, confused and are not able to cope outside institutions. You must try to make institutions as much like home as possible (Denhom 1983). Patients should be shown not only where their beds, the toilet and dayroom are, but also the office or where nurses are generally to be found, the light switches in the dayroom and how to turn on and off radios and televisions. They should be encouraged to bring something from home, for example, a bed cover (it may have been made for their wedding 50 or 60 years ago), photographs, a picture, a vase or a cushion.

Part of the mechanism that we use in hospital to help emphasize the institutionalization is to depersonalize the patient. One of the ways in which we remove the person's grasp of who he is and thereby make him secure is to call him 'Pop', or 'Gran' in the case of a female patient. This is an element in increasing their loosening grasp of the psychomotor social skills. If other people do not even think them worth being called by name, why should *they* bother? It is also very important to allow patients to keep their own clothes and for as many as can get up and dressed, to do so each day.

Another area in which you can be a very useful monitor relates to the patient's medical treatment, in the supervision of drugs that the patient is taking. Research, as reported by Williamson and Chapin (1980), shows that much greater care is needed both in the use of particular drugs and the combinations of drugs that often produce or increase the patient's difficulty in coping. Though, of course, nurses cannot prescribe, they are the members of the caring team most likely to notice the effects on mood or changes in mental state caused by drugs (see Chapter 30).

In attempting to preserve the social skills or, indeed, in enhancing them, one of the important times and activities is eating. The process of eating is a very complex one and if there is fragility in the patient a great deal of care needs to be given. Davis and Snaith (1980) have pointed out that mealtimes in hospital are often organized for the good of the institution rather than as a means of aiding patients. Personalized trays and helping in choice of food, as well as sensitive serving of that food, while not feeding patients unless it is absolutely necessary, are all ways in which patients can be helped.

Toiletting is another area which causes much difficulty and sometimes not a little embarrassment. It is difficult if the patient takes a lot of time to find the toilet. Many people, not just the elderly, do not like to be rushed when they are in the toilet. Even more, there is the need for nurses to spend time and care in preserving the dignity and privacy of patients. It is far too easy to assume that, like small children, old people will not mind if the toilet door has no lock on it or, even worse, not shut when the toilet is being used. Nurses should not shout the length of the ward asking a colleague to bring another pair of pants or trousers. Patients often have days when they are aware of not having reached the toilet in time or, indeed, may always be so but merely cannot talk about it. Clothing that is difficult to manage, like combinations or long-johns or buttoned trousers with braces and belts, many nurses would think better replaced by clothing of more modern design, but that is a decision that would have to have much thought put into it for styles people have worn always are important to them. The advent of Velcro has been of inestimable value. Trouser buttons or zips being replaced and, indeed, the seam being lengthened to the crotch can suddenly make a man with dexterity difficulties independent again — at least in that sphere.

Obviously, one of the most important principles that has been implicit in what has been suggested is acceptance. You must demonstrate acceptance of the patient and that acceptance must be hugely laced with understanding. It is so easy to give patients a feeling that they have been bad, or at least a nuisance, not by saying anything but by the way you look or walk. It is salutary to realize that some of our own habits, if made open to public gaze, would equally be thought odd.

Understanding without kindness is of no use at all. Reassurance is needed that, whatever catastrophe has occurred, it is not really to be viewed in that light. Rather, the patient needs to be told in a kindly way that all is well and that all will always be alright, that care does not depend on tests or competitions.

If a patient does have a difficulty, then some teaching help needs to be given, after having made sure that the problem is not a 'one off' caused by something extraneous. One must reject the notion that the elderly cannot learn. Erber *et al.* (1980), Baraclough and Fleming (1984) and others have carried out research which demonstrates that behavioural procedures can be taught.

Such teaching needs to be done on a one-to-one basis, it is very time consuming and requires infinite patience. There is much literature on behaviour modification, for example, Weinman (1981), Miller (1983), Norton (1983). In his article, Burton (1981) recommends the use of rewards as reinforcements to build up appropriate patterns of behaviour. There are many people who raise ethical questions about the propriety in involving the elderly in withdrawal of 'privileges' or, indeed, in using a token economy as means of modifying the behaviour. Personally, this author would be much happier in using a much lower key method of verbal praise but I am equally sure that shouting or showing great displeasure or irritation is not useful and is, indeed, demeaning to both patient and nurse. The preservation of the dignity of the patient is always a vitally important principle of care. Certainly, by constant rehearsing of what one would like a patient to do, to be supportive, encouraging and praising, is effective. The other aspect is not to do things for the patient he can do for himself, for that is a self-defeating exercise. Of course, it must also be remembered that many people, men in particular, frequently have been accustomed to having a very great deal done for them at home and so when he says, 'I can't do that', he may be speaking the truth. All teaching has to take into account the skills already available as well as those threatened; persuasion can be very effective.

PATIENT PROFILE

Mr Burns, an 82-year-old widower, was visited by his daughter on her usual weekly visit. She was alarmed to find her father sitting in his pyjamas beside an uncleaned fire. Though the house was cold, Mr Burn's face was flushed and he complained of a sore chest but insisted with the next breath, 'I'm fine'. The house was untidy, with unwashed dishes in the kitchen. When asked if he had eaten breakfast, he replied, 'I can't remember'. The daughter helped her father back to bed and called the doctor. Mr Burns was admitted to hospital. A diagnosis of pneumonia was confirmed and antibiotics were commenced. Mr Burns continued to be confused during the first part of his stay. He tried repeatedly to get into a bed in the same position as his but in a different bay. The nurses were constantly asked, 'Where is the toilet here?' and after going to the toilet Mr Burns frequently forgot to do up his fly. He spoke a lot to staff about his wife as if she were still alive and, indeed, he would say, 'I'll tell Nelly about this when she comes in'. At mealtimes he was careless about his eating habits and often said, 'I've already had dinner, take this stuff away'. As the treatment of his medical condition continued he improved, as did his mental state. Three weeks after admission, Mr Burns was able to return home, his usual neat, polite self.

ORGANIZATION OF NURSING CARE

Subjective Evidence (What the Patient Says)

Mr Burns showed that his distant memory was intact by saying:
- 'I'll tell Nelly about this when she comes in'.

Conversely, he illustrated his inability to remember recent information by constantly asking:

- 'Where is the toilet here?'

The patient showed an irritation with his confusion and attempted by the irritation to hang onto control by demanding:

- 'I've already had dinner, take this stuff away'.

Objective Evidence (What the Nurse and Others Observe)

- Mr Burns repeatedly attempted to get into the wrong bed, though it looked the same, and was in a similar position in a different bay, to his own.
- After successfully going to the toilet, the patient tended to forget to do up his trouser fly.
- At mealtimes, Mr Burns was careless in his eating habits and, indeed, would refuse food thinking he had already eaten, which made motivating the patient to eat difficult.

Assessment (Nursing Diagnosis)

- Social skill deficit.

Plan of Nursing Care

- Encourage the patient to get up and dressed; if he cannot manage all of this himself then assist him.
- Put something like photographs or a vase from home on his locker so that he will be helped to recognize his own bed.
- Reassure the patient that he can feed himself and encourage him by staying with him and helping him, if necessary, to achieve this.
- Walk with the patient, showing him where different facilities are as often as is needed to assure him that he knows the layout, but be very patient if he fails and show him again.
- Give him a daily newspaper which will help him remember which day it is and what is happening.

Expected Outcome

- Will be able to get up and dress himself properly. He will also be able to keep himself tidy throughout the day.
- Will be able to find his way about the ward without having to ask.
- His bed will be readily recognized and so he will stop trying to get into the wrong one.

- Eating habits will resume the previous standard and the timing of meals will be remembered.
- The patient's irritation will diminish as his confusion lessens.

NURSING CARE OF PATIENT WITH SOCIAL SKILLS (PSYCHOMOTOR) PROBLEM (EXAMPLE)

07.30 hours	Encourage Mr Burns to get up. When this has been achieved, walk with the patient to the toilet pointing out other things on the way so that he will feel secure.
08.00	Supervise dressing and washing — help should be offered only as necessary. Time must be given as well as lots of reassurance.
08.30	Breakfast — food of choice should be given and great care taken to help the patient eat as neatly as possible without hurting the patient's self-esteem.
09.00	Medicine round — supervision to ensure that the drug is properly taken.
10.00	Walk round the ward to ensure the patient's orientation is increasing.
11.00	Coffee — which should be supervised and help perhaps given to ensure that no catastrophe occurs.
11.15	A daily newspaper should be given to the patient and a nurse might need to point out the date and headlines.
12.30	Lunch — supervision and help to ensure increasing dexterity. Irritation, if shown, must be accepted and reassurance given.
13.00	Medicine round.
13.15	Toiletting should be supervised so that the toilet is found and also that clothing is properly replaced. Personal hygiene should also be attended to sensitively.
14.00	Sit with the patient and talk about things that are in the day's newspaper and things that have happened in the ward. If there is still difficulty about siting of facilities in the ward, accompany the patient on a tour and point things out again.
15.00	Teatime — involve the relatives who have come in to visit. Encourage them to speak with the patient about home, his family and community activities.
17.00	Medicine round.
17.30	Involve the patient in conversation with other patients.
18.00	Supper — the nurse should give as much or as little help as necessary.

19.00   Supervision of those parts of the toiletting cycle that the patient still has difficulty with.

19.30   Give advice to the relatives as to how to help or merely monitor the patient's behaviour and mental state when he goes home. Emphasis of how this must be done in a very sensitive way should be underlined.

21.00   Medicine round.

21.30   Hot drink — when the nurse should talk about the day's activities; for example, who had come to visit, or who they were, and how they fitted into the family, how often the patient normally saw them.

22.30   Supervision of the patient's oral and personal hygiene, getting undressed and comfortably settled in bed.

ASSESSMENT OF SOCIAL SKILLS (PSYCHOMOTOR)

Dress

- Ability to select appropriate clothing.
- Can dress self appropriately.
- Can dress with ease/difficulty.
- Requires dressing 'aids'.
- Requires specially adapted clothing.

Mobility

- Can move freely/with difficulty.
- Can walk freely within ward/home.
- Can leave the ward/home.
- Can move freely in the local community.
- Can use public/private transport.

Domestic Functioning

- Can make bed, dust, clean, wash laundry.
- Can budget, take care of own finances.
- Is aware of/can arrange domestic 'time table'.

Personal Nutrition

- Can cook, serve meals, clean kitchen.
- Can feed self.
- Can assist others/entertain.

Personal Hygiene

- Can wash, shave, use cosmetics.
- Can care for dentures.
- Can care for nails and hair.

Toilet

- Can prepare self for toilet.
- Can use toilet.
- Can wash/clean up after toilet.

REFERENCES

Baraclough C. & Fleming I. (1984) Not too old to learn. *Community Care* **500**, 16–17.

Bowder B. (1980) Fawcett 1 — human dumping ground. *New Age* **9**, 14–16.

Burton M. (1981) The behavioural approach to nursing the elderly. *Nursing Times* **77**, 247–8.

Davis A.D.M. & Snaith P.A. (1980) Mealtime problems in a continuing care hospital for the elderly.*Age and Ageing* **9**, 100–5.

Denhom M.J. (ed.)(1983) *Care of the Long-Stay Elderly Patient.* Croom Helm, Beckenham.

Erber J., Feely C. & Botwinick J. (1980) Reward conditions and socioeconomic status in the learning of older adults. *Journal of Gerontology* **35**, 565–70.

Fottrell E., Spy T., Mearns S., MacLean I. & Fogarty M. (1980) Asset stripping — the declining mental hospital. *British medical Journal* **6207**, 89–90.

Kuypers J.A. & Bengston V.L. (1973) Social breakdown and competence: A model of normal aging. *Human Development* xvi, 190.

Miller G.E. (1983) Teaching psychiatric patients. In Wilson-Barnett J. (ed.) *Patient Teaching.* Churchill Livingstone, Edinburgh.

Norton C. (1983) Training for urinary continence. In Wilson-Barnett J. (ed.) *Patient Teaching.* Churchill Livingstone, Edinburgh.

Sheldon F. (1982) Supporting the supporters: working with the relatives of patients with dementia. *Age and Ageing* **11**, 184–8.

Slack S. & Simon R. (1980) The specialist nurse support core and the elderly mentally infirm. *Nursing Times* **76**, 45–6.

Weinman J. (1981) *An Outline of Psychology as Applied to Medicine.* John Wright & Sons, Bristol.

Williamson J. & Chapin J.M. (1980) Adverse reactions to prescribed drugs in the elderly: A multicentre investigation. *Age and Ageing* **9**, 73–80.

FURTHER READING

Burton A. (ed.) (1982) *The Pathology and Psychology of Cognition.* Methuen, London.
Zarit S.H. (1980) *Aging and Mental Disorders: Psychological approaches to assessment and treatment.* The Free Press, New York.

Chapter 29
Trust

Trust may be defined as a solid and continuous belief that a person or thing may be consistently relied on. It relates to ones confidence in and reliance on the integrity and honesty of another person or persons. As with other concepts dealt with in this section of the book, trust is on a continuum which ranges from complete trust to serious distrust (paranoia).

It might be useful to think in terms of different types of trust: fundamental trust, which we have in a close friend or colleague; informal trust, which is based on casual friendship and contact; formal trust which is based on the professional and/or social status of the other individual, for example the doctor, nurse or solicitor; experiential trust which is built up over a long period of time and which becomes part of our 'personality'. The development of trust begins at an early age and is especially noticeable during the first two years of life and relates particularly to the close bond which exists between mother and child. During this period the child develops a number of expectations of the mother, for example that she will feed him when he is hungry. Increasingly, the infant becomes more confident and reliant on the mother for the satisfaction of a range of physical and psychological needs. In short, the child begins increasingly to 'trust' the mother and, in due course, a range of other individuals.

FACTORS RELATING TO TRUST

Previous Personality

The extent to which the person has developed a strong trusting relationship with significant others during his formative years (particularly the first three) will determine the extent to which he trusts or distrusts individuals in subsequent years. We have all met individuals who are very 'trusting' and those who are particularly cautious, even suspicious, of others until they get to know them very well. It is likely that the wide range of levels of trust that exists in a given group of people reflects their personality, which, in turn, reflects the levels of trust which they developed as a child.

351

Previous Experience

Even those of us who have, by nature, a high level of trust in others will become less trusting if we have a series of experiences in which our trust has been misplaced; for example, if a child who has developed a strong trusting relationship with his immediate family finds that, on entering school, he is frequently 'let down' by those in whom he places his trust, he will undoubtedly be less trusting in the future. If these negative experiences are repeated frequently enough, the individual will undoubtedly become much more cautious (even suspicious) in his development of relationships with other people.

Personal Relationships with Others

The continued development of trust is dependent on having opportunities in which to develop mutually trusting relationships with others. Exposure to close personal relationships with other individuals and groups gives us the opportunity to 'test out' the extent to which they can be trusted. Thus, our environment must give us opportunities in which we can practise placing trust in others. (Readers are referred to Chapter 27.)

Ability to Communicate

Our ability to communicate generally and to give and receive 'messages' which indicate trust, is essential. In order for two people to develop a trusting relationship it is essential that each of them 'know' that the desire and willingness to be trusting is mutual. Any impediment to communication skill is a serious barrier to development of a trusting relationship. A very important communication deficit which diminishes our level of trust is partial or total deafness. It is well known that the incidence of 'paranoia' amongst the partially or totally deaf population is much higher than for those who have no hearing deficit. Part of the problem here lies in the inability of the person with a hearing deficit accurately to interpret the communications of others; for example, he may wrongly interpret the difficult to understand voices of two nearby people as being a personal attack on him. (Readers are referred to Chapter 15.)

Expectations of Others

It is a truism that those who trust are trusted. In other words if we meet and communicate with other individuals in an open, free and trusting manner we increase the likelihood of a trusting relationship developing. Conversely, if we are cautious in our relationships with others, the development of trust is inhibited.

PRINCIPLES OF CARE

Be trusting and positive in your initial contacts with patients, assume that you can be open and reasonably frank with them and that a trusting relationship will develop if given time to do so. Of course, one should never automatically assume that complete and utter trust on the part of the patient will exist from the outset. We all need time to get to know and learn how to trust others, we should never take the existence of complete trust for granted. During our early contacts with our patients we need to make judgements as to whether or not a trust problem exists. If you feel that a trust problem does exist, this needs to be taken account of by using the following types of general strategies.

Be unconditional in your acceptance of the patient and avoid the unnecessary imposition of conditions concerning your relationship. If a trust problem exists, the patient will feel a strong need to play the dominant role in the relationship. As far as is possible this should be permitted in order to avoid the conflict which results when two individuals each try to play the dominant role in a relationship.

As soon as is possible identify at least one staff member who is distrusted least by the patient. As is the case with all non-physical problems, nursing care is firmly dependent on the existence and development of a close one-to-one relationship. Although the development of this relationship may take weeks or even months, it is an essential component of any successful nursing care programme.

All staff, particularly those who are attempting to form a close relationship, must be entirely and completely honest and consistent in their dealings with the patient. Any attempt to be anything other than completely honest will soon be detected by the patient and this will merely confirm that he should trust no-one.

Competitive activities, particularly if these involve a group, should be avoided in the short term. Remember, that any defeat in a competitive activity will be regarded as a *personal* attack and/or defeat by the person with a trust problem. Initially, interactions should be of the non-competitive one-to-one type in which the patient has a large degree of control of the situation.

Be alert to the singling out of specific individuals by the patient as people whom he particularly distrusts. In the short term it might be as well for the patient to be allowed to avoid these persons, in the longer term the extent to which he begins to trust them may be a measure of your success.

Allow the patient to have a large degree of privacy and personal space. Initially, he will wish to spend a large amount of time on his own and will ensure that all of his possessions are kept under secure lock and key. He will feel threatened if his 'personal space' is invaded by staff or other patients, this points to the necesssity to avoid close contact and/or touching the patient as far as is possible. We must demonstrate a high level of competence and sensitivity when delivering nursing care which involves intimate contact or any other form of touching the patient with a trust problem.

Remember that any whispering or verbal communication which he cannot clearly interpret may be regarded by this patient as an attack on him. As far as is possible, conversations which do not relate to him should take place in another room, those which do relate to him should include him, and additional time should be taken to explain our activities to him.

Any sensory deficit, partial deafness or blindness for example, should be treated if and when possible. All barriers to communication, such as those relating to hearing, add significantly to an existing trust problem.

As the development of a closer one-to-one relationship continues it is essential that the way in which we as nurses perceive the patient's trust problem be openly discussed with him; for example, we might say something like, 'How are you getting on with the others?' or, 'I see you carry your things around with you all day' or, 'I have the feeling that you have difficulty trusting me'. It is only when a relationship is fairly strong that we can begin to ask questions of a 'probing' type. If these are asked too early, they will invariably result in strong rejection by the patient.

In the longer term our task is to expose the patient to experiences which his trust in us and others has justified. In addition to facilitating the immediate health care process, these experiences may well be generalized by the patient and give him a basis upon which to develop positive trusting relationships with others in the longer term.

PATIENT PROFILE

Mr Croal is aged 67 years and lives alone in a ground floor flat in a rural village. Although physically frail, he suffers from no specific physical or psychiatric illness. He has no relatives or close friends and lives a relatively isolated life, spending most of his time alone at home. Apart from two or three weekly visits to the local shop and post office he has little contact with the 'outside world' and never has visitors to his house.

This man was recently treated by his general practitioner following the onset of lobar pneumonia. The treatment, which included two visits to the GP and the prescription of antibiotics, was entirely successful. Subsequently, the GP suggested to his health visitor colleague that she should visit Mr Croal on a regular basis. On her first visit to Mr Croal, the health visitor was told by him (through the letter box) that he had not requested this visit and that she should 'go away'. One week later the health visitor returned and was told by Mr Croal, 'I am perfectly OK; I don't need anyone'. Following the delivery of a letter to Mr Croal from his general practitioner outlining the purpose of the health visitor's visit, the health visitor finally did obtain entry to Mr Croal's house. Her first visit was conducted in the outer lobby of the house and lasted for less than one minute. During this time Mr Croal made it quite clear that he thought the health visitor was interfering with his privacy and more concerned about her job than for him personally.

During the past six months the health visitor has made six further visits, the last one taking place in Mr Croal's living room and lasting 30 minutes.

During the last six months Mr Croal has become increasingly physically frail and is having some difficulty in doing his housework. Although still fairly able to cook and look after himself from a personal point of view, his house has become dirty and untidy.

ORGANIZATION OF NURSING CARE

Subjective Evidence (What the Patient Says)

- 'I have not requested this visit, go away.'
- 'I am perfectly OK; I don't need anyone.'
- 'You are interfering with my privacy and more concerned about your job than for me personally.'

Objective Evidence (What the Nurse and Others Observe)

- Has no close friends and lives an isolated life.
- Spends all of his time alone at home apart from three visits each week to the shop/post office.
- Never has visitors to his house.
- First health visitor visit conducted in the lobby of the house and lasted for less than one minute.

Assessment (Nursing Diagnosis)

- Lack of trust.

Plan of Nursing Care

- Increase frequency and duration of health visitor visits.
- Discuss with Mr Croal his isolation from other people, particularly from his neighbours and friends of many years ago.
- Encourage him to increase the number of visits made outside his home;

for example, try to reactivate his interest in reading and visits to the local library.

- Be punctual, consistent and scrupulously honest in personal dealings with Mr Croal.
- Closely monitor the development of new interpersonal relationships, particularly with the home help who has recently started to visit Mr Croal.
- Encourage Mr Croal to make medium- and longer-term plans which include contact with other individuals and groups.

Expected Outcome

- Will make visits to places outwith the home, other than the shop or post office, at least once per week.
- Will initiate conversation with one or more neighbours.
- Will indicate a willingness to extend the duration and frequency of the health visitor's visit.
- Will discuss the existence of a trust problem and participate in decisions about reducing this.

NURSING CARE OF PATIENT TRUST PROBLEM (EXAMPLE)

The following description of the 'care' of Mr Croal over a 24-hour period illustrates how that care will have been planned and developed by the health visitor and Mr Croal during their prolonged and successful contact. It is important to remember that the success which is indicated below has resulted in substantial time and effort being invested in Mr Croal by himself, the health visitor and a number of other people including his home help.

07.00 hours	Mr Croal gets up at his usual time and begins the day by using the bathroom and washing, shaving, etc. He knows that his home help will not visit on that particular day but that the health visitor is due to see him between 09.00 and 10.00.
7.30	He begins to tidy up the house, knowing that it will take some time and that the major cleaning tasks will be done later in the week by the home help.
8.30	Breakfast, which is deliberately light because of his plan to visit the local old folk's club later that day and have a midday meal, is over by 09.00, when he waits for the arrival of the health visitor.
9.30	The health visitor arrives and is shown into the living room

and offered a cup of tea. They discuss general events which have taken place since the last visit (10 days previously) and, in particular, discuss his concern about allowing a relative stranger (the home help) to have free movement within his house. This subject opens the way for discussion of Mr Croal's trust problem and the way in which he sees the successes of the past few months as having diminished it.

The health visitor stays for 45 minutes and reviews Mr Croal's general activity during the past 10 days and makes specific plans with him for the next 10. Although the relationship between Mr Croal and the health visitor still contains a high degree of caution on his part, considerable progress has been made since the early visits.

10.15 Following the departure of the health visitor, Mr Croal prepares for his daily visit to the local shops. Rather than make one or two visits per week, he is now making a deliberate point of visiting the shops daily and, where possible, making casual conversations with his neighbours who also shop there.

11.15 On return from the shops he prepares for one of his thrice-weekly visits to the local old folk's club where he spends 3 hours with other old people from the village and has a three-course meal.

12.00 On arrival at the club he meets with the staff member who, by arrangement with the health visitor and with the agreement of Mr Croal, has made it her business to form a fairly close relationship with him. Through this relationship Mr Croal has been introduced to and started to make friends with two others who attend the club. At present, this relationship is rather tentative and one-sided with the other two individuals taking a more positive role. However, Mr Croal has indicated to the health visitor that he is feeling decreasingly threatened by the emotional closeness of these individuals.

15.00 Mr Croal leaves the old folk's club and returns home, where he spends the remainder of the afternoon and early evening alone.

20.00 A visitor, a neighbour who lives nearby, calls on Mr Croal to exchange daily newspapers. This arrangement, which was engineered by the health visitor with the consent of Mr Croal, is being used as a means of enabling him to develop new relationships with his neighbours. Although this arrangement has a long way to go and develop it is regarded as a useful and positive starting point.

23.00   Prior to preparing for bed, Mr Croal makes an entry into a diary which has been given to him by the health visitor. The purpose of the diary entry is twofold: first, to enable him to focus on and describe his progress in developing relationships with others and in tackling his specific trust problem; second, periodic review of the diary contents will enable him and the health visitor to measure the progress which they are jointly making.

23.15   Prepares for bed.

The crux of success in maximizing nurse – patient trust is a strong interpersonal relationship which utilizes the principles of the psychotherapeutic relationship (see Chapter 9). The contents and references presented in Chapter 15, Communication, and Chapter 27, Social Skills (Interpersonal), are of particular importance to the development of trust. Additionally, the references given in the Further Reading at the end of this chapter focus on the psychotherapeutic use of interpersonal skills, of which the development of trust is a crucial and central feature. This aspect of the therapeutic relationship was expressed by Rogers (1965) thus:

'1. ... when in the relationship with his client he (the therapist) is genuine and without front or facade.' (p.96)

'2. ... when the therapist is experiencing a warm, positive and acceptant attitude towards what is in the client, this facilitates change.' (p.97)

'3. The third essential condition of change is that the therapist is experiencing an accurate empathic understanding of the client's private world.' (pp.98 – 9)

'4. Unless some communication of the sort of attitudes I have been describing has been achieved, they do not exist in the world of the client and thus cannot be effective.' (p.99)

ASSESSMENT OF TRUST*

Interactions with Others

- *Alone/aloof,* enjoys company.
- Initiates, *avoids interactions.*
- *Avoids,* enjoys *group activity.*
- *Avoids,* enjoys *competitive activity.*

*Those items which indicate a low level of trust are italicized.

Property

- *Overprotective,* reasonably protective of property.
- *Suspects others of interfering with property.*

Acceptance of Information

- Accepts, *repeatedly 'checks' information.*
- *Refuses to accept,* accepts *reasonable decisions.*
- *Unwilling,* willing *to make personal decisions.*

Caution

- *Overcautious,* accepting.
- *Generally 'unsure',* confident.
- *Gives information* freely, *with reluctance*
- *Rigid, flexible.*

Hostility

- *Overbearing/assertive,* submissive/passive.
- *Hostile,* friendly.
- Accepts, *rejects offers of help.*

REFERENCES

Rogers C. (1965) The therapeutic relationship: recent theory and research. *Australian Journal of Psychology* **17**, 95–108.

FURTHER READING

Borsig A. & Steinacker I. (1982) Communication with the patient in the intensive care unit. *Nursing Times* **78**, 111.

French P. (1983) *Social Skills for Nursing Practice.* Croom-Helm, Beckenham.

Hayter J. (1981) Territoriality as a universal need. *Journal of advanced Nursing* **6**, 79–85.

Macilwaine H. (1978) Communication in the nurse/patient relationship. *Nursing Mirror* **16**, 32–4.

Peplau H. (1962) Interpersonal techniques: the crux of psychiatric nursing. *American Journal of Nursing* **62**, 50–4.

Roosa W.M. (1982) Territory and privacy. Residents views, findings of a survey. *Geriatric Nursing* **3**, 241–3.

Volicer B.J. (1974) Patients' perceptions of stressful events associated with hospitalization. *Nursing Research* **23**, 235–8.

White P.H. (1983) Supportive counselling in action. *Geriatric Nursing* **4**, 176–6A.

Wilson-Barnett J. & Carrigy A. (1978) Factors affecting patients' responses to hospitalisation. *Journal of advanced Nursing* **3**, 221–8.

PART 3
FACILITIES FOR THE ELDERLY

The six chapters of Part 3 focus on a range of facilities, resources and staff which contribute to the care of the elderly person. Although all topics mentioned in these chapters, drugs and community facilities for example, will have been briefly referred to in earlier chapters, they are dealt with in more detail in Part 3.

Drug therapy in all its aspects, including the role of the nurse, is of fundamental importance in relation to the elderly and to geriatric nursing care. Indeed, drugs constitute a major element in the treatment available to old people; they also constitute a major *potential* hazard.

Community and in-patient facilities, although presented in separate chapters, should be seen as a *single* and *interchangeable* alternative to independent living by an old person in his own home. Increasingly, there is considerable overlap between the two (rightly so), the hospital-based community psychiatric nurse, and the 'holiday bed' system being two obvious examples. The therapeutic use of the environment, irrespective of its location, is crucial to successful care. Whilst many of the examples in Chapter 33 are 'institutional', the principles apply equally to all environments in which well and ill old people live.

Health education, which constitutes a major means by which nurses can positively influence the health status of the ageing and elderly person, represents a major 'facility' for this group. This subject is an excellent example of the holistic approach to people in which the physical, psychological and social factors are given equal consideration.

Finally, the chapter on geriatric nursing research portrays one of nursing's major contributions to the care of the elderly, it optimizes the use of existing resources, facilities and staff and paves the way in identifying future strategies and needs. That chapter ends by giving direction to research-based care of the elderly, and indicates the direction to be taken by that part of the profession which has taken on the demanding and rewarding task of caring about and for the elderly.

Chapter 30
Drugs and the Elderly

In the context of the work of the professional nurse, drugs include those substances for which a medical prescription is required, and range from the simple analgesics to the complex antibiotics. They range from the relatively safe vitamin supplements to the relatively dangerous sedatives and tranquillizers. The term also includes those 'drugs' which are obtainable without prescriptions. Although in some countries, parts of the United States of America for example, nursing staff are permitted to prescribe a small group of drugs, prescribing is still largely the prerogative of the medical profession in the United Kingdom.

Where prescription of drugs is not part of the nurses role, she must never give them without the appropriate medical prescription being made. In most instances this prescription means that an actual *written* instruction, by a suitably qualified medical practitioner, has been made. Although there *may* be a small number of exceptions to this general rule, in certain emergency situations for example, it should never be broken except in these generally accepted exceptions.

DRUG USE IN OLD AGE

Because of the existence of multiple pathology and chronicity in old age, the likelihood of multiple and prolonged drug prescriptions is common. Thus, the elderly consume a much larger number of drug doses and variety of drugs than most other members of the population. Although the general approach taken by the health care professions, doctors and nurses in particular, is to minimize the quantity of drugs consumed by the elderly, it is inevitable that that group will require more drug therapy than other groups. Because nurses are often the initiators of drug therapy, having reported the relevant problem/s to the medical staff, we have an important responsibility to ensure that drugs are only prescribed when absolutely necessary. This responsibility is particularly relevant in relation to the prescription of sedatives and/or tranquillizers which may conceivably be prescribed for elderly patients at the request of nursing staff because they (the nurses) have a problem in accepting or dealing with the behaviour of elderly patients. In short, before urging our medical colleagues to prescribe drugs such as sedatives and tranquillizers, we must be sure that the problem we are trying to resolve is one which is experienced by the patient and not by us, the nurses.

Reluctance to Use Drugs

Many elderly patients have a long personal experience of a time when virtually no drugs were available. This, combined with the current focus on drug abuse and drug addiction, may cause certain old people to take a negative view in relation to drug prescription. Similarly, because of a lack of knowledge of the nature of some drug therapies, some old persons may self-terminate their drug prescriptions because they now feel 'better' when, in fact, they should continue with the prescription.

The role of the nurse in educating the elderly person and making him more aware of the purpose of his particular prescription is clearly important. It is not sufficient to assume that the elderly person will always understand the nature of the prescriptions, or will always completely trust the judgement of his doctor. For this reason it is essential that we monitor the extent to which patients, particularly non-institutionalized patients, are taking their prescriptions. We must also work hard at helping them to understand the effects and side-effects of their prescriptions in order that they can play a personal part in monitoring these.

Prescription Compliance

The nature of old age and the various physical and psychological changes which accompany it, may mean some old persons have difficulty in complying with their drug prescriptions, particularly if they are living at home; for example, because of the short-term memory deficit which a number experience, some may accidentally overdose by taking double, treble or even more frequent doses. Others still may simply forget to take their prescriptions. Here, community nurses will have to work hard at devising means by which the person can be assisted in recalling whether or not they have taken their medicine. The use of diaries and other memory aids are being researched by those concerned with this problem (see MacDonald *et al.* 1977, Wandless & Davie 1977, Roberts 1978).

Prescription compliance requires a considerable amount of manual skill, the administration of insulin, suppositories, and eye-drops are good examples. It must never be assumed that the person has the ability to administer *whichever* drug is prescribed. Indeed, it is probably best to assume that he is deficient in the necessary skills and, therefore, requires to be carefully taught these.

Finally, the way in which the drug is packaged or otherwise contained is of importance as this can actually prevent the elderly complying with the drug prescription. The best examples of these are childproof containers and drugs which are contained within individual parts of a metallic foil strip. The author's own experience is that many old people have extreme difficulty in opening childproof containers and have equal difficulty in extracting pills or capsules from metallic foil strips. Although both of these types of drug container were designed to resolve specific problems, accidental drug overdose in children for example, they have created additional serious problems in that they both tend to prevent the elderly person complying with the prescription. Chemists are increasingly allowing customers to choose childproof or 'normal' containers when collecting prescribed drugs.

Drug Storage

Drugs require a variety of different forms of storage in terms of temperature, light and atmospheric moisture for example. Many also have a fixed expiry date and are dangerous after that point. These factors, and the advice that discontinued drugs should be disposed of or returned, should be made known to all patients.

The safe storage of drugs is essential in all circumstances, including in private houses where children may unintentionally overdose themselves. The possible dangers to grandchildren and other children should be made known to the elderly person and apropriate advice given with regard to the safe placement of drugs (ideally in a locked drug cabinet). See the excellent article by Skeist and Carlson (1981) which discusses safe storage of medication being used by patients at home.

Non-prescribed Drugs

The elderly are not immune from the dangerous practice of storing prescribed drugs and using them at some later date. Nor are they immune from the dangerous practice of 'swapping' drugs which have been success-fully used by other people; for example, one old person may give a few of his 'chest tablets' or 'water tablets' to a friend who is *apparently* experiencing a similar problem. These misguided, and potentially fatal, attempts at self-medication should be prevented by reminding all patients that they must only consume drugs which have been prescribed by their doctor. The study described by Watson (1977) was designed to persuade people, including the elderly, to return surplus and out-of-date medicines.

ROLE OF THE NURSE IN DRUG THERAPY

Whether or not the patient is being cared for at home, hospital, or in some other institution, we have an important part to play in maximizing the effect of drug therapy. In hospital this role includes close monitoring, and usually administration, of all drugs consumed by the patient. In the community this monitoring role often operates either via the patient himself or, frequently, with the assistance of relatives who live with or visit the old person. In either case the responsibilities of the nurse are central to successful medical management of the patient and his illness. These responsibilities may be summarized as detailed in the following sections.

Observation and Reporting

Facts which may influence drug prescription, or prescription change, should be determined and recorded as part of the continuous process of nursing care delivery. Those facts which are relevant to the nature and course of the medical condition, those which relate to the effects and side-effects of the drugs, and those which are thought to relate to the general drug prescription policy should be made known to the appropriate medical staff. This responsibility does, of course, depend on you having a detailed knowledge of the patient's medical history, the particular illness from which he suffers, and of the effect and side-effects of the drugs being used.

Patient Allergies and Previous Drug History

New or previous drug allergies should be recorded in a conspicuous colour on the patient's chart and this information made known to medical staff; because of our continued and prolonged contact with patients and their relatives, we are often the first to obtain this kind of information. Indeed, it should never be left to 'accident' but should form part of the information which we collect about patients and which will form an important part of the decisions about medical strategies generally and drug prescription in particular.

Be Aware of Normal Drug Dose Ranges

Although the first and possibly major responsibility for being aware of the normal dose of a particular drug lies with the prescribing physician, you have a crucial role to play in this area. All nurses, particularly those who are administering the prescribed drugs, must be aware of the normal adult dose of the drug and, if the person receiving the drug is elderly, know whether or not the elderly require a 'special' dose of the drug. This information can be obtained from drug manuals or manufacturers literature, either of which *must* be available on the ward, or from the pharmacy. Such literature will normally state whether or not the elderly require doses which are different from that prescribed for other adults. It is *not* being suggested that we carry this information around in our heads, rather it is being suggested that we *must* have access to, and make full use of, the literature on the subject.

As is the case with all drug prescriptions which are being administered by nurses, you must feel free to draw any apparent or suspected over-prescription to the attention of the medical staff concerned. If this is a clear overprescription, for example 100 mg instead of 1 mg of a particular drug, the initiative in drawing this to the attention of the prescribing physician is usually welcomed. However, one does need to be more careful when suggesting, for example, that a prescription of 10 mg may be more than the recommended dose, when the manufacturers literature suggests that 5 – 8 mg is the normal dose for an elderly person. This is the kind of situation which is dependent on the positive multidisciplinary relationships which exist between those who prescribe medications (physicians) and those who frequently have to administer them (nurses).

Be Aware of Physiological Changes Affecting Drug Therapy

The differing drug doses which are required by the elderly, as compared with non-elderly adults, are partly related to changes which have occurred in the physical make-up of the elderly person. The way in which the person responds to the drug, the intensity and duration of the response, and the possible interactions with other drugs are affected by four major factors which are: first, absorption of the drug from the point of administration; second, the distribution of the drug within the body; third, the ability to metabolize the drug; and, fourth the ability to eliminate the drug.

ABSORBTION

Most, although by no means all, drugs are given by the gastrointestinal route. Apart from those drugs which are designed to act upon the gastro-intestinal tract (that is act without being absorbed into the bloodstream) most are dependent on being absorbed from the intestine into the blood-stream. A number of changes in the gastrointestinal tract effectively diminish the extent to which the drugs are absorbed. The general ability of the digestive system to break down and absorb all substances which enter into it is reduced by a number of factors. These factors include a reduction in the acid and mucus-secreting cells in the stomach, a reduction in the digestive enzymes generally, reduced peristaltic activity, and a reduced blood flow to the gastrointestinal tract generally. Reference to the manufacturer's literature will enable you to give appropriate advice to patients where necessary.

DISTRIBUTION

The distribution of the drug throughout the body of the older person is usually slower than in younger adults. The drugs, which enter the liver via the portal circulation, then enter the systemic circulation where they may be bound to proteins, to blood, or to tissues. They may enter cells, be distributed in body fluids or accumulate in certain organs or tissues in high concentrations.

It should be assumed because of the changes in systemic blood flow, cardiac output, percentage of body fat, and other anatomical and physiological changes, that most (if not all) drugs will function differently in an elderly person as compared to a younger adult.

METABOLISM

The metabolism of drugs, a process that converts the drug into a form which can be more easily excreted, may also be affected by the ageing process. Any diminution in the rate at which the metabolism of the drug occurs, will clearly have consequences for the intensity and duration of the blood levels of the drug. The rate of metabolism is likely to be decreased if the enzymes, and the liver which produces them, have a decreased function due to malfunction from diseases such as cirrhosis of the liver. In some older persons antidepressants and tranquillizers often have an increased effect which may be due to reduced speed of metabolism by the liver. With many such drugs, the margin between the therapeutic and toxic dose is very narrow, causing older persons to develop side-effects easily.

ELIMINATION

Elimination of the drug is the final phase and results in it being excreted from the body, usually via the kidneys or the gastrointestinal tract. The quantity and quality of the nephrons (the working unit) of the kidney decreases with age. The resulting partial inability of the kidney to eliminate drugs as rapidly as would be the case in a younger adult may result in a prolonged and increased drug level in the body.

All these factors need to be taken into account when drug prescriptions are made (and when nursing staff are 'checking' prescribed doses of drugs.) In all instances the manufacturer's literature will have taken these factors into account, this being reflected in the statements about effects, side-effects, contraindications and special precautions made in the literature with regard to the elderly person. For further general information on this subject you are referred to papers by Mullen and Granholm (1981) and by Hayter (1981).

Be Aware of Effects and Side-Effects

A major part of the nurse's role is to report on the effects and side-effects of all drugs that she administers to her patients. This can only be done effectively if you are fully familiar with the nature and features of the illness which the drug is designed to cure, reduce or prevent. It can only be done if you are also familiar with the full range of effects and side effects that the drug is likely to produce. It is *not* being suggested that you carry all of this information around with you in your head. However, it *is* being suggested that you make yourself fully familiar, by using the manufacturer's or some other form of literature, with the effects and side-effects of each and every drug you use. In many instances there will be 'special' effects and/or side-effects which relate to the elderly in particular. If this is the case, the literature will inform you. If in any doubt whatsoever, feel free to contact the prescribing physician, the pharmacy, or any other source of accurate and factual information. Remember, for many elderly patients the margin between successful drug therapy and hazardous side-effects (or even death) is small.

Be Aware of Abnormal Drug Interactions

Over the decades in which drug therapy in the elderly has developed into a sophisticated area of medicine, a number of significant reported drug interactions have become known because of the astute observations of nurses and other health care workers. In some instances these undesirable interactions are difficult to determine in terms of frequency, on other occasions they might be easier to predict. The abnormal interaction may be such that it would be extremely unwise for the two or more drugs to be given simultaneously, on other occasions it may be safe to do so, providing certain reasonable precautions are taken.

As with doses, effects, side-effects and contraindications we as nurses must be familiar with known drug interactions. This information is most likely to be found in the manufacturer's or other forms of literature which should be available on all wards in which these drugs are being used. An excellent article by Hussar (1982) considers 118 drugs which, when used in combination, may have undesirable interactions. The range of interacting drugs begins with aspirin which, when taken in combination with alcohol, can increase the risk of gastrointestinal irritation and bleeding. The list of drugs considered in that particular paper ends with vitamin K which, when taken in combination with certain anticoagulants, can antagonize the action of the anticoagulants and, in some cases, is used as an antidote in managing overdoses of, or excess responses to, these anticoagulants.

Ensure Correctness of Prescription

Nurses, particularly those who are involved in administering prescribed medications, have a major role to play in ensuring that the physician who prescribes medications does so in a manner which is clear, consistent with established practice, does not conflict with the normal dose or frequency of administration range, and which is not clearly contraindicated in the manufacturer's literature. Any such deviation should be brought to the attention of the prescribing physician and, depending on the form of deviation, appropriate action taken. If a massive overdose of a drug (100 mg instead of 1 mg) were being prescribed, for example, you should refuse to administer the medication until the prescription was discussed with a further physician. Alternatively, if the dose of the prescribed drug were marginally different (10 mg rather than the normal 7 mg from that recommended by the manufacturer's literature) you may wish to bring this to the attention of the prescribing physician. If, after you have talked to him about the drug dose and he has confirmed that this was indeed what he wished the patient to have, you should record the conversation with the doctor in the patient's note.

It is not being suggested that nurses should 'challenge' the knowledge and expertise of their medical colleagues, rather, it is being suggested that we, as nurses, and givers of many prescribed medications, have a serious and firm obligation to ensure that the medications we give are reasonable, accurately prescribed, and what the prescribing physician *really* intends us to give. If in doubt, check with the prescribing physician, the pharmacy, the manufacturer's literature or with a colleague.

Educate and Inform the Patient/Family

As with all aspects of care the patient, and where possible the family, should be fully involved in, and informed of, appropriate aspects of drug therapy. Examples of the kind of information which can be given are: the problems which the drugs are designed to prevent, reduce or minimize; name of each drug and its purpose; dose of each drug and its frequency; effects and side-effects of each drug; and names of substances which may be harmful if taken in combination with the drug. Finally, the patient should be allowed, indeed encouraged, to play a full part in the medication process. This is particularly necessary if he is presently, or shortly, to be expected to self-medicate. It is both thoughtless and dangerous to take full control of a person's medication programme, for example if he is in hospital, and then expect *him* to take full control without any experience, education or understanding of the process. Meguerdichian (1983), in an excellent paper on self-medication in a health-related facility, described how approximately 25% of residents were successfully taught about dosage, route, action and side-effects. In another paper Macauley *et al.* (1980), in a research-based study of patient-administered drugs in a municipal hospital, achieved a high level of success. Finally, in a photographically illustrated paper, Griffin (1980) demonstrated how a patient who had a paralysed left arm following a stroke, was taught how to prepare and inject her insulin using only one hand.

As nurses we have tended to be overinvolved in control of our patients' medication, to the extent of making them dependent on us. It would, of course, be unwise to expect all of our patients to be fully self-sufficient in terms of handling their own medications. However, we need to allow them to take as much control as is possible given the environment in which they are living, ensuring that there will be no danger to others, and that the self-medication will be carried out effectively and without danger to the patient.

Administer Prescribed Drugs

In most countries, including the United Kingdom, *virtually* all drugs administered by a trained nurse have been prescribed by a physician. Where this is the case, the nurse must be careful to administer *only* those drugs which have been officially and formally prescribed by a physician. In most instances the recipient of the drug (the patient) will be willing and cooperative, but there are instances when you meet with a refusal. Although it is the legal right of our patients to refuse drugs which we offer to them, it is necessary for us to be *reasonably* persuasive and/or take steps to establish the reason for the refusal. If a patient refuses to take prescribed drugs then we should: first, try reasonable persuasion and, for example, offer the drugs a second time a few minutes later; second, if there is a firm refusal, we should talk to the patient and try and establish why he is refusing the drugs; third, if no clear reason is given for refusal, we should try further reasonable persuasion which might include explaining the reasons for the drug being prescribed, the nature and function of the drug, the consequences of not taking it, and our personal view of the necessity for taking the drug; fourth, if the refusal continues, this should be recorded in writing in the patient's notes or another appropriate place, the prescribing or attending physician should be notified, and the patient closely observed for the effects of non-compliance with the drug prescription.

Remember, we as nurses cannot force our patients to take drugs which have been prescribed for them. However, in most instances it is expected that we will encourage our patients to comply with the drug prescriptions which have been made by their physicians and in their best interests.

Monitor and Observe

Having administered the drugs with which you are quite familiar in terms of effects and side-effects, you now need to observe the patient for these. Observation, coupled with conversation with the patient about the effects and side-effects of the drug, enable you to make meaningful and objective reports on the patient's progress. These reports will enable the prescribing physician to modify the prescription and, if necessary, make appropriate alterations in the drug, frequency, dose or combination of drugs. Finally, as nurses we play an important role in the decision-making process which results in the discontinuation of drug therapy. Our observations and subsequent reports on patients and their conditions will cause physicians to examine the need for drug prescriptions and, as is quite often the case, discontinue the drugs following our reports.

DRUG-RELATED ACUTE CONFUSIONAL STATE

Acute confusional states (see Chapter 8, pp. 77–8) can be caused by a variety of drugs and, therefore, attention will be drawn to this important aspect of drugs and the elderly.

The drug-induced mechanisms which are likely to result in acute confusional states include: reduced cerebral blood flow; reduced arterial oxygen supply; hypoglycaemia; increased intracranial pressure; dehydration; nutritional deficiencies; liver and kidney failure; and any febrile condition. Additionally, general anaesthetics, alcohol, and any tranquillizer or sedative may result in the onset of an acute confusional state. Since prescriptions of the latter two are often made at the request of, or are dependent on nursing reports, we have a special responsibility to ensure that these are kept to a minimum or, where they are prescribed, to be alert for the onset of acute confusional states.

It is essential, because of the large range of drugs which the elderly are prescribed, and our obvious inability to carry around appropriate infor-mation relating to all of them in our heads, that we have constant and adequate access to the manufacturer's literature regarding them. Similarly, we should have access to other forms of expertise on the subject such as that available from the pharmacist, prescribing physician and other experts in the subject area.

REFERENCES

Griffin A. (1980) How to prepare and inject insulin with one hand. *Geriatric Nursing* **1**, 112–3.

Hayter J. (1981) Why response to medication changes with age. *Geriatric Nursing* **2**, 411–6, 441.

Hussar D.A. (1982) Interactions involving drugs used in the care of geriatric patients. *Geriatric Drug Interactions* 11–23. Sandoz Pharmaceuticals.

Macauley C., Murray L. & Ellis H. (1980) Patient-administered drugs in a municipal hospital. *Geriatric Nursing* **1**, 109–11.

MacDonald E.T., MacDonald J.B. & Phoenix M. (1977) Improving drug compliance after hospital discharge. *British medical Journal* **2**, 618–21.

Meguerdichian D. (1983) Improving self medication in a HRF. *Geriatric Nursing* **4**, 30–4.

Mullen E.M. & Granholm M. (1981) Drugs and the elderly patient. *Journal of gerontological Nursing* **7**, 108–13.

Roberts R. (1978) Self-medication trial for the elderly. *Nursing Times* **74**, 976–7.

Skeist R. & Carlson G. (1981) Storing medications safely. *Geriatric Nursing* **2**, 429–32, 441.

Wandless I. & Davie J.W. (1977) Can drug compliance in the elderly be improved? *British medical Journal* **1**, 359–61.

Watson P.J. (1977) A medicine return campaign. *British Journal of Addiction* **72**, 83–9.

FURTHER READING

Alafano G. (1982) Meaning of the medication: Clue to acceptance or rejection. *Geriatric Nursing* **3**, 28–30.

Bliss M.R. (1981) Prescribing for the elderly. *British medical Journal* **283**, 203–6.

Cotterell M. & Miller M. (1980) Nursing implications of drug therapy. *Geriatric Nursing* **1**, 271–6.

Gotz B.E. & Gotz V.P. (1978) Drugs and the elderly. *American Journal of Nursing* **78**, 1347–51.

Holmes S. (1984) Chemotherapy and the gastrointestinal tract. *Nursing Times* **80**, 29–31.

Mayers M.H. (1981) Legal guidelines. *Geriatric Nursing* **2**, 417–21, 441.

Moir D.C. & Dingwall-Fordyce I. (1980) Drug taking in the elderly at home. *Journal of clinical and experimental Gerontology* **2**, 329.

Pakov J. & Stephenes B. (1981) Special considerations for the community based elderly. *Geriatric Nursing* **2**, 422–8.

Potterton D. (1984) Drugging the elderly. *Nursing Times* **80**, 20–1.

Rajda M.J. (1984) Drug reduction works. *Journal of gerontological Nursing* **10**, 19–21.

Royal College of Nursing (1983) *Drug Administration, a nursing responsibility.* Royal College of Nursing. London.

Royal College of Physicians (1984) Medication for the elderly. A report of the Royal College of Physicians. *Journal of the Royal College of Physicians* **18**, 7–17.

Smith D. (1983) Outpatient care of the diabetic. *Journal of gerontological Nursing* **9**, 422–7.

Vancura E.J. (1979) Guard against unpredictable drug responses in the ageing. *Geriatrics* **34**, 63–5, 69–70, 73.

Williamson J. & Chopin J.M. (1980) Adverse reactions to prescribed drugs in the elderly: A multicentre investigation. *Age and Ageing* **9**, 73–80.

Wolanin M.O. (1981) Nursing therapy, drug therapy, or both. *Geriatric Nursing* **2**, 408–10.

Chapter 31
Community Facilities

During the past 20 years a rich variety of community care facilities for the elderly person has developed in response to the very real need of the elderly in the community. Not so many years ago, the elderly person who required help with a health care problem would either have been admitted to hospital, and possibly given more care than was required, *or* would have been cared for at home with minimal help and support. The developments taking place in recent years have resulted in the availability of wide-ranging levels of care, with occasional, but regular, visits from a health visitor or general practitioner at one extreme, to hospitalization in an acute assessment unit at the other extreme.

The purpose of this chapter is to demonstrate this variety of community care facilities whilst bearing in mind that the availability of these will vary considerably from area to area; for example, older persons living in an urban community may have access to the full range of facilities, on the other hand those living in rural communities might have a more limited access.

Since some of the personnel who are involved in delivering community care have a role which is virtually identical to that which they have in delivering the same type of care in a hospital setting, these groups will be referred to briefly. Their role will be more fully discussed in Chapter 32.

MEDICAL PERSONNEL

In the United Kingdom most community medical care is performed by the family doctor/general practitioner. It is normal for all individuals in a given geographical area to be registered with a general practitioner of his or her choice. Although all general practitioners deal with the health care problems which are referred to them by old people, or by their relatives on their behalf, a number of these doctors take additional steps to monitor the health status of all of their elderly patients including those who do not report with health care problems. This additional monitoring takes two forms, *screening* and *case finding*. Screening may be defined as the search for precursors of disease in those who do not have symptoms of disease and who believe themselves to be in good health. Conversely, case finding is a form of prevention in which established diseases are sought out in order to achieve early diagnosis and treatment. For an excellent review of the problems and progress in screening and case finding you are referred to the brief and readable text by Taylor *et al.* (1983).

Domiciliary visits (made by hospital-based consultants rather than by the family doctors themselves) are usually made at the request of the family doctor. These visits made by consultant physicians, surgeons, psychiatrists and other consultants have the distinct advantage of enabling the doctor to take the patient's immediate environment into consideration when making decisions about the type of treatment to be offered, and in deciding whether or not the person should be treated at home or elsewhere.

Medical out-patient clinics are usually, but not always, conducted at the local general, or some other, hospital. Here, the patient visits the specialist following referral by his general practitioner. In this way, hospital-based specialists can either follow up their treatment of patients after discharge, or can supplement the treatment offered by family practitioners on this out-patient basis.

General practitioners and other members of the primary health care team, including community nurses and others, work from a facility usually referred to as a health centre or medical centre. The way in which the work of the medical and other staff in such a centre is handled can be found in Faulkner (1983).

NURSING STAFF

District nurses, health visitors and community psychiatric nurses are the three largest groups who provide nursing care in the community.

The district nurse, who will be an experienced general nurse with an additional training in district nursing, carries out nursing procedures on a regular basis in the patient's home. She might either provide the nursing care to a patient who is being treated at home and has not been hospitalized, or continue the nursing care of a discharged hospitalized patient. There can be no doubt that, but for the availability of district nursing care, many old people would have to be hospitalized. Caring for the elderly forms an increasingly large part of the work of the district nurse, 50% of cases dealt with by them involved elderly people in 1978 (see Department of Health and Social Security and Welsh Office 1978), and have most probably increased since then.

Health visitors, experienced general nurses with an additional health visiting qualification, provide a health advisory and health monitoring service to families and individuals. In principle, the health visitor visits all families, not only those which contain an ill person. Her function is to detect early signs of ill health, give support to those families who are caring for an ill person, and, if necessary, mobilize the assistance of other health care personnel. Health visitors have an important role to play in giving support to families who are caring for a chronically ill person, for example someone suffering from senile dementia. Although a major part of the work of the health visitor relates to families with newborn babies, they also have a major responsibility for monitoring the health status of old people and for alerting other health care professionals when necessary.

Community psychiatric nurses are involved in visiting mentally ill patients in their own home. These patients may be mentally ill but never have been hospitalized, others may have been hospitalized and are now recovering at home. Although the mentally ill elderly, those suffering from dementia in particular, will form only a part of the caseload of the community psychiatric nurse, they do constitute an important and time-consuming part. These nurses often play a vital role in maintaining elderly mentally ill patients at home as an alternative to hospitalization, they also give much-needed support to the families of such patients. They are frequently involved in establishing priorities with regard to admitting patients to psychogeriatric beds, which are usually in short supply.

DAY HOSPITALS

Day hospitals, for both physically and mentally ill persons, have been increasing in number over the past ten years. The day hospital, which may be part of, or attached to, an existing hospital or, more commonly, be a purpose-built or converted facility provides its patients with a 'partial' hospitalization. Most day hospitals, which are staffed by a full range of medical, nursing and other staff, are usually open between 09.00 and 17.00 Monday to Friday. Some patients will attend for eight hours per day, five days per week, whilst others may only attend for one, two, three or four days.

The day hospital, which provides a full range of therapeutic activities, is an important and essential alternative to total hospitalization for many old people. Indeed, the day hospital can be seen as providing care which is shared between the hospital and either the patient himself, or the patient and his family. Transportation to and from the day hospital may be either by ambulance, relatives, or, in some instances, by public transport.

DAY CENTRES/SOCIAL CENTRES/LUNCH CLUBS

These centres provide an important social facility for many old people who would otherwise be isolated. They also provide the means of obtaining companionship, peer group support, and contact with staff who are genuinely interested in their individual welfare. A typical centre will offer meals at a reasonable cost, a range of recreational and occupational activities, possibly washing, drying and other facilities and, most importantly, a feeling of being wanted and belonging.

MEALS ON WHEELS

A number of housebound frail elderly people have extreme difficulty in maintaining even a reasonable nutritional status. The meals on wheels service, usually run by the local social services and dependent on considerable voluntary help, delivers hot nutritious meals at a reasonable cost to the housebound and/or frail elderly. Although the frequency of delivery of meals may vary from two to five times weekly, it does constitute an important part of the maintenance of reasonable nutritional status for many old persons. This service, and others, such as the home help arrangement, provide an additional and effective means of making an unofficial and informal check on the general health status of the elderly person.

LAUNDRY SERVICES

Some health authorities/local authorities have arrangements whereby the soiled laundry of incontinent persons can be collected, washed and returned. For families caring for an incontinent patient, this service frequently enables him to be cared for at home rather than be hospitalized.

SHELTERED HOUSING

Sheltered housing usually takes the form of a number of specially adapted or purpose-built individual houses which are available only for elderly and/or infirm people. These self-contained housing units are linked up to a house which is occupied by a paid resident warden or supervisor. The role of the supervisor is to keep a general check on the health, activities and problems experienced by the residents. A regular daily check on all residents may be made by the warden, alternatively residents communicate with the warden by means of a call-button system or telephone. The job of the warden is not 'to do for' the residents, rather it is to be there in case of emergency. Residents are responsible for organizing their own homes, housekeeping and general independence.

NURSING HOMES

Nursing home places should be available for 25 per 1000 elderly in the community, thus constituting a major institutional alternative to long-term hospitalization. This type of care, which can either be organized by local authorities, voluntary organizations or private (for profit) commercial concerns, is usually offered as a long-term alternative to living at home.

When this type of facility was first developed in the late 1940s it was anticipated that most of the residents would be relatively independent and fit from a health viewpoint. Over the years the average age of residents has increased (70% to 80% of new residents being aged 75 years and over) and an increasing proportion of residents are physically and/or mentally infirm. Although these homes are nearly always staffed by personnel who have little or no professional health care education, many of the residents are likely to experience actual or potential health care problems which require intensive medical or nursing intervention. Ovenstone and Bean (1981) made a medical, psychiatric and social assessment of 272 residents admitted to residential care homes in Nottingham in the year ending 31st January, 1978. They found that more than half, who were assessed within one month of admission, had medical conditions which had not been previously diagnosed. They also found that half the sample suffered from dementia, and that only 23% had no detectable mental illness. They reported that 18% of the group were totally independent; the majority, 77%, were moderately disabled, and the remaining 6% were severely impaired.

The findings of Ovenstone and Bean (1981), and many similar conclusions, indicate that a substantial amount of medical and nursing care is now required by the residents of nursing homes. That professional nurses should become more involved in the work of nursing homes, including those run for profit, was suggested by Slack (1983) in a discussion of the 'twilight zone' of private nursing home care.

That the National Health Service (NHS) is becoming increasingly interested and involved in nursing home care for the elderly is evidenced by the opening of three NHS nursing homes in England. These homes, which have trained nurses on the staff, will be heavily dependent on the professional nursing care input and on the ability of nurses to recognize the needs of patients in relation to requiring an input from other health care staff (see Dopson 1983).

HOME HELP SERVICE

A home help is someone who provides a 'home making' or 'helping in the home' service, one to four hours per day for example, for a number of days per week. This help is to supplement the abilities and skills of the frail old person who may be expected to contribute to some of the work of running the house. The home help may do such things as house cleaning, bed making occasionally meal preparation, shopping and pension collection. In general, she performs a multitude of small tasks which enable the old person to enjoy the independence of living at home rather than in an institution.

The home help service is usually funded and organized by the local authority, with the elderly person contributing something to the cost according to his or her financial means.

SOCIAL WORKER

The social worker, who is equally involved with in-patient and out-patient social work, is concerned with the social, environmental and financial aspects of care. The role of the social worker in guiding the patient and other health care professionals through the maze of financial, bureaucratic and communication difficulties which face the elderly person living at home is absolutely essential. In some instances the role of the social worker may relate to determining the need for, and obtaining, a variety of aids and appliances which enable the person to continue living at home. The role of the social worker in providing support and advice to other members of the family, particularly as these relate to means of obtaining other appropriate types of assistance, is another important area.

FAMILY SUPPORT GROUPS

A wide variety of mutually supportive groups for the families of those caring for mentally or physically impaired elderly persons exist. The very existence of these groups underlines the severe strain which is placed on the families of patients who suffer from dementia, cerebrovascular accidents, incontinence and a variety of other chronic and distressing problems. These groups, initiated by health care personnel or by the families themselves, are an invaluable means of giving support to family care givers. Vargna (1979) describes a means of giving group psychotherapeutic help to the wives of patients suffering from Alzheimer's Disease. Hirschfeld (1983) attempted to achieve:

'(1)   the identification of factors crucial to managing a person with senile brain disease in the home;
(2)   an understanding of the kind and size of the burden involved;
(3)   an assessment of the behaviour leading to successful management of overwhelming stress;

(4) increased knowledge of the strategies which enable families to manage life with senile brain disease.'

PHYSIOTHERAPISTS

Physiotherapists play an important role in maintaining the physical independence of patients who live at home but who suffer from an illness which interferes with their general mobility. As well as initiating exercises to correct and/or prevent muscle deformity and wasting, the physiotherapist may use the natural environment of the patient's home to enable him or her to maintain independence.

OCCUPATIONAL THERAPISTS

Occupational therapists will also use the natural environment of the patient's home to maximize independence and will, for example; help the individual cope with such tasks as dressing, drinking, cooking, washing and house cleaning.

The responsibility of the nurse, whether working in the hospital or the community, is first, to be fully aware of the entire range of health care and supportive facilities which are available for the elderly population in any given community. Second, nurses must be aware of the administrative means by which the services of each of these facilities can be utilized. Third, all nurses must be able to make clinical judgements as to when these services should either be utilized, or when patients should be assessed as to their need for these services.

The wide range of alternatives to hospitalization, means that a 'package' can be put together to suit the needs of almost any old person. As nurses we must make very fine clinical judgements about the extent to which patients need these services, bearing in mind that too much will cause unnecessary dependence, and too little may result in hospitalization and increased general deterioration.

REFERENCES

Department of Health and Social Security and Welsh Office (1978) *A Happier Old Age.* Her Majesty's Stationery Office, London.

Dopson L. (1983) Having your own front door. *Nursing Times.* **79,** 10–12.

Faulkner H. (1983) *An Experience of Caring.* Help the Aged, London.

Hirschfeld M. (1983) Homecare versus institutionalization: family caregiving and senile brain disease. *International Journal of Nursing Studies* **20,** 23–32.

Ovenstone I.M.K. & Bean P.T. (1981) A medical social assessment of admissions to old people's homes in Nottingham. *British Journal of Psychiatry* **13**, 226–9.

Slack P. (1983) The twilight zone. *Nursing Times* **79**, 8–10.

Taylor R., Ford G. & Barber H. (1983) *The Elderly at Risk*. Age Concern, Mitcham.

Vargna D. (1979) Group treatments for wives of patients with Alzheimer's disease. *Social Work in Health Care* **5**, 219–21

FURTHER READING

Allibone A. & Coles R. (1984) There's no place like home. *Nursing Mirror* **158**, 22–3.

Arcand R. & Williamson J. (1981) An evaluation of home visiting of patients by physicians in geriatric medicine. *British medical Journal* **283**, 718–20.

Ashton P. (1984) The community psychiatric nurse and the elderly. *Nursing Times* **80**, 49–50.

Brocklehurst J.C. (1982) A geriatrician's view. *Health Visitor* **55**, 356.

Challis B. & Davies B. (1980) A new aproach to community care for the elderly. *British Journal of Social Work* **10**, 1–18.

Cormack D.F.S. (1981) Nursing care of the elderly in Scotland. *Journal of gerontological Nursing* **7**, 749–58.

Davidoff D. & Slater P.F. (1982) Domestic care dependency in the aged: A total community survey in Israel. *Journal of the Royal College of General Practitioners* **32**, 403–8.

Davies B. & Challis D. (1980) Experimenting with new roles in domiciliary service. *The Gerontologist* **10**, 288–99.

Day L. (1981) Health visiting the elderly in the 1980's. Do we care enough? *Health Visitor* **54**, 538.

Doyle D. (1982) Domiciliary terminal care demands on statutory service. *Journal of the Royal College of General Practitioners* **32**, 285–91.

Fitton J. (1980) Health visiting the aged. *Health Visiting* **53**, 521–5.

Fitton J. (1984) Health visiting the elderly: nurse manager's views. *Nursing Times* (Occasional Paper) **80**, 67–9.

Fitzgerald A. (1981) Maintaining the elderly mentally frail in the community. *Nursing* **1**, 1097–8.

Gooding H. (1982) Developing a preventative service for the elderly. *Health Visitor* **55**, 593–7.

Luker K.A. (1981) Health visiting and the elderly. *Nursing Times* (Occasional Papers) **77**, 137–40.

Luker K.A. (1982) Screening the well elderly in general practice. *Midwife, Health Visitor and Community Nurse* **18**, 222–9.

McNeil T. (1982) Home health care for seniors. *Canadian Nurse* **78**, 36–8.

Mortimer E. (1984) Part of a team. *Nursing Mirror* **158**, 28–30.

Neil M. (1982) It's nice to know that someone cares. *Nursing Times Community Outlook* **78**, (Supplements), 243.

O'Brien C. (1981) Adult day health care and the bottom line. *Geriatric Nursing* **2**, 283–6.

Partridge C.J. (1982) Access to physiotherapy services. *Journal of the Royal College of General Practitioners* **32,** 634–6.
Tinker A. (1984) Health and housing. *Nursing Times* **80,** 57–9.
Willis P. (1983) A day in the life (of a C.P.N.) *Nursing Times* **79,** 109–10.

Chapter 32
In-patient Facilities

In-patient facilities for the elderly come in a variety of shapes and sizes. Those where care for the physically ill elderly is managed are usually referred to as 'geriatric' wards, units or hospitals; those for the mentally ill elderly are usually referred to as 'psychogeriatric' wards, units or hospitals.

The facilities may be a ward within a general or psychiatric hospital, a specialist unit (collection of wards) within a larger hospital, or a small specialized psychogeriatric or geriatric hospital which is totally concerned with the care of the elderly.

Whether the facility is a ward, unit or hospital; geriatric or psychogeriatric, the range of facilities, resources and staff is similar if not identical. In all instances the facility may care for patients on a variety of in-patient bases.

FULL-TIME IN-PATIENT BASIS

Most patients are admitted on a 24-hour per day, seven day per week basis. The hospitalization may be in an assesment ward, usually for a short term such as 2-3 weeks, during which time an intensive assessment of all aspects of health status will be made. Although a considerable number of patients may die in, or be discharged home from, this ward, a number will be transferred to one of two longer term in-patient facilities. Rehabilitation wards are used for those patients who have been fully assessed and found to require longer-term rehabilitation prior to discharge to their own home, or to some other form of community care facility; for example a patient who is recovering from a cerebrovascular accident may need to relearn a number of self-care and mobility skills prior to being discharged. The rehabilitation ward provides a high level of expertise in this area, and is concerned with intensive and active treatment which will help the patient reach the desired goals. The long-term or continuing care ward is used for those patients who require longer-term care, rather than active and *intensive* rehabilitation. This is not to say that patients in long-term/continuing care wards should not be actively encouraged to maintain an optimum level of independence (the *real* meaning of the word rehabilitation), clearly they must.

384

Any of these three types of full-time in-patient wards can use their beds in a variety of ways which enable patients to be hospitalized on a non full-time basis.

'Shared' Beds

A shared bed is one which is used by more than one patient on a rota basis; for example, one bed may be used by two patients who use it for alternate two-week periods. Such an arrangement is clearly useful when a family, or patient, is partially able to cope with living at home providing that equal support is given in terms of shared bed hospitalization.

Monday-to-Friday Beds

For many patients it is inappropriate to consider complete hospitalization as being the only alternative to living an independent or semi-independent life in their own homes. For such patients, and their families, the availability of a hospital bed on either a Monday-to-Friday basis, or some other suitable arrangement, is all that is necessary. If a ward operates exclusively on a Monday-to-Friday basis, it means that the staffing requirements of the unit are considerably reduced by no longer having to cover Saturdays and Sundays.

Holiday Beds

Many elderly people are only able to live at home, either on their own or with relatives, because of the tremendous support which is given to them by relatives. Holiday beds are used by patients on a 1, 2 or 3 week basis in order to give them a 'holiday' away from their own home and/or relatives, or to give their relatives a 'holiday' away from looking after a dependent relative. This type of arrangement, and other similar flexible arrangements for the use of in-patient beds, plays an important part in helping patients and relatives cope with what are often very demanding and difficult personal situations. The physical structure and the therapeutic use of the environment of the in-patient facility will be discussed in Chapter 33. As important as the physical structure of the environment in which the elderly are cared for, are the quantity, quality and range of health care personnel available to such patients. The remainder of this chapter will discuss the role of those staff who come into relatively close contact with patients.

HEALTH CARE TEAM

As with all patient groups, the success of treatment and care is heavily dependent on good multidisciplinary team work. Some years ago this team may have consisted primarily of nurses and doctors. However, in the past 10 to 15 years the needs of the elderly have been (rightly) recognized as requiring an input from a variety of other professionals who have much to offer the elderly ill person. As nurses, we must fully understand the roles of all members of the health care team, how to communicate with them, and what to communicate to them. Nursing staff are recognized as being the key figures in facilitating the smooth flow of information between all members of the health care team. The ward, which is constantly and continuously staffed by nurses, is undoubtedly the hub of all patient activity, with the individual patient being the central point of this hub.

Nursing Staff

The nursing staff group consists of the ward sister/charge nurse (a registered nurse who has been promoted to this grade), staff nurses who are also registered nurses, enrolled nurses, nursing assistants and possibly nurses in training.

CHARGE NURSE/WARD SISTER

The charge nurse/ward sister performs a dual role in terms of administrative leadership, and in ensuring clinical excellence in the delivery of nursing care. This role is a demanding one which can only be performed well by nurses of the highest calibre, by those with complete dedication to the care of the elderly, and by those with a wide experiential and professional training in the disease processes and nursing care of the patients for whom they are caring. In many instances the focus of health care attention for elderly persons is *care* rather than *cure,* highlighting the centrality and importance of the role of the charge nurse/ward sister in achieving and maintaining high quality health care for this group. In maintaining these professional standards this nurse has a clear responsibility to ensure that her nursing team is appropriately balanced in favour of professionally trained, high quality, dedicated and skilled nurses who have a clear preference for caring for elderly patients.

STAFF NURSE

The staff nurse, who has also undergone a three-year training to become a registered nurse, has a major responsibility for implementing the clinical care policies and standards which have been set by the ward sister/charge nurse. The staff nurse is a clinician and is the clinical, as opposed to administrative, team leader. She is closely involved in the delivery of care and, when necessary, taking over the leadership and administrative duties of the ward sister/charge nurse. The active involvement of staff nurses in all aspects of geriatric nursing care is essential to achieving and maintaining the high quality of care which the elderly need and deserve.

ENROLLED NURSES

Enrolled nurses have a two-year training which, partly by design and partly by its two year duration, has a narrower and more practical application than the three-year training of the staff nurse. The practical, rather than practical with additional theoretical, training of the enrolled nurse enables her to function under the direction and/or general supervision of registerd nurses.

NURSING ASSISTANTS

Nursing assistants, who may have no formal training other than 'in house' study day or short study block training, can only work under the very direct supervision of trained nurses.

NURSES IN TRAINING

Student nurses, who are undergoing a three-year training in order to become registered nurses, and pupil nurses, who are undergoing a two-year training in order to become enrolled nurses, form the final part of the ward nursing team. As with nursing assistants, nurses in training can only work under the very direct supervision and/or guidance of trained nurses.

Staffing Levels

The complexity and intensity of the nursing care requirements of elderly people are such that they can *only* be properly cared for by a professionally trained nursing team assisted by some untrained staff who can only work under the very close guidance/supervision of trained nurses.

Although there is no formula which can be used to determine the required staffing levels of all wards in all circumstances, the following is offered as a general guideline. *Daytime* staffing levels in a ward with fifteen patients might be a ward sister/charge nurse, two staff nurses, two enrolled nurses and a nursing assistant on each shift. One nurse in training might be used as an alternative to the nursing assistant providing that work experiences can be arranged under the supervision of trained staff and regarded as teaching sessions for the nurse learner. If more than one nurse learner is on the ward at any given time, then an additional registered nurse will be required to supervise the work and training of these learners. During the *night-time* a reasonable *minimum* staffing level might be one registered nurse and one other nurse. These suggestions are offered in relation to all three types of ward (assessment, rehabilitation and continuing care) bearing in mind that the nursing activity is of similar intensity and requires similar expertise in *all* three types of ward.

Medical Staff

The medical staff, lead by a consultant geriatrician (or consultant psycho-geriatrician), work closely with the nursing staff team. The multidisciplinary partnership between nurses and medical staff is dependent on a mutual understanding and appreciation of each others role. Successful care of the elderly is also dependent on the recognition of a considerable amount of overlap between health care professionals.

The geriatrician, a doctor of medicine who has chosen to specialize in the care of the elderly, has a responsibility to provide *medical* care and to direct and coordinate the work of the paramedical staff groups who are under his direct control. The geriatrician has the responsibility for admitting patients to hospital, prescribing and providing medical care, and making the final decision with regard to the patients need for further hospitalization or discharge. The extent to which the provision of medical care, and the general medical management of the patient is dependent on close cooperation between nursing and medical staff, cannot be overemphasized.

The consultant geriatrician will be supported by junior medical staff at senior registrar, registrar and houseman levels. If the unit or ward is associated with a medical school, it may be regarded as a training area for those junior medical staff who are pursuing a career in the care of the elderly.

Paramedical Staff

Paramedical staff are those groups directly responsible to medical staff for their work. Doctors refer patients to their paramedical staff and may additionally provide specific prescriptions for them.

SPEECH THERAPIST

The speech therapist works with patients with any sort of speech problem which can be minimized by intensive speech therapy. She usually works with patients on an individual basis, but works with groups on some occasions.

Although some aspects of speech therapy are dependent on the use of appropriate technology, much of its success is dependent on nurses continuing the work of the speech therapist on an informal and regular basis. The close contact which exists between the speech therapist and nursing staff, will enable the latter group to learn enough about the speech therapy technique being used with an individual patient to enable treatment to be continued by nurses.

SOCIAL WORKER

As the name implies, the main function of the social worker is to be concerned with actual or potential *social* problems of the patient and his family. The importance of the role of the social worker is that she will be concerned with the wider social, economic, occupational and residential problems of the patient. Because not all patients are referred to or seen by a social worker, nursing staff must determine which patients have problems requiring social work intervention, and refer these patients to the medical staff who will subsequently refer them to the social work department.

PHYSIOTHERAPIST

The prime concern of the physiotherapist is the ability of the patient to move, perform psychomotor tasks, and generally to lead as independent a physical existence as possible. Physiotherapists either work in a central location within the hospital, patients travelling to that location, or visit the ward to see their patients. In suggesting to medical staff that patients should be prescribed physiotherapy, nurses must make judgements about their own ability to provide this sort of service to patients. Alternatively, the work of the physiotherapist may be combined with the work of nurses who will use their frequent/informal contact with patients to maximize their mobility, activity and independence.

Physiotherapists, like occupational therapists and speech therapists, are normally able to work with patients for a short period daily (or perhaps less often). You should therefore seek opportunities to participate in the continuation of the treatment which has been initiated by these groups. It is pointless, for example, to have a physiotherapist visit a patient periodically to 'teach her how to dress herself' if you are to reduce the patient's level of independence by doing virtually everything else for her at other times.

OCCUPATIONAL THERAPIST

The occupational therapist has traditionally been involved with arts and crafts of the basket making, woodworking, pottery, painting and knitting type. However, in recent years occupational therapists have diversified their work to include a much wider range of therapeutic activities including music and movement, reality orientation, maximizing skills of daily living, and a variety of activities which also include psychotherapeutic and socio-therapeutic techniques.

The work of the occupational therapist is increasingly overlapping with that of nursing staff who are well placed to continue her work, and to work with her as a fellow member of the health care team.

DENTIST

The dentist is an essential ingredient of multidisciplinary work with the elderly. Because most elderly persons have dentures and/or considerable problems with gums and teeth, the role of the dentist is to maximize the quality of patients' general mouth care and status.

Dental or denture problems are commonly first reported by patients to nursing staff, or, more usually, first noticed by nurses. A common example of such a problem is ill-fitting dentures, something which is relatively easy to remedy providing the dentist is involved. Nurses must therefore report any actual or potential dental problem to the medical staff who will then refer the patient to the dentist.

OPHTHALMOLOGIST

As with the dentist, patients are referred to the ophthalmologist by the medical staff. Similarly, visual problems and deficits are usually either reported to the nursing staff by patients or, more commonly, first discovered by nurses.

Ideally, routine checks of mouth and eyes should be made by the dentist and ophthalmologist in order to detect problems at an early stage.

AUDIOLOGIST

Hearing deficits, a relatively common problem in old age, can often be reduced by appropriate treatment by the audiologist. This treatment, often in the form of hearing aids, is dependent on substantial support being given to patients by nurses. Many elderly patients have extreme difficulty in becoming used to their hearing aids, a problem which can be overcome by sympathetic and understanding nursing staff.

CHIROPODIST

The chiropodist is an expert in dealing with problems relating to patients' feet. Many patients with problems such as corns, bunions and ingrown toe nails would be quite unable to walk were it not for regular treatment by a chiropodist.

As with other paramedical staff, patients are normally referred by a doctor who usually has the problem drawn to his attention by nursing staff.

Other Staff

The presence and role of other staff on the geriatric ward may vary from unit to unit. *Domestic staff,* who work under the direct supervision of the ward sister, but who are responsible to the domestic supervisor, are usually present on the ward continuously in the daytime. Apart from having a general responsibility for keeping the ward clean, domestic staff usually take responsibility for cleaning up the result of incontinence or sickness. In some areas this is a 'bone of contention', with domestic staff feeling that the cleaning up of urine, faeces or vomit is a 'nursing task'. The author's very firm view is that all aspects of cleaning are the responsibility of the domestic staff, providing that the cleaning does not involve direct patient contact.

Volunteers are used on some units to assist the domestic staff and other groups who have no direct patient contact. In other units they are used to 'assist' with nursing care, a role which brings them into direct patient contact; for example, volunteers may read newspapers to patients, generally fetch and carry, entertain patients, and perform some of the tasks which are normally performed by nursing assistants. If volunteers, who must be mature and interested people, are willing to give their time on a regular basis over a long period of time, there is no doubt that their help can be of value. However, you must be very selective about the kind of role which you allocate to volunteers who must *never* be regarded as substitutes for health care staff.

As nurses, we can contribute to the multidisciplinary nature of the care of the elderly in three major ways. First, by assisting with and continuing the work of other members of the team. Examples of this are the distribution of medications ordered by the medical staff, and the continuation of the work of the speech therapist who is teaching a patient who is recovering from a cerebrovascular accident to talk. Second, by closely monitoring the extent to which the patient requires the services of other members of the team; for example, we must regularly examine our patients' feet and mouths in order to ascertain whether or not they should be referred by the doctor to a chiropodist or dentist. Third, nurses play a major part in coordinating the work of the health care team and focusing their collective efforts on care of the individual patient.

The purpose of this chapter has not been to present a comprehensive and detailed account of the range and function of all members of the health care team. Rather, it is intended to illustrate the importance of teamwork in caring for the elderly person, and to demonstrate the centrality of the nurse to that *collective* effort.

FURTHER READING

Chenitz W.C. (1983) The nurse's aide and the confused patient. *Geriatric Nursing* **4**, 238-41.

Gray P.L. (1982) Gerontological nurse specialist: Luxury or necessity. *American Journal of Nursing* **82**, 82-5.

Hays A. (1982) Caring for the hospitalized elderly. *American Journal of Nursing* **82**, 930–1.

Horrocks P. (1982) Hospital treatment for the elderly. New directions. *British Journal of geriatric Nursing* **1**, 3–5.

Jordan S. (1983) The nurse in long term care. *Geriatric Nursing* **4**, 171.

Klus G.W. & Thoreson E.H. (1980) The nurse's aide. *Nursing Homes* **29**, 2–5.

Lowe K. (1982) Hospital care of the elderly. *Nursing* **1**, 1099–1101.

Nichols K. (1984) The nurse and the psychologist. *Nursing Times* **80**, 22–4.

Nichols K.A. (1981) Psychological care in general hospitals. *Bulletin of the British psychological Society* **30**, 90–4.

O'Connor C.E. & Carr S. (1981) Interdisciplinary collaboration between nursing and dental hygiene. *Journal of gerontological Nursing* **7**, 233–5.

Penrose J. (1983) Does he take sugar? *Nursing Times* **79**, 52–4.

Pomerantz P. (1982) Considerations in the physicians approach. *Geriatric Nursing* **3**, 311–15.

Redfern S.J. (1983) Nursing care of the elderly in hospital. *British Journal of geriatric Nursing* **2**, 8–11.

Smiler I. (1982) Foot problems of elderly diabetics. *Geriatric Nursing* **3**, 177–81.

Woodhams P. (1984) Nurses and psychologists — the first hand experience. *Nursing Times* **80**, 34–5.

Chapter 33
Therapeutic Use of the Environment

Nowhere is the therapeutic use of the environment more important than in relation to the elderly person. This importance is highlighted by the fact that the environment *may* be potentially damaging to the health of the elderly person, a long-term relationship frequently exists between the person and the environment, and the environment can positively be used as a therapeutic tool (as in reducing disorientation for example). Finally much is known, and can therefore be applied, about the therapeutic use of the environment in caring for older adults. Because of the rich variety of environments in which our patients are cared for, it would be impossible to provide a 'recipe' for everyone. However, this chapter is intended to introduce the general principle that the environment can be used therapeutically. You will have to apply these principles to your own environment and, more importantly, become aware of the therapeutic opportunities which result in the *particular* environment in which you work.

Much of the rest of this book has been concerned with the therapeutic role of nursing staff, other health care personnel and relatives, so this chapter will be confined to features of the environment other than the people in it. It is not, of course, being implied that the people in the environment are unimportant; they are probably more important than any other aspect of the environment. However, in the interests of avoiding repetition, this chapter will concern itself only with the 'non-people' aspects of the therapeutic use of the environment.

The therapeutic potential of the environment is equally important whether the person is living at home, in an institution or in any type of community facility. Although many of the examples used in this chaper relate to an institutional setting, the principles can be applied equally to any environmental situation; for example, the availability of water or of some other fluid suitable for drinking in a hospital ward, will apply to any environment in which the elderly person is living or being cared for. Similarly, the availability of orientation aids in the psychogeriatric ward is equally important in other environments in which a person with an actual or potential disorientation problem lives.

LOCATION

The location of the setting in which the person lives, particularly in relation to its nearness or distance from the population generally, needs to be carefully considered. This applies to an elderly person living alone in a flat which is some distance from shops and other facilities; it applies to the increasingly popular tendency to congregate elderly people in facilities which effectively isolate them from other age groups, sheltered housing and retirement villages are examples; it also applies to the siting of wards, units and hospitals for the elderly, ideally these facilities should be within a reasonable distance from the main centre of population. Remember that most of the visitors received by elderly persons, will themselves be old, often without personal transport, and liable to be 'put off' by the prospect of a long journey. If the facility in which the person is cared for is some distance from the main population, then it is absolutely essential that a good and frequent bus service be available. As far as is possible the location of the environment should not include hills or stairs as these make mobility for the elderly, and for their relatives, difficult if not dangerous.

BUILDING AND ASSOCIATED FACILITIES

A full range of ancillary facilities must be available within reasonable reach of the individual or group of elderly persons (see Chapter 32 for a discussion of the full range of facilities). If facilities such as occupational therapy, physiotherapy and recreational therapy are not within easy reach, it is likely that the elderly person will refuse to suffer the physical and mental 'wear and tear' which travelling to some distant department will involve. Although nurses are becoming increasingly involved in the general planning and design of these facilities, it is still the case that senior administrative staff input is far greater than that of the clinicians who have experience of, and will be working in, them. All nurses who are working with the elderly should feel an obligation to think about, and comment on, geriatric nursing facilities during the planning phases. It is the author's experience that this sort of input is invariably welcomed by senior nursing, planning, building and medical staff.

GROUNDS

All facilities which have a long-stay patient population, including those catering for the elderly, *must* have spacious and attractive grounds. If these are not available, and if easy access to them is not provided, it is possible that patients may spend many months (even years) 'imprisoned' in their wards.

Remember, not all patients are able to go on bus trips, shopping expeditions and the like.

As far as is possible, the grounds should contain a reasonable range of recreational and entertainment facilities which can be used by patients *and* their relatives. A shop, tearoom, bowling and putting green, and a garden with seats are essentials.

WARDS

Wards should be spacious with a suggested maximum of 20 patients. Overcrowding of wards, although it does facilitate the admission of an 'extra' patient, is destructive and damaging to patients, their relatives and the nursing staff who have to work within them. Overcrowding is a dangerous and antitherapeutic activity which must be strongly resisted by those who *care* about the elderly. A typical ward might consist of a sleeping area, sitting-room, dining-room and television/radio/record player room. Additionally, adequate toilets, bathroom, kitchen and storage facilities should be within reasonable distance. In discussing the influence of the environment on continence in the elderly Irvine (1983) suggested:

'It goes without saying that the lavatory must be clean, warm and inviting. There must be sufficient toilet paper, preferably with a roll or dispenser on each side to assist patients with hemiplegia. Appropriately placed handrails are very important. In well designed buildings for old people there is always a lavatory within 10 metres (40 feet) of patient areas.'

PRIVACY

Privacy in the bathroom and toilet area is of the utmost importance and must be carefully considered and guarded at all times. *Every* patient who uses the bath or toilet *must* have complete privacy. Any 'shortcuts' in nursing care which interfere with privacy (and which may occur because of 'staff shortage') must be reported to senior nursing and/or medical staff immediately. There is no excuse for 'making do' week after week, or month after month, or year after year in the hope that things will magically get better; *they will not.*

Privacy also applies to the number of beds which are in a given area; the arrangements the author has seen have ranged from every patient living in a single room, to up to 30 patients living in one large 'Nightingale' type of ward. I have seen many patients in single rooms, although having plenty of 'privacy', living miserable and lonely existences because they lack basic companionship and company. I have also seen patients in the large Nightingale type of ward, whilst having plenty of companionship and company, being utterly miserable because they lacked the privacy to which they were accustomed and which they yearned for. Some patients may be willing to sacrifice a little privacy for the sake of companionship; these patients enjoy living in two-bedded or four-bedded rooms. Other patients are willing to sacrifice some companionship and company for privacy; such patients may well enjoy living in a single room. However, it is essential that we remember that no one type of arrangment will suit *all* patients, and that we should have a variety of arrangements to suit the individual needs of our patients.

SITTING-ROOM

The sitting-room should be clean, spacious and as much like a domestic environment as is reasonable, possible and *safe.* The use of domestic-style wallpaper, curtains and other soft furnishings, flowers and ornaments will add to the attractiveness of the sitting-room. With the development of modern, high-density pile, manmade and rubber-backed floor coverings, it is now possible to have a near-domestic-style floor covering which is quite resistant to urine and other stains.

The view from the sitting-room window should be carefully considered and used as a therapeutic tool. The windows should be large, have a very low window sill, and must be uncluttered by large curtains, blinds and other objects which diminish the view.

Full and free access to water or other fluids suitable for drinking must be available. At best, this will mean a drinking fountain or some other suitable drinking facility within the sitting-room; examples are a large fruit juice container or individual drinks containers at a suitable temperature. Although very little research has been done on the subject, this author is convinced that many of our patients (particularly those who are disoriented) who are cared for in wards without direct access to fluids, are dehydrated because *we* have failed to provide them with a suitable quantity of fluid.

As with all aspects of the environment, repairs to the worn or damaged parts of the sitting-room should be carried out as quickly as possible. Nothing is better designed to lower the self-esteem of our patients, distress their relatives, and lower the morale of nursing staff than having to work in an untidy, ill-repaired, broken down and damaged environment.

ORIENTATION CUES

All parts of the environment should contain, or be labelled by, appropriate orientation cues. These orientation aids range from individualized lockers/ bed cover colours, to the labelling of all rooms and doors with letters at least half an inch high and no more than five feet from ground level. The route to toilets can be clearly marked, for example with a floor marking or with easily seen directions. Additionally, the toilet door will be of a different colour from *all* other doors in the ward.

All lockers, beds and individual wardrobes should be clearly marked with the users name, using large block capital letters. A photograph of the patient's relatives, friend, neighbour or some other well-known person could be placed on (or, if necessary fixed to) each patient's locker.

Contact with the 'outside world' and people in it, such as relatives and friends, is of great importance. This can be achieved by having reasonable access to writing materials and a public telephone. It is *essential* that each ward has a good supply of daily newspapers and current magazines.

An orientation board and 'Big Ben' clock in every major room (sleeping area, dining-room, sitting-room and quiet room) is also essential. In short, all aspects of the environment should be examined closely in order to establish whether or not they are likely to cause disorientation and, if so, how this can be reduced by manipulating the environment and making therapeutic use of it. (See Chapter 23, pp.278–89 for a wider discussion of this subject.)

SLEEPING AREA

Bed

All patients will spend up to one-third of their day in bed, some much more, and other patients may spend all of their time in bed. For these reasons, and because being confined to bed can be a traumatic experience, this part of the environment requires particular attention.

Patients must have reasonable access to, and be able to use where possible, an individual bedlight, locker, bed table, personal radio and an alarm bell. It is appreciated that some patients are unable to use all or any of these facilities personally. However, it is also known that some patients are unable to use these facilities because we as nurses fail to adjust the environment to take account of the patient's individual problem; for example, we need to think about the height of the locker top and whether or not our patients can reach it comfortably, the author's experience is that many lockers are too high for patients to reach with ease. Similarly, we need to think about which side of the bed to place the locker, particularly if the patient has difficulty in using a particular arm or hand. The height of the bed should, ideally, be adjustable in order that it can be lowered to make it easier for the patient to get into and out of bed, and heightened for the convenience of nurses who are working with the patient.

Isolation from other patients is one of the major problems associated with prolonged bedrest. Additional space around the beds of patients who are confined to bed should be made available for chairs to be used by visitors and/or other patients who wish to visit. Thus, whilst all patients need a reasonable amount of bed space in the interests of privacy, those who are confined to bed need additional space in order to achieve a balance between privacy and the prevention of isolation.

The following aspects of the environment, ventilation, noise, lighting, and temperature, although discussed in relation to the patients sleeping area, are equally relevant to all parts of the environment in the ward area.

Ventilation

Good ventilation, by prudent use of natural and artificial forms of ventilation, is necessary in order to introduce fresh, and remove stale, air. Adequate ventilation is also necessary in order to reduce the odours which are often a natural consequence of caring for a number of ill elderly people in an enclosed environment. Because a number of patients will be incontinent of urine and/or faeces, either in bed or in other parts of the ward area, it is *absolutely essential* that an adequate movement of fresh air should be made.

Additionally, the use of artificial aids such as air cleansing and odour-removing systems may be made. The removal of odours by use of adequate ventilation will be assisted if soiled linen and clothing is treated and disposed of effectively and efficiently. The sluice room, if poorly ventilated, can be a major source of unpleasant odours. The role of the domestic staff in keeping the toilet, sluice and other areas clean and free from smell is crucial, as is their role in undertaking prompt and efficient cleaning of all floor areas, including carpets, which have been soiled.

There is no reason why every environment in which elderly people live, irrespective of the numbers of those who are incontinent, should not be free from unpleasant odours. Remember, a smelly environment is unpleasant to visit, difficult to work in, and distressing to those who have to live in it.

Noise

The noise levels in an environment are usually more intrusive for those who have to *live* in it, than those who *work* in it. During our relatively short (approximately 8 hours) stay in a ward, and because we are often involved in making the noise, it is easy to overlook the antitherapeutic effect which this will have on our patients. Staff conversation, the rattle of trolleys, the noise of cutlery on tables, patient conversation, radio, television, record player and cleaning equipment all contribute to noise levels which are often unnecessarily high. Care should be taken to protect those who find the noise levels unacceptable; as a general rule noise in the ward should be kept to a minimum.

Lighting

Lighting in all areas should be clear without being glaring, be appropriate to the time of day or night, and (as far as is possible) be adjustable to suit individual needs. Individual reading lights for patients who are in bed, and for those who are in the sitting room but find the 'normal' lighting insufficient, should be provided. The use of natural lighting, particularly during the summer months, can bring a welcome relief from constant exposure to the artificial form.

Temperature

A room temperature of 21°C (70°F) should be aimed for throughout the year. Higher temperatures can cause excessive sweating and resultant dehydration, lower temperatures can result in exogenous hypothermia (the type which is caused by low environmental temperatures). Additionally, the temperature for individual patients can be controlled by removing or adding appropriate layers and types of clothing.

Centralized forms of heating and cooling systems need to be carefully monitored and adjusted if the temperature is to be kept within reasonable limits. This author once visited a ward in the United States of America in which an air conditioning system had been poorly adjusted and the temperature of much of the ward area was well below 15.5°C (60°F). He has also visited wards in the winter where the poorly adjusted heating system was causing the temperature to be in excess of 26.5°C (80°F). An ample supply of wall thermometers, ideally one in every room, can be used to monitor the temperature.

DINING-ROOM

A dining-room, separate from the sitting area, should contain enough space for tables and chairs without having the appearance of being overcrowded. Individual tables should be large enough for either two or four patients, and be set with the same kind of materials as one would set a table with at home, including a tablecloth. As an aid to orientation it might be desirable to encourage disoriented residents to use the same table and seat for each meal. Additionally, it might be useful to have a name tag for each patient in his or her usual place. It is not being suggested, of course, that patients should be forced to sit at a particular table or in a particular seat. Rather, it is being suggested that these aids should be used to help them recognize their preferred place.

Because the dining area is normally only in use for approximately 3 hours per day, it might be wise to consider using it for an additional purpose at other times of the day; for example, if the tables and chairs are of the type which can be removed and stored at the edge of the dining-room, the area may be used as a games, occupational therapy, physiotherapy or entertainment area at other times during the day.

STORAGE SPACE

Adequate storage space, including wardrobe, should be available for patients' clothing and other property. Ideally, an individual wardrobe for each patient will be available.

Additionally, adequate storage accommodation for all equipment (including wheelchairs, walking aids, medical equipment, linen, food and spare equipment) will be situated nearby.

MOBILITY

Aids and facilities which will enable patients to move around the ward areas are necessary in *all* areas to which patients have access. Doorways will be sufficiently wide to allow patients walking with aids, and those being pushed in wheelchairs. Bathrooms and toilets must be sufficiently large to allow two nurses to give assistance to patients. Handrails in the bathrooms, toilets and other areas are essential. Ramps, rather than steps, should allow access from and entry to the ward.

PERSONAL CLOTHING, POSSESSIONS AND EVENTS

Personal (rather than communal) clothing is necessary in order to allow the elderly person to express his individuality and maintain his self-esteem. If a hospital laundry system is to be used for patients' private clothing, then an adequate and unobtrusive marking system will be necessary in order to identify personal items of clothing.

A number of personal possessions other than clothing *must* be retained by the patients; toilet items; photographs, jewellery and books, for example. Whenever possible other personal items such as small pieces of furniture, bed clothes and wall decorations should be retained and used. These personal items, including clothing, are of fundamental importance to all of us and play a large part in enabling us to maintain our own individuality and personality. Without them we are reduced to becoming an anonymous person lacking in individuality and personality.

Individual hobbies and interests should, as far as possible, be catered for. *Some* patients will enjoy bus trips. *Some* patients will enjoy bingo. *Some* patients will enjoy community singing. *Some* patients will enjoy listening to pop music. The retention of the facilities and materials for personal preferences in hobbies and interests will enable the individual to follow his or her own particular interest.

PETS

Although it might be difficult, if not impossible, for all residents in a particular facility to have their own individual pet, it may be possible to cater for a variety of tastes by having a small number of ward pets; for example, it would be possible to have a small aquarium, a budgie, a cat and a dog in a ward. For people who have enjoyed any, or all, of these pets in the past, their presence might make the difference between an empty and a full life.

SAFETY

Finally, the environment must be *reasonably* safe although not being unnecessarily restrictive. It would be easy to make an environment totally safe by restraining patients to some form of 'geriatric' chair. However, a reasonable compromise is to allow maximum freedom within the environment, whilst making reasonably sure that the environment is free from such dangers as loose or frayed carpeting, low coffee tables, flights of stairs, hot radiators, polished linoleum and very hot water or food.

In some instances, particularly where the patients are disoriented, it may be necessary to make the environment safe by preventing individuals from leaving the safety of the ward and coming to grief on the open road or being frozen to death. Although it has become fashionable in recent years to dispense with locked wards in psychogeriatric and other areas, this often reduces the safety of the patient and adds to the anxiety of the nursing staff. If locked wards can make confused patients safe, and add to the freedom which they have within the locked environment, then this author is in favour of them.

The physical environment in which our patients live can either be therapeutic and work to their advantage, or be antitherapeutic and work to their disadvantage. As nurses we are 'the keepers of the patients' environment' and must examine every aspect of it and be sure that we recognize and make therapeutic use of the environment whether it relates to the individual patient in his own home, to the hospitalized patient, or the individual living in some other type of health care facility.

REFERENCE

Irvine R. (1983) Continence in the elderly. *Nursing Times* **79**, 45 – 8.

FURTHER READING

Chamberlain M.A. & Stowe J. (1982) Bathing in hospital. *British medical Journal* **284**, 1693 – 4.

Coates V. (1984) Inadequate intake in hospital. *Nursing Mirror* **158**, 21 – 2.

Fletcher S. & Macauley C. (1983) The shopping mall as a therapeutic arena. *Geriatric Nursing* **4**, 105 – 6.

Gould D. (1984) What's on the menu? *Nursing Mirror* **158**, 15 – 18.

Hay J. (1984) Incontinence pants: One system. *Nursing Mirror* **158**, 28 – 30.

Heaman D. & Moore J. (1982) A pet show for remotivation. *Geriatric Nursing* **3**, 108 – 10.

Holzapfel S.K. (1982) The importance of personal possessions in the lives of the institutionalized elderly. *Journal of gerontological Nursing* **3**, 156 – 8.

King M. (1984) Aids for incontinence. *Nursing Mirror* **158**, 30 – 6.

Kolanowski A. & Gunter L. (1981) Hypothermia in the elderly. *Geriatric Nursing* **2**, 362 – 5.

Kolanowski A. & Gunter L.M. (1983) Thermal stress and the aged. *Journal of gerontological Nursing* **9**, 12 – 15.

Louis M. (1983) Falls and their causes. *Journal of gerontological Nursing* **9**, 142 – 9, 156.

Marr J. (1983) The capacity for joy. *Nursing Times* **79**, 58 – 61.

Marshall M. & Overstall P. (1983) Mattress to prevent pressure sores. *Nursing Times* **79**, 54 – 9.

Moorat D. (1983) Accidents to patients. *Nursing Times* **79**, 59 – 61.

Odentunde Z. (1982) 'Fell walking'. *Nursing Mirror* **154**, 33 – 6.

Oliver C. (1983) Old and cold. *Nursing Times* **79**, 8 – 9.

Richards M. (1982) Osteoporosis. *Geriatric Nursing* **3**, 98 – 100.

Roosa W.M. (1982) Territory and privacy. Residents' views; findings of a survery. *Geriatric Nursing* **3**, 241 – 3.

Rosswurm M.A. (1983) Relocation and the elderly. *Journal of gerontological Nursing* **9**, 632 – 7.

Rowden R. (1983) A sense of harmony. *Nursing Times* **79**, 9 – 11.

Saddington N. (1983) Winter of discontent? *Nursing Times* **79**, 10 – 11.

Seigel H. (1982) Assessing an environment for safety first. *Journal of gerontological Nursing* **9**, 509 – 10, 515 – 18.

Wells T. & Brink C. (1980) Urinary incontinence: Helpful equipment. *Geriatric Nursing* **1**, 264 – 9, 276.

Chapter 34
Health Education

There is an increasing awareness of the need for health education for all age groups. Unfortunately, this is often associated with a 'don't' image (Faulkner 1984), with emphasis on the evils of smoking, drinking (alcohol), overeating and promiscuity. These are signs of an affluent society, and are warned against by health educators in terms of risk to quality and longevity of life.

All individuals have a wide range of physical, social and psychological needs in order to maintain optimum health. This is particularly true of the elderly who may be slowing down physiologically due to ageing, socially due to retirement and physiological constraints, and psychologically due to a combination of these factors.

EDUCATION FOR PHYSICAL HEALTH

Although it is not possible to halt the degeneration of bodily function in old age, individuals can be helped to maintain optimum health by understanding the needs of their bodies. The nurse herself needs to understand any constraints for a particular individual in meeting his body's needs, in order to offer pertinent and realistic advice.

It is, of course, as important that the elderly are educated towards health as other sections of society, but the emphasis will obviously be different from that used towards young people whose habits are less set; for example, Joe, at 75 years old, is unlikely to see any need to give up smoking if he feels well and has indulged for the last 50 years, but he does need to understand the effects of ageing so that physical health is not neglected.

Physical Environment

Although physical, social and psychological health are separated out for convenience, each impinges on the other. Many elderly people have a restricted income which can affect physical health, especially the environment in which they live. Houses which have no central heating may cause physical problems if rooms are not kept warm. At best, chest conditions can be exacerbated and, at worst, hypothermia can occur in an individual.

Education for the elderly on living in a warm environment may be more concerned with advice on social and voluntary services than with the physiology of degenerating temperature regulation. Physical help can be given on effective breathing, the availability of vaccination against influenza and the rights to free prescriptions.

There are difficulties in educating the elderly especially when finance is involved. Many would rather be cold than accept what to us is their right, but to them is charity. Furthermore, many will not discuss their finances and may be existing on insufficient money when they are entitled to supplementary pension.

It can also be that an elderly person will continue to live in the family home even though it is too big for one person and impossible to keep warm on limited funds. It is easy for the nurse to see such a situation in a purely practical light where, in fact, social and psychological factors may also be involved.

Educating the elderly in this context requires a sensitive approach and an ability to understand the individual's perception of a situation. It is then possible to teach that individual the benefits of maintaining body temperature, and help make the best use of available resourses.

Diet

Individuals' eating habits are usually established early in life but may change in the elderly for a number of reasons. It might be that overeating occurs as a compensation for loneliness or boredom or that diet is inadequate due to an unwillingness to bother to cook, inability to shop and cook, or inadequte income.

Education on diet for the elderly should start from where the patient is in terms of ability, understanding and finance. This requires the skills of assessment and an ability to use language common to both the nurse and the patient. Abercrombie (1979) cites a case of a patient stating that he ate a 'normal diet', which later turned out to be bread, margarine, and treacle, when he was asked which foods he normally ate.

The elderly person who overeats is often aware of the dangers inherent in obesity. Here the problem may be social, and need a social solution. More common is the problem of inadequate diet. Again, elderly people need to be made aware of the meals-on-wheels service, elderly people's clubs and other social services, though some benefit from advice on how to make the best use of limited resources. As with all health education, the aim should be towards informed choice and each individual should remain free to dispose of his income as he chooses.

Relatives and health professionals often become irritated with elderly people who pay into numerous small insurance schemes when income is small. However, from the pensioner's point of view, it may be that the insurance men who collect the premiums are a welcome break in a lonely life, and as such more important than food.

Fluid Intake

Since many elderly people have problems with incontinence, this affects attitudes to fluid intake. The individual might rationalize that limited fluid will reduce the problems of needing to get up at night, and of dribbling in the day. At best, this will result in concentrated urine which can exacerbate the problems of frequency, and, at worst, dehydration will occur with all its attendant problems.

Health education here will need to concentrate, not only on the need for adequate fluid intake, but also on aids to avoid embarrassment such as incontinence pads and knickers. The elderly are more likely to take advice about fluid if they also feel protected. It is hard to accept that bodily functions are no longer under personal control.

Alcohol can become a problem with the elderly. As with other lifestyle habits, patterns will have been set earlier in life. However, these patterns may change in old age for a number of reasons. Whisky, for example, is a warming drink, it takes the edge off hunger and loneliness. Unfortunately, it is all too easy to become dependent to the extent that spirits will be bought at the expense of food.

Of course all elderly people are not alcohol dependent, but where this does occur, help is needed as with any alcoholic, in dealing with the underlying problems. Many physicians believe that a tot of whisky is good for the circulation. In this respect alcohol is different from smoking in that there are safe consumption levels whereas any level of smoking is seen to be harmful (Elliott *et al.* 1983).

It can be seen that education for physical health in terms of a warm environment, adequate nutrition, and fluid, are dependent on a number of factors. Education for the elderly needs to take into account not only knowledge and motivation of the individual, but should also take into account associated factors, both psychological and social.

SOCIAL FACTORS AFFECTING HEALTH

Retirement is frequently seen as a life crisis in that an individual's pattern of living undergoes a total change. This change can be perceived in terms of a move from useful to useless, and is accompanied very often by a drop in income.

Health education seeks to uncover the 'hidden potential of old age' (Gray 1982) and promote a more positive attitude to post-retirement years. For too long, retirement has been seen as the start of an irreversible decline (Health Education Council 1984), rather than the chance to realize potential not possible while a wage earner.

Many firms recognize the need to plan retirement, and put on courses for their workers and spouses. Similarly, the Health Education Council (HEC) is promoting positive health education models in pre-retirement with its project started in 1982.

Unfortunately, retirement may be accompanied by physical disability which will affect social life. Many elderly people, for example, have problems with sight and/or hearing. In a familiar environment, an individual may have no difficulty in manoeuvring round furniture that has been in the same place for years. Visual problems may only arise in strange places and as such may be avoided.

A lowered income will also have social implications both in terms of outings and entertainment, in that if one cannot afford to feed visitors, pride may dictate that invitations are turned down.

Family Support

Family and friends may be concerned as they see such social isolation, especially if an elderly person lives alone and is hampered by physical constraints. There is possible resistance to 'newfangled' devices such as the telephone which would allow help to be summoned in an emergency. Health education in these circumstances needs to include not only the elderly, but those who care for them and are concerned for their welfare.

Current policy (Her Majesty's Stationery Office 1981) is that, where possible, the elderly should remain independently in the community for as long as possible rather than being cared for in long-stay institutions. To this end, the social services provide many services such as meals-on-wheels, shopping, cooking, voluntary visitors and good neighbour schemes. Education for the elderly and their relatives needs to include knowledge about what is available and who is eligible.

Education of Carers

Education for carers requires that the perspective of the elderly is understood. It is natural to be concerned that over 25% of pensioner households are without modern conveniences (Department of Health and Social Security 1978) but this concern might not be shared by the elderly inhabitants who do not know, or wish for anything else. Health professionals are often over-zealous about cleanliness and the need for daily baths. One only has to think of elderly patients admitted to hospital who do not have bathrooms and yet remain clean. They often have a miserable time being bathed daily to meet the needs of hospital staff. Similarly, individuals who do not wash are not more likely to do so if provided with modern facilities.

These points are important because well-meaning carers, both family, friends and nurses, are often keen to remove an elderly relative from less than ideal circumstances when in fact there is no need. If an individual is happy and relatively well in his own environment, he is often better to stay there than to be removed to a more hygienic setting.

Need for Independence

Many elderly people living alone are persuaded to move in with one of their children and the family. Health education is important here since this situation may be fraught with potential problems which have not been fully explored and understood. Once the move is made it is often irreversible, to the cost of all concerned.

At a physical level, problems of vision become apparent as the elderly person trips over unfamiliar objects. Frequency or incontinence, which has been contained by a handy bucket in a corner of the living-room, becomes severe if a slow ascent of stairs has to be made to pass urine. Poor hearing causes irritation to a family, while their pace of living may be too fast for an elderly person who is slowing down.

Other difficulties arise between the generations over personal habits, friends, music and television. Extreme tension can occur, especially if the elderly person cannot have his own sitting-room. That these problems are real are shown by the increase of granny-bashing described by Renvoize (1979).

Health education to deal with social factors affecting the elderly need to concentrate on independence with support wherever possible. In many areas there are informal networks of friends, neighbours, and family, who, if they understand the problems of the elderly living alone, can make sure that there is adequate back-up for living independently.

Support often comes from people who are elderly themselves, but are perhaps more able than their neighbours. Such peer support is beneficial to both the helper and the helped in that activity is encouraged and both are likely to appreciate a more leisurely approach to life. Health professionals should encourage and support such informal networks by education and guidance on the services available (Rossiter & Wicks 1982).

Day Centres

For the elderly who cannot live independently, moving in with a son or daughter may be a necessity. Carers in this situation should learn of the support which is available to both reduce tension between generations and provide peer interaction for the elderly.

Many areas have day centres for the elderly who are collected from home several mornings a week and returned in the evening. During the day the elderly develop hobbies and activities as they are able. Meals are provided along with services such as bathing, chiropody and hairdressing. This service not only helps to keep people alert and interested but can mean that life for the family may be easier, especially if both partners work.

If tensions are going to be reduced in the family, breaks from each other's company are vital, for in today's nuclear families, old and young have often grown apart in terms of culture and patterns of living. Support for the family will help an arrangement of care to survive.

Carers need to learn of breaks available for holidays; for example, voluntary organizations often arrange holidays for the elderly, while many health authorities will take elderly people into care for a few weeks so that the family have a holiday with a peace of mind.

It can be seen that social factors affecting health in old age are quite complex in that financial constraints and poor living conditions may be seen to warrant removal of an individual from his home. The educators need to view the situation from the elderly person's point of view rather than from their own, usually, middle-class view.

If the elderly person is well and reasonably happy in an albeit substandard home, he needs to learn about the support available in his area so that health is maintained in his own environment. Independence should only be given up if really necessary. Education should include support for both the elderly and his carers.

PSYCHOLOGICAL FACTORS AFFECTING HEALTH

Humans are naturally gregarious; they need others to meet needs of love and affection, to confirm self-image and for mental stimulation. Old age is often accompanied by loneliness which is a psychological problem for those who do not have adequate support networks.

Education for mental health needs to include means of avoiding depression and anxiety for both the elderly and those who care for them.

Depression

Growing old is not easy for many people since it involves the acceptance of unpalatable facts. Children who were once dependent have moved away and no longer need parental help and advice. An all-absorbing job may have been given up and left a void. Physical attractiveness is on the wane, and degenerative changes may be slowing the body and mind. Also, quite commonly, a married couple are thrown into each other's company for long periods of time only to find out they have little in common.

Hopefully, education before retirement will have reduced the impact of these effects. New hobbies and fresh interests should give a positive attitude to life which leaves little time for sadness over what is lost.

Those who care for the elderly need to understand the signs and symptons of depression so that positive steps may be taken to maintain mental health. Interests need to be fostered so that brooding over the past does not occur. Most elderly people are reasonably active and can be encouraged to look forward and be useful in some way.

It is a mistake to let the elderly take on a 'helpless' role when it is not necessary, since this can underline a feeling of uselessness which may lead to depression. Problems arise in a family where the elderly have different standards, but it is better to let an individual help rather than giving the impression that they are a hindrance.

Bereavement

One of the problems of becoming elderly is an increase in the possibility of suffering a bereavement; a much-loved partner dies leaving an enormous gap in a elderly person's life. Added to this may be the loss of peers and friends. It is natural to grieve after bereavement, but for the elderly the reminder that all men are mortal may be particularly poignant. In such a situation, loss may lead to both depression and anxiety about one's future.

It is possible to believe that the old will not mind the idea of their own death since their 'useful life', as they see it, is over. However, one only has to read accounts of people celebrating their hundredth birthdays to see that this is not so. These centenarians often talk of 'years to come.'

Copperman (1983) points out that helping people cope with grieving is part of preventive health care. Abnormal grief can lead not only to depression but to physical illness and death (Parkes 1972). With help, an individual can work through the grieving process. Many health authorities involve district nurses in bereavement visits if a partner has died at home. This is not only supportive for a relative but can mean early detection of emotional problems.

Sexuality

Health education on sexuality is usually aimed at the young to discourage promiscuity. Education for the elderly may be required to allow them to continue an active sex life well into old age; for example, the possibility of impotence in men increases with age, especially if physical problems exist such as prostatectomy or stoma. The problem with impotence is that once a man fails to have an erection he may be loath to attempt love-making again for fear of failure and the resultant humiliation.

Education needs to take into account the couple's attitude to sexual practice; for example, a wife who is shocked by anything beyond actual intercourse will not respond well to the suggestion that she helps her husband masturbate, even though health professionals know that this is one way to help overcome impotence.

There is no reason why a loving couple should not continue to have a rewarding love life. Furthermore, after bereavement, there is no reason against another marriage or partnership which will bring mutual benefit to both. This is a relatively neglected area of health education, perhaps because there is an inherent belief that sexual expression is the prerogative of the young.

SUMMARY

Health education for the elderly is not simply a matter of encouraging healthy habits. In fact, most habits of life style are set early in life. For the elderly, a healthy life may be seen to require that services and finance available are utilized, that carers are educated on the importance of independence, and that each individual is accepted as a potentially useful member of society.

Physical, social and mental health should mean that the elderly lead a positive and useful life, accept bereavement and mortality, and continue to make new and loving relationships, and maintain links with family and friends.

Health professionals, in educating the elderly should aim to discard negative, stereotyped images of old age including the notion that sexuality is not part of an old person's life. They will then be able to reinforce a positive self-image in their clients.

REFERENCES

Abercrombie M.L.J. (1979) *The Anatomy of Judgement.* Penguin, London.

Copperman H. (1983) *Dying at home.* John Wiley & Sons, Chichester.

Department of Health and Social Security (1978) *A happier old age.* A discussion document on elderly people in our society. HMSO, London.

Elliott K., Faulkner A., Randell J. & Ward L. (1983) *The facts about smoking.* Health Education Council, London.

Faulkner A. (1984) *Health Education and Nursing.* Nursing Times **80**, 45, 6.

Gray J. (1982) *Better health in retirement.* Age Concern, London.

Health Education Council (1984) *A programme of education for health in old age.* A consultation document. Health Education Council, London.

Her Majesty's Stationery Office (1981) *Growing Older.* HMSO, London.

Parkes C.M. (1972) *Bereavement.* Tavistock, London.

Renvoize J. (1979) *Web of Violence.* Penguin, London.

Rossiter C. & Wicks M. (1982) *Crisis or Challenge?* Study Commission on the Family, London.

FURTHER READING

Brower H.T. (1981) Groups and student teaching: Putting Health Education into practice. *Journal of gerontological Nursing* **7**, 483–8.

Coombs K.L. (1978) Preventive care in the elderly. *American Journal of Nursing* **78**, 1339–41.

Diekelmann N. (1978) Pre-retirement counselling. *American Journal of Nursing* **78**, 1337–8.

Donahue F., Girton K., Baumler J., Moerhlin B. & Strayer L.(1981) A drug education program for the well elderly. *Geriatric Nursing* **2**, 140–2.

Ferguson C.(1983) Fitness in old age. *Nursing Times* **79**, 302–5.

George G. (1982) If patient teaching tries your patience, try this plan. *Nursing 82* **12**, 50–5.

Klein M.(1980) Putting down roots in retirement. *Geriatric Nursing* **1**, 114–19.

Marshall D. (1981) Towards a stimulating retirement. *Geriatric Nursing* **2**, 143–5.

Meguerdichian D. (1983) Improving self-medication in an H.R.F. *Geriatric Nursing* **4**, 30–4.

Shomaker D.M. (1980) Integration of physiological and sociocultural factors as a basis for sex education to the elderly. *Journal of gerontological Nursing* **6**, 311–18.

Turton P. (1983) Health education and the district nurse. *Nursing Times* **79**, 222–9.

Chapter 35
Geriatric Nursing Research

Although much has been done in very recent years, more geriatric nursing research needs to be done. Additionally, more of the research which has been done, needs to be implemented.

Although the main research focus of this chapter is on work done in the United Kingdom, it is recognized that geriatric nursing research is developing internationally, particularly in the United States of America. Whilst some of the work done in countries other than your own may not be applicable to your circumstances, much of it is transferrable.

This chapter, will not attempt to cover all relevant research, rather it will provide an overview of selected studies. Hopefully, it will stimulate interest in the subject and help you identify areas in which further work is urgently required. It will also examine a few of the findings and recommendations of some researchers and explore the extent to which these have (or have not) been implemented.

First of all, some questions. What is geriatric nursing research? Do we need it? What are we going to do with the results as they emerge?

Nursing research should help us to find the best ways of providing the best care for our patients; for example this may be in terms of the equipment used, organization of nurse management, planning ward layout, determining priorities of care, devising nursing care plans, improving communications and actually studying nursing practice. Nursing care of the elderly takes place in hospital, in the home and in various places offering sheltered accommodation such as local authority and private nursing homes.

Do we need research? Are we satisfied that we are giving our patients the best care available? What is the 'best care'? Does care mean making sure our patients are fed, watered and clean or is it something more than that? There are still too many places where the elderly receive what might be termed 'basic nursing care' — the facilities are basic, the number of trained nurses on duty is at the 'basic' (absolute minimum) level so the care given is only that necessary to maintain a 'basic' life. An anonymous nurse teacher (Anonymous 1983) describes her shock at finding that care given by nurses to geriatric patients in the United Kingdom National Health Service could still be so abysmal and degrading when all nurse training is supposedly

412

geared towards the idea of 'total patient care.'

Incidents of inadequate nursing care of the elderly in hospital are described by Redfern (1983). In that paper Redfern discusses some factors that might lead to lack of care:

The elderly are undervalued in our society.

They are viewed in negative terms by themselves and society as they no longer work or contribute materially to our society.

Both geriatric nursing and medicine are seen as low-status occupations. Possibly geriatric nurses are not given enough responsibility.

Long-term care is not personalized and there is a rigid adherence to ward routines. Baker (1978) terms this the 'routine geriatric' style of nursing.

There is a lack of communication between nurses and patients.

Nurses working in the geriatric field have a lack of knowledge. Very little post-basic training is given or taken up.

It is obvious from such work that many elderly patients are not receiving our 'best care'. However, the question still remains, will nursing research allow us to give *better* care? It is officially recognized that it should (Report of the Committee on Nursing — Briggs Report 1972, para 370: 'Nursing should become a research-based profession'). So, if nurses want to be viewed as belonging to a profession with a say in its own future, some autonomy in the way care is delivered to patients and worthy of respect from other professionals the profession must become research-based. More importantly perhaps, nurses must be seen to act on the findings of that research.

Nursing the elderly can be seen as one aspect of nursing where there are most opportunities for nurses to show how well-planned and managed nursing care can improve the condition of patients; for example, Storrs (1982) describes the dramatic change in a group of dependent, incontinent and confused elderly patients when vigorous attempts were made to improve the quality of care.

RESEARCH FINDINGS

There are many books and articles on the 'how to's' of research, so it is not necessary to consider methods of research in depth in this chapter. Before embarking on any research, or perhaps attempting to implement research findings, it is important to consider any ethical implications.

Hirschfeld (1979) and Denham (1984) both mention the question of ethical standards and issues. Hirschfeld, for example, asks us to question what right we have to interfere in an old person's autonomy in order to create 'desirable' behaviour. Should we expect patients to conform to our ideal of behaviour patterns; maybe Mrs Smith would rather sit quietly in a corner thinking about her past than join in with an enforced bingo session. Conversely though, patients who demand individual treatment in very forthright manners are often labelled as 'difficult'. The ideal patients to nurse are sometimes seen as those who happily comply with hospital routines. We need to think whether we are unconsciously manipulating patients to act as we want them to, and so taking away their right to choose how they want to act and live.

Denham (1984) discusses some of the ethical problems involved with research and the elderly, particularly the problem of obtaining informed consent to participation in research projects. There are obvious difficulties in obtaining consent from confused elderly patients, and consent often has to be obtained from close relatives.

Nursing research is only just becoming accepted by nurses in the United Kingdom. As mentioned previously, we do not have a large fund of geriatric nursing research to call on and most of the work already done probably needs repeating so that the findings and any implications are shown to stand up to critical assessment.

The pioneering work in the field of geriatric nursing was done by Norton in the early 1960s (Norton *et al.* 1975). Many of her recommendations for geriatric nursing are still very relevant today. The aims of the research were:
1   to improve nursing techniques in the management and care of the elderly sick;
2   to provide greater comfort for the patient and increase his/her independence;
3   to reduce the work of nurses both in time and effort.

The research included observational studies and practical experiments. Five headings or proposals were considered: incontinence; pressure sores; clothing; furniture and equipment, and nursing techniques.

The research report describes the problems of nursing the elderly in hospital and attempts to show how the problems may have arisen. The researchers found many of the problems more complex than anticipated and that studying and attempting to solve them were not just questions of practicalities, but of principles: 'The principles of assessing and meeting the needs of individual patients.'

To summarize some of the findings: basic nursing time was mostly devoted to patients who were doubly incontinent; much of the nursing care was arduous and unpleasant; there was a need to assess and group patients according to their condition and capabilities. Two groups were set containing:
1   those requiring encouragement and aid to independence;
2   those requiring concentrated nursing care so that basic nursing routines

could be planned (a) to meet the needs of the patients, and (b) to distribute the pressure of work more evenly throughout the day.

Many nursing problems were found to be due to use of unsuitable furniture and equipment. Many of the elderly were found to have dressing difficulties and a need for specifications for special hospital garments was felt. Many factors were found to be involved in the development of pressure sores. A scoring system was devised as a way of evaluating which patients were most at risk from the future development of pressure sores.

Another major nursing research study into the problems of geriatric nursing care was done by Wells in the mid 1970s (Wells. 1980). The objectives of that research were to examine geriatric nursing care and to investigate methods of implementing improvements. Wells work marks the next step in geriatric nursing research from the work of Norton. Wells found in a search of the literature that there had been no advances in geriatric nursing care and that, in fact, there was 'no aggregate of knowledge or methods distinguishable as geriatric nursing'.

To summarize some of her findings: an improvement in ward design was needed; ward sisters should be included on planning committees; wards should be adequately supplied with suitable furniture and equipment and nurses should be taught how to use equipment to the best advantage of the patients; the nursing staff allocation was not related to patient nursing care needs; nursing knowledge was limited. Nursing auxiliaries had very little knowledge about causes and care of common problems in the elderly. The knowledge of trained staff was confused and questionable. It was noted that there was no in-service training programme and this was seen as an important need. Clothing was inadequate and unsuitable. Nurses were not taught how to dress disabled patients.

Auxiliary nurses were found to give most direct care. Nursing work was not focused on patients' needs but on routines — nursing care was depersonalized. Nurses kept no record of individual patient's needs. Sustained nurse/patient verbal communication was infrequent, of limited quality and often meaningless. Good nurse/patient communication was felt to be important as a measure of the effectiveness of nursing care. Wells recommended that in order to improve nursing care of the hospitalized elderly, a clinical nurse expert prepared to induce change was needed. This nurse should give nursing care, teach and pursue nursing research. She suggested that few ward sisters or charge nurses had enough knowledge to be 'change-agents.'

Norton's earlier work, started in 1959, showed that the needs of individual patients were not being met. She specified a number of practical ways in which nurses could change their patterns of nursing to give improved care. Thirteen years later in 1972, Wells found that despite this earlier work, nurses still did not focus on the individual patient and that nursing care was depersonalized and fixed on rigid ward routines. Twelve years on in 1984, how much has the picture changed? What has nursing research achieved in the past decade?

Firstly, let us consider some of the results coming from the United States of America, the country from which most of the published nursing research emanates. Kayser-Jones (1981) reviewed recent gerontological nursing research and found that there had been a gradual increase in the amount of work done but could find 'no large-scale, well-defined research programs that systematically investigated the promotion, maintenance and restoration of health for the elderly'. She found evidence to show that students of nursing received only limited teaching on the theory and clinical practice of nursing the elderly and suggested that this was why so few nurses took up gerontological nursing research. Kayser-Jones also studied the effect of nursing research on the quality of health care available to the elderly. There has been little nursing research on community nursing care although nurses are uniquely qualified to identify the health needs of the elderly. Nurses have not made major inroads in developing preventive and continuing care programmes which are currently very limited in the United States of America.

Looking at the care of the institutionalized elderly, Kayser-Jones found past research had focused mainly on the psychosocial needs of patients, for example on factors relating to morale; use of reality orientation and group therapy with confused elderly patients. Few clinical studies had been done on the physical and medical nursing needs of patients, for example, incontinence, confusion and immobility. Paradoxically, studies on nursing care actually given show that nurses spend most time catering to the physical and medical needs of their elderly patients and give little attention to their psychosocial care and personal needs.

Let us move on from this overview of American research to a more detailed look at some recently published papers.

Measuring Nursing Care

For nurse managers, sensible allocation of nurses to where they can give the most effective nursing care is very important. Several studies have been made which have looked at ways of measuring nursing care and patients' needs.

Norwich (1980) made a study of geriatric nursing care in order to produce geriatric dependency measures. The care given was found mostly to relate to feeding, toiletting and dressing. It was found that, in practice, not all the demands and needs of the patients could be met. Activities relating to the rehabilitation of patients and to the provision of a more social environment were low on the list of nursing priorities.

Smith *et al.* (1980) studied a group of self-care geriatric patients and investigated the views of the patients and nurses on the nursing care needed. Nurses felt that physical care was most important whilst patients rated the nurse's role as teacher as most important. The study showed that nurses have difficulty in establishing when a patient wants to be independent.

The use of the nursing process as a way of assessing and measuring nursing care has been studied by several workers; for example, Wade and Snaith (1981) describe the use of a patient state form to consider various aspects of care in order to obtain patient workload estimates. Rhys Hearn (1979) has developed a nursing workload package based on nursing time requirements to estimate the care needs of elderly patients (Rhys Hearn 1979, Magrid & Rhys Hearn 1981).

Psychosocial Studies

Whilst some progress has been made on the most appropriate methods of delivering psychosocial care to elderly patients, most work reveals that this aspect of care is least likely to be attended to by nurses. Somewhere along the line, nurses are made to feel very strongly that nursing care of the elderly involves physical and medical care of the body and that any time spent caring for the individual emotional and psychological needs of patients is not a priority but a ' bonus' if the workload permits.

Wells (1980) in her study showed how limited communication was between nurses and patients. There has been a fair amount of work recently which has looked at the problems of communication in nursing (for example, Faulkner 1980, Macleod-Clark 1981). Poor communication can be seen to be at the heart of many of the problems of geriatric nursing. Macleod-Clark (1981) suggests that content and length of communication between nurses and patients is an indicator of the quality of nursing care.

Confusion in the elderly is a major nursing problem. Nurses often find this aspect of geriatric nursing depressing as there appears to be no way of preventing progressive mental deterioration. One therapeutic technique for helping the elderly confused is reality orientation. This therapy is designed to help withdrawn, confused and depressed old people find their bearings and improve their quality of life (Teasdale 1983). Teasdale notes that a number of research reports question the value and effectiveness of reality orientation but comments that as there is no standard handbook on reality orientation, therapists do not use the same techniques. He states that reality orientation is an attitude towards caring for the elderly which requires flexible, adaptable and optimistic approaches. Obviously more work needs to be done by nurse researchers to find out the value of various techniques.

Low morale amongst the institutionalized elderly is frequently recognized. In an experimental study by Chang (1979) it was found that giving patients control over their daily activities was the strongest contribution to a high morale.

Equipment and Ward Conditions

Many nurses and nurse researchers (for example Norton *et al.* 1975, Wells 1980) have criticized the equipment and ward conditions that they have to work with. Wells (1980) suggested that ward sisters should be included in planning committees and that nurses should have more say in the type of furniture and equipment supplied to the ward. However, there is little evidence of nursing research interest in this field.

An example of one effective research study is that of MacLean *et al.* (1982), who reported on restraints used on elderly agitated patients found to be in common use in North America. From their assessment they were able to give recommendations for proper use of certain types of restraint.

Personal clothing for elderly long-stay patients is recognized as being important by nurse researchers. The Disabled Living Foundation (1983) have recently published a booklet entitled 'A Guide to the Introduction of a Personalised Clothing Service'. It would be worthwhile for someone to publish a report on the impact of the introduction of such a service on patients and nursing staff.

Incontinence

There are many articles written by nurses on the problems of dealing with incontinence. This is not surprising as researchers have found that toiletting and washing patients take up most nursing time. There have been improvements in the ways in which we can manage our incontinent patients, whether there have been such improvements in the ways we do manage the problems of incontinence is another matter.

Two recent national reports published in the United Kingdom indicate that more action is needed to cope with the problems of incontinence. The Royal College of Nursing (1983) report *The Problem of Promoting Continence* emphasizes the need to improve the education about incontinence given to all health professionals and stresses the urgency of establishing a social policy for the care of incontinent people in the United Kingdom. The Incontinence Action Group (1983) have also recently published a report *Action on Incontinence.* This again suggests the need for better education and asks for the provision of more posts for continence nurse advisors.

Pressure Sores

Again, there have been many articles written by nurses on the problems of pressure area care. Norton (1975) first suggested a constructive nursing approach to the problem of pressure sore prevention and the Norton Scale has been widely and successfully used. A recent evaluation of the Norton Scale by Newman and West (1981) found that it was useful in indicating patients most likely to develop late pressure sores, but only of marginal value in assessing, *on admission,* patients at risk of developing early pressure sores.

Equipment used for minimizing the risk of acquiring pressure sores has been looked at in a number of research studies; for example Marshall and Overstall (1983) looked at various mattresses and were able to recommend one particular type as the best for pressure sore prevention.

A new nursing post the 'Tissue viability nurse' has recently been developed (Dowding 1983) and such nurses are beginning to publish more research findings.

Drugs

It is well known that many elderly people have medicine cabinets full of drugs and probably make many errors in self-medication. Shannon (1983) describes a study of self-medication in the elderly. She evaluated a group of patients discharged from a rehabilitation ward who had received self-medication training, and compared them with a group who had received no training. The trained group made significantly fewer errors in self-medication than the control group and Shannon was able to make several recommendations for future practice.

Another study by Whitley and Smith (1981) looked at the withdrawal of night hypnotics in a group of clients in a residential home. They found clients were less confused and the number of falls was reduced at night.

Community Nursing Care

Predictions for a massive increase in the number of elderly living in the United Kingdom during the next few decades have obvious implications for future planning of health care. An increase in the next 10 years of 13% in the over 75s and 31% in the over 85s has been proposed (Edwards 1982). We do need to plan for people to have a healthy old age.

Brocklehurst (1982) suggests that the ideal person to advise and counsel the elderly in the community would be the health visitor. He points out that much disease in the elderly is currently unknown to general practitioners and suggests that health visitors should give health screening to all those over 75 years of age.

Health visitors have become aware of the necessity to identify elderly patients who may be at risk. Read (1982) investigated whether health and social services were reaching those most at need and found that those with the greatest incapacities were being identified. The over 80s should be the priority group for surveillance. The home help and chiropody services were found to be particularly important in preventing incapacity.

Luker (1978) has studied and assessed the care given by the health visitor. She found that visits to the elderly were not structured and could find no clear criteria by which health visitors worked. Fitton (1980) also studied health visitors' visits to the elderly. She found their main preoccupations were with an assessment of the *needs* of the elderly and that clients were viewed in a negative way. She found no use of a nursing process model.

Experimental Nursing Schemes

In 1982 it was decided to set up three experimental nursing homes within the National Health Service (Fowler, Hansard 1982). The homes were intended for use by elderly patients who needed no further hospital treatment; trained nurses were to be in charge of patient care. The priority was to keep the residents active and to give them choice in their patterns of daily life. The concept has been met with great enthusiasm in some quarters (Hooper 1983) but remains to be fully evaluated.

Earlier experimental schemes run on similar lines have shown excellent results. Storrs (1982) describes the results of changes in care given to a group of 40 elderly patients who were moved from a long-stay geriatric ward to a NHS nursing home. In the former ward, the patients were highly dependent; many were confused and incontinent; they were given no choice in many aspects of their care, which were determined by hospital routines; the patients were unwilling to participate in activities, did not converse with each other and were very institutionalized. On moving to their new home the residents (as opposed to patients) were given much more freedom of choice; they were allowed to bring in their own possessions and wear their own clothes; were able to eat what they wanted and to decide when to get up or go to bed; most of them chose to take part in activities offered such as bingo sessions, whist drives, craft classes and various outings. The changes in the residents were dramatic. They became less dependent both physically and emotionally and the rate of incontinence dropped by 50%.

In a later report Storrs (1983) comments on the changes in the nursing staff. Initially the staff found the work very hard and many nearly gave up. The staff eventually became friends and helpers to the residents and found the changes in the residents very exciting and rewarding. Residents were treated as dignified individuals with the right to choose their own way of life.

McIntosh (1983) reports on another scheme to give continuing care to the elderly in an experimental unit attached to a hospital. Care was given by auxiliary nurses under the guidance of a district nursing sister. The aim was to provide non-institutionalized accommodation, giving the residents more choice and encouraging their independence. It was felt important to stick to strict admission criteria in order for the unit to run successfully. Only ambulant, continent patients able to dress and feed themselves were admitted. Many residents were able to achieve greater independence and transfer to other residential homes.

FUTURE RESEARCH REQUIREMENTS

On making this review of geriatric nursing research several factors have stood out. So far, very few major research projects have been completed, we still desperately lack basic knowledge as to how to give the best nursing care. Several small-scale projects have been, and are being, undertaken but most findings from such studies need further testing by other researchers.

This chapter ends by giving some examples of questions that we need to consider.

Care

Why do most nurses on geriatric wards still rely on ward routines instead of giving individual nursing care ?

Education

Why is what nurses are being taught in the classroom not being applied at ward level?

Status

How can we make geriatric nursing, at present a low-status occupation, more acceptable ?

Communication

Many nurses just do not talk with their patients; how can we improve this?

Qualifications

At present, unqualified auxiliary nurses give most care to our elderly patients; is it important that more qualified nurses should be giving that care?

Priorities

What is the best method for assessing priorities of care?

Ward Organization

Is it in the best interests of nurses and patients to put all those requiring long-term care in the same ward?

Equipment

Do nurses know how to make the best use of specialized equipment, for example, chairs, walking frames, incontinence appliances, pressure sore equipment and hoists? Should nurses have more say in ordering and even designing such equipment?

Reality Orientation

How should nurses apply this method? Is it the best way to cope with the confused elderly?

Community Care

What sort of support should nurses give the elderly in the community? How do we decide where the elderly infirm will receive the best nursing care?

Future

We have a rapidly expanding geriatric population; how prepared is the nursing profession to cope with the increase?

REFERENCES

Anonymous (1983) The bottom of the pond. *Nursing Times* **79**,32–3.
Baker D.E. (1978) *Attitudes of nurses to the care of the elderly*. Unpublished PhD Thesis, University of Manchester.

Brocklehurst J.C. (1982) Health visiting and the elderly — a geriatrician's view. *Health Visitor* 55, 356–7.

Chang B.L. (1979) Locus of control, trust, situational control and morale of the elderly. *International Journal of Nursing Studies* 16, 169–81.

Denham M. (1984) Ethics of research. *Nursing Mirror* 158, 36–8.

Disabled Living Foundation (1983) *A guide to the introduction of a personalised clothing service.* Disabled Living Foundation, London.

Department of Health and Social Security (1972) *Report of the committee on Nursing.* H.M.S.O. London.

Dowding C. (1983) Tissue viability nurse — a new post. *Nursing Times* 79, 61–4.

Edwards M. (1982) *Nursing Times* (In the News) 78, 994.

Faulkner A. (1980) Communication and the nurse. *Nursing Times* 76, 93–5.

Fitton J. (1980) Health visiting the aged. *Health Visitor* 53, 521–5.

Fowler N. (1982) *Hansard,* February 4th.

Hirschfeld M.J. (1979) Research in nursing gerontology. *Journal of advanced Nursing* 4, 621–6.

Hooper J. (1983) An NHS home of their own. *Health and Social Services Journal* July 21st, 870–1.

Incontinence Action Group (1983) *Action on Incontinence.* King's Fund Project Paper 43.

Kayser-Jones J.S. (1981) Gerontological nursing research revisited. *Journal of gerontological Nursing* 7, 217–23.

Luker K.A. (1978) Goal attainment — a possible model for assessing the role of the health visitor. *Nursing Times* 74, 1257–9.

McIntosh J.B. (1983) Experimental care for the elderly. *Nursing Times* (Occasional Paper) 79, 56–7.

MacLean J., Shamian J., Butcher P., Parsons R., Selcer B. & Barrett M. (1982) Restraining the elderly agitated patient. *Canadian Nurse* 78, 44–6.

Macleod-Clark J. (1981) Communication in nursing. *Nursing Times* 77, 12–18.

Magrid S. & Rhys Hearn C. (1981) Characteristics of geriatric patients as related to nursing needs. *International Journal of Nursing Studies* 18, 97–106.

Marshall M. & Overstall P. (1983) Mattresses to prevent pressure sores. *Nursing Times* 79, 54–9.

Newman P. & West J. (1981) The value of the Norton scale. *Nursing Times* 77 (Supplement), 81–4.

Norton D., McLaren R. & Exton-Smith A.N. (1975) *An investigation of geriatric nursing problems in hospital.* Churchill Livingstone, London.

Norwich H.S. (1980) A study of nursing care in geriatric hospitals. *Nursing Times* 76, 292–5.

Read S. (1982) Elderly people at home — do health and social services reach those most in need? *Health Visitor* 55, 600–3.

Redfern S.J. (1983) Nursing care of the elderly in hospital. *British Journal of Geriatric Nursing* 2, 8–12.

Rhys Hearn C. (1979) Staffing geriatric wards. Trials of a 'package'. *Nursing Times* 75 (Supplement), 45–8.

Royal College of Nursing (1983) *The Problem of Promoting Continence.* Rcn Publications in association with Squibb Surgicare Limited.

Facilities for the Elderly

Shannon M. (1983) Self-medication in the elderly. *Nursing Mirror* 157: *(Clinical Forum)* i–viii.

Smith C.E., Buck S., Colligan E., Kerndt P. & Sollie T. (1980) Differences in importance ratings of self-care geriatric patients and the nurses who care for them. *International Journal of Nursing Studies* 17, 145–53.

Storrs A. (1982) What is care? *British Journal of Geriatric Nursing,* 1, 12–14.

Storrs A. (1983) A change of direction. *British Journal of Geriatric Nursing* 2, 5.

Teasdale K. (1983) Reality orientation — a programme for the elderly. *Nursing Times,* 79, 49–52.

Wade B. & Snaith P. (1981) The assessment of patients' need for nursing care on geriatric wards. *International Journal of Nursing Studies* 18, 261–71.

Wells T.J. (1980) *Problems in geriatric nursing care.* Churchill Livingstone, London.

Whitley M.W. & Smith H. (1981) Elderly clients and withdrawal of night hypnotics. *Nursing Times* 77 (Supplement), 35–6.

Index